Praise for *The Hashimoto's Healing Diet*

"*The Hashimoto's Healing Diet* should be in the tool kit of anyone looking to go beyond the autoimmune protocol and learn how to layer the dietary principles from Chinese medicine into their wellness journey. If you are looking for deeper self-assessment and troubleshooting, this book is for you."

— Mickey Trescott, certified nutritional therapy practitioner, author of *The Autoimmune Cookbook,* and co-author of *The Autoimmune Wellness Handbook*

comprehensive book to heal Hashimoto's that we have all been waiting for. What from the numerous books on thyroid diet and health is that Marc is an experienced practitioner who has years of clinical experience to guide his suggestions, inspirations, He opens up the much needed dialogue between the gut microbiome and immune system that is missing in most autoimmune healing conversations. This is the book I will be recommending to all my clients."

— Jessica Flanigan, clinical nutritionist and author of *AIP One Dish* and *The Loving Diet*

"Marc is a masterful storyteller. He eloquently weaves the concepts of Chinese medicine into an innovative approach to treating autoimmune diseases that every patient (and every doctor) needs to know. His 'Food as Medicine' excerpts were powerful—chrysanthemum flower tea for headaches, watermelon tea for edema, and aloe for constipation. Answers for common and oh so stubborn Hashimoto's symptoms, finally!"

— **Dana Trentini**, founder of Hypothyroid Mom and co-author of *Your Healthy Pregnancy with Thyroid Disease*

"This is it! This is what the millions of people challenged with Hashimoto's have been searching for. *The Hashimoto's Healing Diet* is a blueprint for healing through proven nutritional strategies. Marc combines ancient wisdom with practical dietary interventions to help you heal for good. Do yourself and your thyroid gland a huge favor by following Marc's guidelines. Your road to recovery starts at your next meal."

— **Sachin Patel**, founder of The Living Proof Institute and functional medicine practitioner coach

"A delightful read full of important informational gems for those of us moving through the sometimes complicated journey that is Hashimoto's. The information is presented in an easy-to-follow format, especially for those of us dealing with brain fog. Marc weaves meaningful and relatable case studies (appropriately called 'Hashimoments') throughout the book, allowing the reader to feel validated, heard, and supported. A rare treat, not to be missed!"

— **Danna Bowman**, founder of Thyroid Nation, host of *Thyroid Nation Radio*, and co-founder of Thyroid Refresh™ and Thyroid30™

"This is not your average book about *diet*, but much, much more. Marc has a unique ability to communicate complex subjects in a non-threatening, even entertaining way—which weaves together modern, cutting-edge scientific research with Traditional Chinese Medicine in a way I've not seen done before. A very refreshing perspective for those interested in the inner-workings of autoimmunity and other immune-related conditions. I highly recommend this book for anyone looking to take control of their own personal health, and have fun while doing it!"

— **Michael Roesslein, M.Sc.**, co-founder of Rebel Health Tribe and producer of The Human Longevity Project

"Marc has always proven himself to be an ardent student and practitioner of functional medicine. In a friendly and even comforting tone, he leads the Hashimoto's reader through cutting-edge foundations to improving health and well-being. What really sets his book apart, however, is his ability to integrate Traditional Chinese Medicine with modern functional medicine. You'll find Chinese herbal remedies for common Hashimoto's related issues and explanations of symptoms through Chinese medicine's use of elements and nature. The result is an uncanny insight into the holism of Chinese medicine that works together with our modern, scientific understandings of thyroid autoimmunity."

— **Datis Kharrazian, D.H.Sc., D.C., F.A.C.N, C.N.S.**

"Marc Ryan does Hashimoto's patients a great service in weaving the powerful tenets of Traditional Chinese Medicine with humor, candor, and a highly digestible writing style. His message speaks to the interconnectedness of our bodily and planetary systems, while at the same time honoring the dynamic nature of true well-being. As patterns of deficiency and/or excess ebb and flow in our bodies, what we give them should follow suit. This may be the most evolved approach to 'food as medicine' that I've encountered—and the most ancient."

— **Ginny Mahar**, co-founder of Thyroid Refresh™ and Thyroid30™

The
HASHIMOTO'S
HEALING
Diet

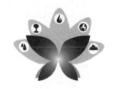

ALSO BY MARC RYAN, L.AC.

How to Heal Hashimoto's: An Integrative Road Map to Remission

The above is available at your local bookstore, or may be ordered by visiting:

Hay House UK: www.hayhouse.co.uk

Hay House USA: www.hayhouse.com®
Hay House Australia: www.hayhouse.com.au
Hay House India: www.hayhouse.co.in

MARC RYAN LAc

The
HASHIMOTO'S
HEALING
Diet

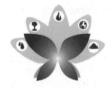

Leabharlanna Poiblí Chathair Baile Átha Cliath
Dublin City Public Libraries

Anti-inflammatory
Strategies for Losing Weight,
Boosting Your Thyroid and
Getting Your Energy Back

HAY HOUSE

Carlsbad, California • New York City
London • Sydney • New Delhi

Published in the United Kingdom by:
Hay House UK Ltd, Astley House, 33 Notting Hill Gate, London W11 3JQ
Tel: +44 (0)20 3675 2450; Fax: +44 (0)20 3675 2451; www.hayhouse.co.uk

Published in the United States of America by:
Hay House Inc., PO Box 5100, Carlsbad, CA 92018-5100
Tel: (1) 760 431 7695 or (800) 654 5126
Fax: (1) 760 431 6948 or (800) 650 5115; www.hayhouse.com

Published in Australia by:
Hay House Australia Ltd, 18/36 Ralph St, Alexandria NSW 2015
Tel: (61) 2 9669 4299; Fax: (61) 2 9669 4144; www.hayhouse.com.au

Published in India by:
Hay House Publishers India, Muskaan Complex, Plot No.3, B-2,
Vasant Kunj, New Delhi 110 070
Tel: (91) 11 4176 1620; Fax: (91) 11 4176 1630; www.hayhouse.co.in

Text © Mark Ryan, 2018

Interior photos: Olesia Farberov • Interior illustrations: Maklin Ryan

The moral rights of the author have been asserted.

The information given in this book should not be treated as a substitute for professional medical advice; always consult a medical practitioner. Any use of information in this book is at the reader's discretion and risk. Neither the author nor the publisher can be held responsible for any loss, claim or damage arising out of the use, or misuse, of the suggestions made, the failure to take medical advice or for any material on third-party websites.

A catalogue record for this book is available from the British Library.

ISBN: 978-1-78180-919-8

Printed and bound in Great Britain by TJ International, Padstow, Cornwall.

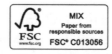

To Mother Earth—
and all the Earth Mothers that sustain and support us

Acknowledgments

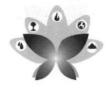

Drawings: All drawings are original works of art by Maklin Ryan.

Photography: Photographs and recipes are by Olesia Farberov.

Work Space: Thank you to Stephanie and Gary O'Dell for providing me with an amazing work space in Rimrock, Arizona, that provided daily inspiration for this book and helped me to really immerse myself in the energy of the earth element and its phases.

Editing: Thanks to Sally Mason-Swaab for her patience and guidance, and Lisa Bernier for her copyediting.

Layout Design: Bryn Starr Best

Thought Leaders: Thank you to my many colleagues in this movement to improve care for thyroid and Hashimoto's patients. Dr. Datis Kharrazian, Deke Kendall, Dr. Sarah Ballantyne, Stacey Robbins, Dana Trentini, Mickey Trescott, Bob Flaws, Li Dong-yuan, and many more who toil daily to help educate and empower patients worldwide.

My Clients and Patients: Thank you for entrusting me with your care and for inspiring me to improve my craft on a daily basis to help solve the puzzle that is autoimmunity and Hashimoto's thyroiditis.

Contents

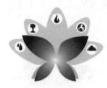

Foreword

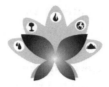

When Marc asked if I would write the foreword for his book, I was truly delighted. Not only because I, too, am a Hashimoto's patient (now in remission), but also because, having grown up in Asia where I spent 22 formative years, Traditional Chinese Medicine (TCM) has a special place in my heart and my own healing journey.

When diagnosed with Hashimoto's in 2008, in Shanghai, China, my allopathic doctor had nothing to offer, not even thyroid medications. Why? Because my TSH, T4, and T3 markers were "in a good range." My TPO antibodies on the other hand, were skyrocketing high at over 1,000. Since there are no pills to lower the antibodies, I was sent home with no solution or hope. I felt like I was losing the person I once was to a fatigued, moody, anxious, hair-losing, sleepless, constipated, puffy, heavily PMS-ing Magdalena I never knew.

A friend pointed me to a wonderful TCM doctor in Shanghai. She immediately diagnosed me with spleen deficiency and put me on an herbal protocol. The herbal blend was highly personalized, and the freshly made concoction was delivered to the house weekly. Mind you, back then, there were no books, online resources, or practitioners specializing in Hashimoto's. I therefore didn't make many dietary changes apart from limiting gluten. To my delight, my TPO antibodies dropped to 500 in a matter of weeks and I started feeling better. With such results, I was armed with hope and encouragement to go deeper.

There is a thin, often undistinguishable line in Asia where food ends and medicine begins. My first serious boyfriend was Malaysian Chinese, whose mom would make a daily vegetable broth, slow cooking it in a Crock-Pot, infusing it with Chinese herbs, roots, berries, and leaves. At any early signs of a looming cold, she would make a concoction that would halt the cold in its tracks.

My colleagues in Hong Kong, when challenged with seasonal allergies, acid reflux, onset of colds, or headaches, instead of running to the nearest pharmacy would head for a Chinese herbal medicine store to get a dose of herbs.

Because this stuff works. TCM works if you learn and commit to applying it.

Marc Ryan takes both the ancient traditional Chinese masters' teachings and paleo for autoimmunity (AIP) to the next level—and shows why one diet will not work for everyone, or one diet might not work in the long term. I have found the exact phenomenon in my community—each person's genetics and current deficiencies need to be honored. This is huge: If you have been that "healthy person" who is "eating so well," yet you feel stuck and resigned, this book might have the answers.

Let me be honest: the beginning parts of Marc's book might feel dense at first. The concepts might be unfamiliar to you. The bodily systems and terms used are different from what allopathic medicine has taught you. Do not worry though; whether you are experiencing liver qi stagnation or spleen qi deficiency, the symptoms are clearly laid out so that you know where to start, how to proceed,and what foods to use to guide you to health.

Marc is my favorite kind of teacher: science-based, practical, concrete, and thought-provoking with his sharp words. He says, "I don't want to write another book that adds another 50 supplements for you to take." His ultimate mission is to guide you to healing by uncovering and personalizing a food protocol.

Yet, he is kind, , and reflective. In "Hashimoments," he inspires you by helping reframe the thought process most Hashimoto's patients struggle with, like losing hope or feeling alienated and overwhelmed. One of the questions that struck me was *"What can you do without?"*

If you've just recently been diagnosed with Hashimoto's, this book is for you. It could be that by just applying the Elimination phase and incorporating some of the delicious and medicinal foods such as tangerine peel, radishes, or squashes, you put Hashimoto's into full remission. Commit, and wondrous things will happen.

If you have been struggling with Hashimoto's for a long time, this book is ever so much for you. Marc goes into the areas many practitioners omit—personalizing nutrition based on your unique deficiencies and addressing systemic infections such as SIBO, *H. pylori*, Yersinia, EBV, and Candida to name a few. I have experienced it firsthand; no matter how hard you try to heal with a diet, these sneaky infections are often the passive aggressive kinds, sabotaging your energy, mental sharpness, healthy weight, and ability to eat a wide variety of foods—and ultimately, put Hashimoto's into remission.

Be grateful for Hashimoto's, because it has come knocking on your door for a reason. What you will learn about your body and the signals it's sending you will stay with you for life. If you commit 100 percent, align nutrition with your energetics, and take action, your body will respond lovingly. After all, it was built to thrive. Just give it what it's calling for.

Let Hashimoto's be the best teacher that ever showed up. Just as Marc's book—let it be vocal, daring, and enlightening to your path.

Magdalena Wszelaki

Hashimoto's patient, in full remission

Author of *Cooking for Hormone Balance*

Preface

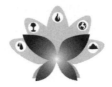

I wrote this book as a follow-up to my first book, *How to Heal Hashimoto's: An Integrative Road Map to Remission.* If you read that book and you're back for more, welcome back! I'm excited for you, and for our continuing journey. And if this is our first time meeting, welcome! I'm excited for you as well; we have lots to cover. The goal of both books is to help people overcome the suffering caused by the debilitating effects of Hashimoto's thyroiditis.

My grandmother used to say, "The quickest way to a man's heart is through his stomach." And I believe that the quickest way for you to achieve long-term, lasting results in getting your Hashimoto's into remission also happens to run through your *stomach* and the rest of your digestive tract.

The connection between diet and autoimmune disease is clearly on many people's minds. In fact, the most searched term on my website is *Hashimoto's diet.* The stomach is also the most common place for problems with people I work with, and it's the place where autoimmune disease originates and progresses. Therefore, I believe it is also the place where healing and remission can be leveraged and achieved.

Furthermore, it is my hope that this book will put to rest once and for all the notion that "diet doesn't matter," which I have heard umpteen times by members of the medical profession who haven't been trained in nor have the intellectual curiosity to inquire how important diet is.

In the words of a three-year-old I know, "Diet matters infinity!" I have set out in this book to make a case for that notion and to provide reams of evidence-based research, clinical data, and personal and professional experience to demonstrate that this is true.

HOW TO GET THE MOST OUT OF THIS BOOK

This book is organized into three parts. The first part explores the physiology of the digestive tract and all the interconnected systems. The second part looks at the specifics of the Hashimoto's Healing Diet. This section gives you a simple, adaptable approach to diet and helps to guide you on what the appropriate diet is for your unique set of circumstances

Finally, the third part shows you how to modulate the diet for specific health complaints. This section provides guidance for diets that will support healing from many different issues such as acid reflux, constipation, and even tooth and gum disease.

In addition, I have added some additional information in the form of sidebars—things I've learned in practice, and some actual case studies from people who have used these strategies successfully. These include Food as Medicine sidebars, which, as the name implies, show you how to use everyday foods to heal. Hashimoments are positive thoughts and affirmations that I created for my online community. These have been added to boost your spirit and give you inspiration as you work through all this material. Clinical Pearls are things I have learned after being in practice for many years. These are quick insights designed to help you get better results. And finally, as mentioned, I have shared Case Studies from some of the people that I have worked with. These were shared with me by people who gave me their permission to share their names and stories because they wanted to provide inspiration to others.

If you read my first book, you know that I believe it's important for you to understand how things work. And here's why: many doctors and practitioners, despite years of training, do not have a great understanding of physiology, especially physiology outside of their area of expertise.

They also don't seem to care to understand how the various systems of the body affect one another. And they rarely keep track of how one drug or intervention may affect other parts of the body that they are not treating.

This mystifies me, and it puts the onus on you to learn this so that you can make an informed decision on whether or not to accept their treatment recommendations. This matters because everything that is done to your body results in consequences.

I'm not exaggerating—every intervention, every drug, every surgery, every food, and every supplement matters. They all have physiological consequences. Some have a more profound impact than others, but over time, even smaller impacts can develop into larger changes.

If you understand how these systems work and interact with one another, and how different interventions can impact your body, at least in a general way, then you are going to be able to determine whether or not doing something makes sense for you. And you will also be much better prepared to ask the right questions of your doctor.

In researching and writing this book, I was faced with an enormous amount of conflicting information and a very complicated number of variables. I spent a lot of time trying to figure out how to radically simplify this, and I have done my best to lay it all out for you in an easy-to-follow manner.

I think the most important takeaway I got from this process is that *one diet will not work for everyone and often does not even work for one person in the long term.* Your body goes through cycles and changes, and you must be able to adapt to those cycles and changes.

In addition, there are often unintended consequences to rigidly staying with one type of diet because this also has physiological consequences. For example, I have observed that some people who stay on the AIP (autoimmune paleo) diet, which is quite restrictive, actually develop *more* food sensitivities, not fewer. (There is a reason for this, which I explain in detail in the second part of the book.)

If that happens to you, you must adapt. And when other things happen in your life, such as stressful events or treatments for certain complications (like those I mentioned above), your body goes through additional changes as a result. In my opinion, your diet needs to adjust accordingly.

Most books on diet and diet programs are designed to appeal to large numbers of people. I think this is partly to maximize sales and also because it takes a lot of knowledge and experience to be able to understand all the different things that can happen.

For example, very restrictive diets can degrade populations of good bacteria in your gut and diminish your body's ability to tolerate foods. Diets high in protein can put extra stress on your kidneys. Vegan diets can sometimes lead to deficiencies in certain vitamins (like B12).

So in this book, I have worked to help you understand that diets should be dynamic. The way you eat is not something that you should blindly follow and never deviate from. You must be able to adapt and make changes when necessary.

One of the blessings for me of having Hashimoto's and living through it as well as working with and interviewing over 2,000 people with this disease is that I have seen many different permutations of it. That is a decent sample size, and it has given me insights in what could happen and also what may work in various situations.

Finally, this book is not a cookbook, and it's not a gimmicky quick fix. It is designed to be a reference guide that you can turn to whenever you need it. Think of it as a dietary manual for your body that you can refer to again and again as you go through the cycles and changes of your life with Hashimoto's.

Next, I want to share a little about my own story so that you can see where I'm coming from. I also want to give you the basics of the diet to provide you with an overview of what it is and how and why it works. But before we get to that, here's a thought about visualizing the healing that you want.

HASHIMOMENT:
Visualize the Healing You Want

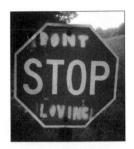

One of the central functions of our brains is to look into the future. Psychologists and neuroscientists have only recently begun to understand this.

Our behavior, memories, and the way we see the world are all shaped by our relationship to our future.

We don't learn by perfectly recording the past and never changing it; instead, we are constantly reshaping and reinventing our memories and imagining new stories about what is to come.

Even our emotions are guides to future behavior. Therapists are now exploring new ways to treat depression by treating the way we use past experiences to project what will happen in the future.

For many people who suffer from anxiety and depression, it is the fear of a bleak future that causes their suffering.

This can be broken into a couple of segments: imagining future scenarios and estimating future risks.

Anxiety and depression are often caused by imagining some sort of undesirable future experience and by imagining that the future risk is higher than it actually is.

This gives us tremendous insights into how to visualize.

First, you want to focus on a positive, healing vision. Concentrate on clear, detailed scenarios of what you would like to happen.

When we apply this to healing Hashimoto's, certain things come to mind: abundant energy, joy, mental clarity and focus, our immune systems calming down and not attacking, our thyroids regenerating and working beautifully, our adrenals healing and becoming revitalized, our guts healed and nourishing us effectively, etc.

Take some time to write out and clearly imagine the outcomes you want.

Don't obsess about risk. Risk is something that is incredibly hard for even the best computer models to accurately predict. There's no way for you to know what will happen.

So let that go, focus on imagining what you want, and replay this visualization repeatedly with as much detail as you can come up with. Next, think about what small action steps you can take to make this vision a reality.

Finally, look for small victories in the form of gratitude and little daily "wins"—for example, losing a pound or two, having more energy, sleeping better, or making yourself a healthy meal. Being grateful for small victories is a very important way to build larger success. Write them down and take time to celebrate them.

You may be surprised by the future your imagination creates for you!

Introduction

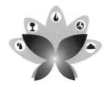

I'm sitting here in Rimrock, Arizona, just outside of Sedona, where I came to write this book on diet. Like my last book, this one is an exploration into both functional medicine and Chinese medicine.

If you aren't familiar with these two approaches to medicine, functional medicine, as the name implies, focuses on improving function in the body. The basic premise is that if your body is functioning optimally, you will be healthy. And it makes sense: form follows function. Good health is dependent on all your organs and glands, muscles, tendons, and bones all working properly.

So, a functional medicine practitioner (like myself) will use common diagnostic tests (like blood, stool, and saliva tests) to determine your baseline health. Then, they will prescribe supplements and diet and lifestyle changes to help your body to function better. After doing that for a period of time, they will retest and reevaluate you to determine whether or not these interventions work.

Chinese medicine, in my view, is the original functional medicine. Since ancient times, Chinese doctors have been concerned with how the different parts of the body interact and function. And much of the emphasis of Chinese medical diagnosis is on specific patterns of dysfunction.

The reason for this is quite logical. Any disease (and Hashimoto's is no exception) goes through different stages of progression. And often as it progresses, more organ systems become compromised (they stop functioning properly). Therefore, the goal is to stop and, hopefully, reverse that progression and restore proper function in the body.

This is what leads to better health and well-being. Because when you are healthy and thriving, everything is working harmoniously. When you're young and healthy, you just take it for granted. It isn't until things break down as you age or become sick that you start to understand how important these various functions are.

I came to Arizona to write for a couple of reasons. First, I wanted to be in a place where I could experience the earth in all its glory. If you haven't been here, there are breathtaking views of the landscape and incredible rock formations. The sky is huge, the clouds are epic. There's wind and monsoon rains in late summer and early fall. It's hot during the day and cool at night, and the nighttime sky is full of stars.

It's quite a bit different from where I live in Los Angeles, and that's another reason why I came. Being in Arizona, away from my familiar surroundings, has allowed me to reflect on our relationship to the earth and to our food and to ourselves. And it has helped me to imagine what it may have been like a few thousand years ago when our ancestors lived simpler lives that relied on the earth for sustenance.

The ancient Chinese, like many indigenous peoples, were close to nature; they studied it and strove to learn from it and emulate its natural cycles. Though these cultures were once considered backward, we are now beginning to see the wisdom of their relationship to the earth around them and their focus on sustainability and respecting and preserving the environment.

MY STORY

Diet and food choices have played an important role in my own story. As many of you know, I have Hashimoto's and my daughter also has it, so we have had to heal as a family, and making lifestyle adjustments has been a big part of that healing.

In the process of discovering my diagnosis for Hashimoto's and another autoimmune disease (ankylosing spondylitis), I asked a number of doctors whether or not diet had any impact on my health. For the most part, I was looked at like a simpleton and was told that diet didn't matter.

In the case of the doctor who diagnosed my Hashimoto's, I was told that in his experience, "It was easier to get an alcoholic to stop drinking than it was to get people to change their diets." And besides, diet didn't do anything for Hashimoto's.

In both cases, their only recommendation was that we wait and see and keep an eye on developments. In other words, we wait until a sufficient amount of tissue was destroyed by my immune system—and only then would we take action.

If you have to live through that, it's a demoralizing and painful descent into misery. In my opinion, it's too late to stop the progression or reverse the destruction by the time they recognize "sufficient" tissue damage. Those of us who are living through this need to take action *immediately* to slow (or stop) the progression of auto-immunity and tissue destruction.

I didn't want to wait for my thyroid to be destroyed. The research I was reading and the people that I was studying (Dr. Sarah Ballantyne, Dr. Datis Kharrazian, and others) were saying that diet mattered—a lot.

The reasons why diet matters are pretty logical: first, most of the immune system lives in the gut (by some estimates as much as 70 to 80 percent), and there is an enormous amount of research supporting the idea that dietary proteins cause immune responses.

In addition, the immune system that is found in the gut is very much intertwined with tolerance to our own proteins. Autoimmune diseases like Hashimoto's are the result of the loss of self-tolerance; our immune system short circuits, and the job it performs naturally (cleaning up old cells and dead tissue) morphs into something more destructive and dangerous.

There are many theories about what leads to this, and it seems to have numerous causes (e.g., Epstein-Barr and other pathogens, genetics, stress, exposure to gluten, lectins and other damaging proteins, and more). But the bottom line is that diet is integral to the disease process and is, therefore, the foundation of any successful treatment of autoimmunity.

And from my own personal experience, I can tell you that I didn't start to feel any better until I went all in with my diet and made some pretty significant changes. At first, I gave up gluten, dairy, and soy and then I tried the autoimmune paleo protocol. This is a diet that eliminates all foods that are potentially inflammatory, such as those I just mentioned as well as grains, nuts and seeds, nightshades (tomatoes, peppers, eggplants, and white potatoes), alcohol, and coffee.

This resulted in a dramatic improvement in my weight; I lost 25 pounds of bloating and inflammation. My overall energy, endurance, and memory and cognitive ability also improved. My TPO (thyroid peroxidase) antibodies dropped from 1200 to 153. As a result, I have become a firm believer in the power of diet and lifestyle changes.

And one thing all of us who have researched and treated people with Hashimoto's have in common is a strong belief that diet can make a huge difference in improving people's quality of life. So, we have to take it into our own hands and use diet effectively because no one else will.

As I mentioned, in Chinese medicine, the digestive system is a part of the Earth phase. The five elements, also known as the five phases, is an algorithm for understanding complex interactions between the different systems of the body. It provides a template for understanding positive and negative feedback loops, these are the mechanisms our organs and glands use to communicate and influence one another.

The earth element is central to our health and vitality. We literally live and die through our bowels. So, taking care of the earth element is absolutely essential if you want to feel your best. And, the truth is that taking care of the actual earth is also absolutely central to our own health and well-being.

IF WE DESTROY THE EARTH, WE DESTROY OURSELVES

One simple biological truth that you cannot refute is that any organism that destroys its environment destroys itself. This is true of every magnitude of species from parasites to large predators. If a parasite kills its host, it must find a new host or it will die. If a big predator kills off all its prey and destroys the balance of its environment, it will die.

And we are currently charting a course on this planet that puts us at risk of destroying our environment.

As any self-respecting scientist will tell you, it's pretty indisputable that we are causing the planet to warm, and this is having a major impact on our environment and on ourselves. And we are also living a huge chemistry experiment with over 4 billion pounds of toxic chemicals being released by industries in the U.S. alone each year.[1]

This is also true of the soil (the earth) that we grow our food in. Dust blowing off of fields that have been tilled repeatedly for years has led to respiratory illnesses in rural America. Thousands of people are exposed to drinking water with levels of pesticides that far exceed the levels the Environmental Protection Agency has deemed safe.

The drinking water of over 200 million Americans is polluted with nitrates from fertilizers. It has been linked with developmental problems in children and poses cancer risks for adults. The United Nations considers the neglect and destruction of soil to be one of the central threats to human health in coming decades.[2]

We have *literally* poisoned the earth on which we depend. This radical altering of our soil and our environment is having an effect on all of our health. Certainly, one of the central themes of ancient Taoist thought and Chinese medicine is that what takes place in the outer world also takes place inside of us.

There is no question that everything is connected. Within our bodies, all the different systems of the body are connected. I demonstrated this in depth in my first book, and we will be exploring that again in this book.

But, this is also true of the larger world. Herbicides, pesticides, and fertilizers poured onto our farmlands end up in our waterways and our oceans. Plastic is now everywhere on the planet; there are even huge floating islands of garbage (consisting mostly of plastic pollution) in the five gyres or surface currents in our oceans.

POLLUTION IS AFFECTING OUR HEALTH

We are only beginning to understand the full extent of all of this pollution on our health. And the great irony of the chemical industry lobbyists and executives profiting off of this is that they are only hurting themselves and their children and grandchildren. All the wealth they accumulate will not keep them from the chemicals that they continue to pour into our environment. It affects us all.

What I'm driving at here is that any study of our digestive health and the earth element must also include a consciousness of planet Earth, and healing the earth element must include some conscious work toward healing the *entire* planet.

Because in the process of thinking about and experiencing the earth, we are also learning about where our food comes from, what chemicals and additives are in our food, the ways in which food can alter our own internal environment, and much, much more.

I'm not telling you this to freak you out or to add to your list of things to worry about. I just want to provide context for why this matters, and how the little things we do can improve our relationship with our world and ourselves. There's a lot we can learn from these ancient masters who were really in touch with nature, the world around them, and (go figure) themselves.

HERE'S THE BIG SECRET

I like to read works from the ancient Taoist masters like Lao-tzu and Chuang-tzu. Their writing is really concise, yet it's also incredibly deep. There's some dispute about when these two men actually lived but general consensus is it's somewhere around the 4th or 5th century B.C., so, roughly 2,500 years ago.

Okay, time-out. Just take a minute and imagine what the world was like 2,500 years ago. No cell phones, no computers. No electricity. It was you and the earth. In most places, you were at the mercy of the weather. In fact, you had to always be aware of it, because your life could depend on it. You had to pay attention to the cycles of the seasons, and you had to know where your next meal was coming from.

There was a legitimate chance that you could starve to death. This is a completely different world from what most of us live in today. "Progress," the industrial revolution, and the industrial food complex have taken you entirely out of that world.

Today, because of the advances of food science and distribution, you can literally (and many people do) eat yourself to death. But, the truth is, we are still the same people, biologically and physiologically, that we were 2,500 years ago.

And 2,500 years is nothing in the scheme of things. It's a blip in terms of the age of the planet, which is estimated to be 4.5 BILLION years old (you want to talk about wisdom!). So the wisdom of these sages still applies. Times infinity!

JUST DO LESS

One theme that appears over and over again in their writing is the simple idea of doing less. OMG! Stop the presses! That's right I said it: *do less.*

Okay, check this out.

In Chapter 48 of the *Tao Teh Ching*, written by Lao-tzu, the sage wrote:

> *Learning consists of daily accumulating;*
> *The practice of Tao consists of daily diminishing. . . .*[3]

Simple words of wisdom.

What does he mean?

In our culture of consumption, we are often conditioned to think about what more we need to be happy or healthy or fulfilled.

But the reality is that accumulating more things doesn't fill that void. Because there is no void, it is all just desire and projection. And if we apply this idea to healing, how often are we told to simplify?

A lot of health advice is about adding this supplement or that medication. And here's why: People are angling to make money off of you. They want to sell you on changing to this diet or this exercise regimen. But here's the thing—some of the most powerful health decisions actually involve doing less.

This can be especially helpful with something like Hashimoto's because there are so many variables.

Simplifying your diet allows you to see what foods you may be reacting to. Simplifying your life allows you to really see how destructive stress can be. Simplifying the number of supplements you take allows you to actually see what is working.

Furthermore, later in the same chapter, Lao-tzu refers to the concept of "Non-Ado." This refers to doing without doing, and comes from the Chinese term *wu wei*. This means acting naturally, without struggle or tons of effort. It's kind of like "being in the zone" where you just feel it.

When applied to meditation, it is very powerful. Meditation can be a fight with your mind for quiet and dominance, or it can be a letting go and acceptance that thoughts will come and go.

Reaching that place of acceptance and flow is how we get the most out of meditation. And they are often fleeting and elusive moments (at least for me). But when I have experienced those moments of flow, time seems to stop and all my cares and worries disappear.

And the truth is, we can't will ourselves to that inner peace, nor can we force serenity.

The same can be said of healing; you can't always will yourself to be better. Sometimes, you really need to begin by simplifying and letting go.

And once we start to get our lives back, we are in a position to help others and be of service. And then we can let go of the private ends that would be served. Here's the thing: those that live to serve private ends, end their lives alone.

I'm here to serve you. Come what may. Hey, what's the worst thing that could happen? Together, we might actually find a way to heal.

MOST CHRONIC DEGENERATIVE DISEASES ARE DISEASES OF EXCESS

According to the Centers for Disease Control and Prevention (CDC), the top 10 leading causes of death in the U.S. are as follows:[4]

#1 Heart Disease

#2 Cancer

#3 Chronic Lower Respiratory Diseases

#4 Accidents

#5 Stroke

#6 Alzheimer's

#7 Diabetes

#8 Influenza and Pneumonia

#9 Kidney Disease (nephritis, nephrotic syndrome, nephrosis)

#10 Suicide (I was sad to see that this made the top 10.)

If you look at this group and think about what causes them, with a few exceptions they are mostly diseases of *too much*: too much cigarette smoking, too much alcohol drinking, too much sugar and fat consumption, too much sitting (and too little exercise).

These are very much diseases of the excesses of modern life. And another way to think about them is that they are also mostly self-inflicted. Right? These things that we are doing too much of are all choices we make and habits we develop.

The top three causes account for 75 percent of deaths, and I think we can add to this list of causes exposure to too many chemicals and carcinogens as another potential culprit in these diseases. (Certainly this is true of cancer and respiratory diseases; air pollution is a known factor in both. And while it's harder to link, the body is all connected and the heart is also impacted and damaged by smoking and air pollution.)

So this idea of doing less is still a wise recommendation, and it still resonates 2,500 years later. It's obvious in its simplicity, but look around you. Clearly, a lot of people are not choosing to do less.

BUT WHAT ABOUT AUTOIMMUNE DISEASE?

That's a fair question. Can we also categorize autoimmunity as a disease of excess or the result of excesses?

If you read my last book, you'll recall that there is no single cause for autoimmunity. Let's review these causes:

In many people there is some exposure to a virus or other pathogen, like Epstein-Barr virus (or other herpes viruses), Coxsackie virus, or other pathogens like Yersinia or Lyme disease. Some have theorized that these viral fragments resemble thyroid tissue, and that is why the immune system attacks the thyroid after fighting the virus. There may also be exposure to environmental toxins (mercury, bisphenol A, etc.), and these actually form what are called "neoantigens." These new antigens comprise the chemical plus our own tissue.

The formation of these neoantigens initiates an immune response, which may result in antibody production against the chemical and the human tissue hybrid. Exposure to the chemical and the production of antibodies against various tissue antigens may result in autoimmune reactivity.

Genetics are also a factor with Hashimoto's. We often see clusters with family members. It is not unusual to find first-degree relatives with thyroid disease with people who have confirmed Hashimoto's.

What's more, exposure to gluten and celiac disease can be factors in the formation of autoimmune disease.[5]

Stress can also play a major role in the expression and proliferation of autoimmune disease and Hashimoto's. In a retrospective study from the journal *Autoimmunity Reviews*, researchers noted that "(up to 80 percent) of patients reported uncommon emotional stress before disease onset. Unfortunately, not only does stress cause disease, but the disease itself also causes significant stress in the patients, creating a vicious cycle."[6]

Taken as a whole, I think you can legitimately argue that "too much" is also a factor in autoimmunity. Too much stress, too many environmental toxins, too much gluten, combined with the bad luck of genetics (which, remember, genes are expressed by our behavior and environment—so these can be influenced by our "too much" lifestyles) and exposure to a pathogen.

So where am I going with all this?

Well, as I was writing this book, I wanted to find a simple overarching theme and I just kept seeing this over and over again. I don't want to write another book that adds another 50 supplements for you take. I will be making some recommendations for things that you should do in specific situations, but I will always begin with first asking: *What can we do without?*

As we explore the role of food and digestive health in Hashimoto's and autoimmune disease, I think the first question we should be asking ourselves is: Where can we do less?

How can we have less stress? What habits need to be addressed and stopped?

What foods do we need to eat less of or eliminate altogether? What drinks do we need to drink less of or eliminate altogether?

How can we be exposed to fewer chemicals and environmental toxins, and how can we minimize the damage from those we are exposed to?

And maybe we can also stop dumping so much garbage and pollution on our planet by choosing to embrace a "do less" life. Because, here's the thing, the Earth will survive us. In 4.5 billion years, it's seen many, many species come and go. Maybe we should be open to what the planet has to teach us.

Just saying.

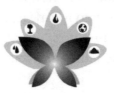

HASHIMOTO'S DIET AT A GLANCE

In researching this book, I came upon a lot of conflicting information and a lot of complicated approaches to diet and healing through diet. But before we get into some of the theory and background of the approach that I have developed, I'd like to give you a brief overview of the basic principles and explain in a relatively simple way how you can apply these ideas.

Here are the basic steps that you will take as you use diet as the foundation of your successful campaign toward remission. As I mentioned already, you must first assess where you are and what you want to accomplish before you choose which dietary approach is best for you.

Step One: Elimination:

If you are a beginner or you have fallen off the wagon and are not eating the way you know you should, do the elimination diet for 30 to 60 days. The details of the elimination phase can be found in Chapter 13.

This diet will allow you to reduce variables, and it will cause your immune system to calm down, allowing you to work on healing your gut. This will jump-start the healing momentum.

This follows our basic approach of simply doing less. There are so many variables with Hashimoto's, and these include food sensitivities and food reactions, secondary infections, stress-induced health issues, blood sugar imbalances, adrenal issues, and lots more.

The process of healing involves conducting a series of experiments with your body. The more variables you have, the harder it is to determine whether or not your experiment worked. If you can't figure out what worked, then you can't build on that success.

So, first, do less and keep track of it all. Keep a journal so that you can accurately assess your progress (or lack thereof). Journaling is a goldmine of data that can be useful to make sure you're hitting your goals.

Once you have eliminated your variables and given your immune system time to calm down, the next step is to reintroduce foods and to work on boosting oral tolerance.

Step Two: Reintroduction/Reboot Oral Tolerance:

Once you have completed the elimination phase, you should start trying to reintroduce foods and work on building oral tolerance (this is covered in Chapter 14).

The importance of not staying on a strict elimination for a prolonged period of time cannot be overstated. Long-term elimination diets can result in the loss of both the diversity in the microbiome and your ability to tolerate various foods. This can have serious health consequences and can make your life absolutely miserable.

Reintroducing food and working on improving oral tolerance should be done when you feel like you have some improvement in your symptoms and your lab results. This should happen relatively quickly, somewhere between 30 to 90 days. If you don't see any improvement after three months, something else may be going on (such as an infection) and this should be investigated and treated.

We will explore this much further in the book, but as I mentioned, too many restrictions and adhering too rigidly to a limited diet may have physiological consequences that can result in more, not fewer, food sensitivities and more stress.

Regardless of where you are in this progression, I recommend applying an approach that I have coined the Tummy Triangle Treatment. It is a very effective way of choosing a treatment plan and approach based on what's going on with you.

——Tummy Triangle Treatment——

I came up with this idea after looking at lots of different variations and lots of variables in both Western nutrition and the Chinese medicine dietary model, and I realized they could all be simplified to three areas. In other words, we can take everything we are going to learn in this book and simplify it to a triangle of pathologies.

And the reason for this is simple. Experience has taught me that these three problem areas show up over and over again, and they lead to each other (and to all other issues). They are the "holy trinity" of digestive imbalance and, therefore, the root cause of the vast majority of digestive problems.

So, in a simple sense, all we have to do is to make sure we address all three of these issues at some point. And sometimes, we may have to vary the proportions of the triangle as circumstances shift.

I have created a simple diagram that reflects these three areas. Each corner of the triangle represents a different issue, and we must always be conscious of which area we are trying to work on in the short term.

And in the long term, we must always remember to return to one area in particular, that of the stomach and spleen, or the Earth phase. Returning here is important because (as we will learn in this book) the Earth phase is the center and good health revolves around it, much like the Earth revolves around the sun.

These three issues are:

1. **Spleen and stomach qi deficiency:** If you aren't familiar with the term *qi* from Chinese medicine, it refers to metabolic activity or energy.

    This term is another way of describing metabolic weakness, like hypothyroidism, adrenal fatigue, too little stomach acid, too few pancreatic enzymes, etc. Weakness here can lead to other deficiencies like anemias and nutrient deficiencies.

    This spleen and stomach deficiency diet is also a foundational diet, and the place where we should return periodically, in order to maintain sustained health of the Earth phase. It is "home base," if you will.

2. **Liver qi stagnation:** This is another term from Chinese medicine and a different way of saying the emotional component of disease (stress, anger, rage, resentment, anxiety, worry, depression, etc.). Dietary interventions can actually make a big difference with some emotional issues and ignoring the role of emotion can undermine any treatment strategy.

    While it should be fairly obvious that your emotional state can have a big impact on your digestive health, I am not aware of any other diet that actually takes this into consideration and instructs you on how to eat when you have emotional challenges.

    Both herbs and foods can have a significant impact on you emotionally, and they can provide a much faster avenue for achieving equilibrium and balance again. And, of course, the opposite is true: fighting at the dinner table and having conflict and drama be a regular part of your mealtime can also have some negative health consequences.

3. **Damp heat:** This third leg of the triangle is also a term from Chinese medicine, and this covers all pathological infections that are so often intertwined with Hashimoto's and hypothyroidism. Epstein-Barr virus, *H. pylori,* Yersinia, Blastocystis, SIBO, Lyme disease, and Candida, as well as internal excesses like phlegm, which leads to nodules, plaque in the arteries, and painful inflammatory conditions.

These are the three cardinal issues of Hashimoto's (and any other autoimmune or chronic degenerative disease). They are present in everyone in some measure, in my opinion.

As we will see over and over again when we look at specific problems, these three issues lead to each other and then can lead to other problems like blood and yin deficiency, blood stagnation, phlegm, and fire (more on this in upcoming chapters). But, basically, these are the core imbalances that lead to everything else.

For example, liver qi stagnation damages the spleen and stomach, weakening them and impairing their function. When their function is impaired, that leads to dampness.

Dampness can bog everything down in the digestive tract. This combined with the qi stagnation tends to result in the development of heat (inflammation) because things don't move. This stagnant heat combines with the dampness and creates damp heat.

And if you think about it, modern life in the Western world is particularly prone to creating a toxic tummy. Right?

Stressful lives, fast food and terrible eating habits, jobs that mostly require sitting all day, and the overuse of common drugs (like antibiotics and NSAIDs). All of this can damage the health of our digestive tract. And the way to heal it (as we will see) is the Tummy Triangle Treatment!

How do we treat this then?

Well, in every situation we must evaluate and determine which treatment principles we should apply. So what does that look like?

The three main treatment principles are as follows:

1. **For spleen and stomach qi deficiency:** Strengthen the spleen and stomach qi with sweet and warm foods and herbs (you will be provided with a list of these foods). Also include foods and herbs that are nutrient dense and tonifying (which means they are targeted nutrition for a given organ or gland).

2. **For liver qi stagnation:** Regulate the liver, invigorate qi, and stimulate the correct functioning of the qi mechanism with pungent, dispersing foods and herbs. You also have to address the underlying emotional component (ignore this and you put up a major roadblock to healing).

3. **For damp heat:** Clear damp heat and/or heat with bitter, cooling foods and herbs. Many of these herbs and foods have broad-spectrum antiviral and antibacterial properties. That's why they work!

Easy peasy lemon squeazy!

In this book, as in my first book, I recommend that you also use the A.P.A.R.T. System that I created for helping you to figure out which issue is predominant, and then we'll formulate a diet and herb solution. (If you aren't familiar with the A.P.A.R.T. System, I will give you quick review shortly.)

And for many of you who are already following the autoimmune paleo approach, this isn't a change in what you eat. It's a change in how you apply foods to your various symptoms and challenges.

Furthermore, if you're just starting out, be warned that this may be a radical change in both what and how you eat. So, go gently, but go all in. You will be rewarded, and the good news is that this solution is relatively simple and elegant!

Before we get to the background, history, and specific health issues, here's a simplified overview of the basic diet that we will apply this Tummy Triangle Treatment approach to.

If this is all new to you, it's a 90-day, two-step approach. As mentioned, the first step is an elimination diet and the second step is the reintroduction of food and working to restore oral tolerance (explained below).

This will give us a group of foods to work with that we can then apply the Tummy Triangle Treatment principles to. This way, you can treat whatever issues you have while addressing your Hashimoto's and autoimmunity.

I have also included an Appendix for those of you who wish to use a vegan and vegetarian approach (see Appendix 2). And if you have been doing the autoimmune paleo diet for some time, you can skip the chapter on the elimination diet and jump to the chapter on reintroductions and building oral tolerance or simply jump to the various dietary variations for specific health issues.

As I mentioned, think of this book as an owner's manual for your digestive tract. There are recommendations for wherever you are and for whatever condition you may need to address. And I have done my best to make it as simple and easy to follow as possible.

Before we get into this in more depth, here's an inspiring case study about someone who followed the program I have outlined religiously, and it resulted in her losing a considerable amount of weight and improving her quality of life significantly.

CASE STUDY

This time last year I was really feeling awful and packing on the pounds. I could drag myself to work and home again, but that was about it. I didn't feel up to anything. I was totally drained. My TSH [thyroid-stimulating hormone] and cholesterol were sky-high. When my internist ordered a thyroid antibody test, the results were very high. I'd never heard of Hashimoto's, but I had 9 of the 10 most common symptoms. I knew I was in for a fight. My internist prescribed thyroid medication, but I didn't feel much better.

Luckily, I contacted Marc Ryan. He evaluated me, designed an action plan, and really got me on the right track. He encouraged me to be proactive and commit to the autoimmune protocol diet, try new supplements, use positive affirmations, de-stress, and start exercising. I made these my life priorities. Marc was so helpful and supportive in assisting me. Marc understood that the entire body is affected by Hashimoto's and needs to be treated as a whole to get Hashimoto's into remission.

Marc is part of my dream team who is encouraging me and monitoring my progress. I've dropped 72 lbs., and my TSH levels, cholesterol, vitamin D, and B12 are all in the normal range now. My TPO [thyroid peroxidase antibodies] went down from 179 to 163. I'm walking three to five miles daily, and I've started a yoga practice. I have tons of energy and love my new lifestyle.

I'm excited for the future and will never go back to my old ways because I never want to feel that bad again. I'm enjoying life and rejoice that I've come so far in this journey.

Briget B.
California

——How to Apply the Tummy Triangle Treatment——

 Tummy Triangle Treatment: If you are still having challenges or have gone through a period that has set you back, return to the basic principles of the Tummy Triangle Treatment (which we will explore in more depth in upcoming chapters).

First, ask the question: **Is my current challenge of an excess or deficient nature?** (Get familiar with the symptoms of each so that you can develop an intuitive sense of which it may be. These can be found in chapters 11 and 12.)

This is another way of asking, "Do I work on strengthening and building up, or do I focus on simplifying and clearing out?" If deficiency is the predominant problem, then you must focus on rebuilding and use nutrient-dense foods and supplements that replenish.

If excess is the predominant problem, you must do less and work on clearing out the causes of inflammation and possibly treat infections and/or focus on resolving emotional issues.

Emotional issues that involve stress and repressed emotions are considered a form of excess in this model. Dampness-, heat-, and phlegm-related conditions are also excess in nature. (Infections can be thought of as excess conditions involving both dampness and/or heat.)

When the condition is excess, ask: **Where can I do less in this situation?** Once you've answered that, take steps to do less. And make the changes to restore balance.

Deficient conditions are those that involve weakness, cold, and fatigue. These are problems related to metabolic weakness and fatigue or exhaustion of certain organs and organ systems.

Give yourself space to recover and heal. Identify which areas are weak and use foods and herbs to strengthen those areas. Get more rest and sleep, and let go of stressful relationships and circumstances if you need to. Listen to your body and your heart.

And the reality is that, sometimes, you may have to treat more than one area and then transition back to another. Life is certain to change; get to know your body enough to know when changes need to be made, and use this book to help you when you aren't sure.

Sometimes, you may need to experiment and/or make a judgment call. That's okay. The great thing about this approach is that it is flexible and gentle, so if you make a mistake, it's pretty easy to course correct and get back on track.

Long Term: The long-term approach should be the flexible movement between these various diets and, hopefully, as you go through this process and you keep track of it in your journal, you will discover your vulnerabilities and your tendencies.

Your vulnerabilities should be guarded against, and the weaknesses and excesses that lead to them should be addressed. In addition, your tendencies will put you in repeated situations that will inevitably cause something to happen.

Finally, be sure to use the A.P.A.R.T. System to evaluate, plan, and treat the challenges that come up.

The A.P.A.R.T. System gives you a ready-made framework for figuring out where you need to focus, and then it guides you in an effective process for resolving whatever issues you need to work on. Throughout the book, I will provide you with recommendations and guidance for each step of this system.

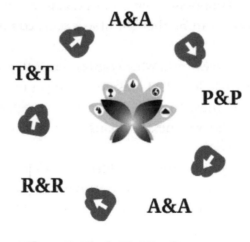

A&A

T&T

P&P

R&R

A&A

The A.P.A.R.T. System

As you may recall from my first book, A.P.A.R.T. is an acronym and each letter has two ideas associated with it:

1. ASK AND ASSESS

The first step is always to ask the appropriate questions and to order or have your doctor order the appropriate tests so that you can develop a working hypothesis for what experiment you want to conduct on your body.

Because let's face it: Regardless of whether it's you or your doctor overseeing this process, you are running an experiment every time you take a medication or a supplement or alter your diet. And you have no idea what the actual outcome of that experiment will be.

This is why we have to do a proper assessment first and then keep track of the results of whatever it is that we decide to try.

2. PRIORITIZE AND PLAN

The next step is to formulate a plan. Not everything is of the same order of importance and not everything should be attempted all at once. If you do too many things, how can you tell what's working?

You first need to make a choice about what question(s) you want to answer and what measurable goal you want to reach or at least attempt to reach. For example, a question could be: Will this diet lower my TPO antibodies? And the measurable goal is, obviously, the blood test results of antibody levels before and after you try this diet.

Be aware that we may not hit all our goals 100 percent, but that doesn't mean we shouldn't try and then learn from that trial. Success or "failure" are both valuable because they give us useful data to work with.

3. ACT AND ADAPT

Once you have your plan, you must put it into action. Take the necessary steps and make the necessary changes to make that plan a reality. A great plan is useless if it isn't executed.

And when you do execute the plan, you must be flexible enough to adapt to changing circumstances as they arise. Things are going to happen, and you may need to tweak your approach or make some changes as you go.

4. REASSESS AND REEVALUATE

After you take action on your plan, you will need to reevaluate. Assess the situation by asking yourself some questions: Did you achieve your goal(s)? Did you alter your test results? Did your experiment yield the results you had hoped for?

Good, bad, or indifferent, this step is very important because it is the moment of truth when the data teaches us. And don't get attached to the results here. If it failed, that's good. Now you know something that doesn't work for you.

If it succeeded, that's also good, for now you have something that you can try again and perhaps even double down on to get even better results. Stop doing things that aren't working, tweak or change your approach, and keep doing the things that are working. Make the appropriate adjustments as you go.

5. TRY AND TRY AGAIN

Finally, remember that using diet to balance and heal is a long-term project. The reason we conduct these experiments is so that we can develop a toolbox of solutions for our various issues and build positive healing momentum.

Keep experimenting and using the A.P.A.R.T. System, keep refining your approach, and when you lose your way or get distracted, come back to the center. Always come back to healing the Earth phase. That should be your default priority and plan.

Next, let's take a few steps back and get some background on this approach and learn why and how it works. We'll look at some theory and some physiology and learn how all of this intersects in the digestive tract.

FOOD AS MEDICINE: *CHRYSANTHEMUM FLOWERS*

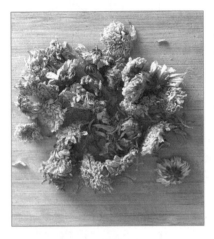

Here's one of my favorite herbs/foods, especially in the middle of a hot summer. It's chrysanthemum flower, or *ju hua,* as it's known in Chinese.

It has a mild sweet and bitter flavor, cooling in nature, and it is traditionally used to dispel heat and wind and to counteract toxins. It's really helpful for relieving headaches and reducing inflammation.

It's also quite beneficial for the eyes. It can improve vision and brighten the eyes, lower blood pressure, and aid in metabolizing fat.

It's helpful for colds and flus and can be combined with mint, forsythia, and mulberry leaf for treating acute upper respiratory issues.

It's also soothing and calming to the liver. In Traditional Chinese Medicine there's a condition called liver heat or liver fire, which can result in headaches and red eyes, and it is often used as part of treatment for that.

Chrysanthemum is also really beneficial for the eyes. It can be taken internally as a tea and is great when combined with goji berries. You can also strain the tea and make an eyewash, and it's very gentle and effective.

Pharmacologically, it has been shown to have antibacterial, anti-inflammatory, and fever-reducing effects. In addition, it helps promote blood flow to the heart and lowers blood pressure. It's also a potent antioxidant and has anti-aging properties.

And to top it all off, it looks beautiful if you put a few flowers in a glass pot!

I make a summertime tea with the following ingredients:

A couple of chrysanthemum flowers
A couple pieces of ginseng
A half handful of goji berries
A pinch of honeysuckle flowers
A pinch of green tea

Boil a pot of water and put all of these ingredients in a glass teapot. Add the hot water and the flowers will bloom, the berries will float, and you'll have a beautiful and delicious pot of tea. Let it steep about 5 to 10 minutes, then serve.

Just delicious, and it cools you off. It's nice served as an iced tea too!

PART I

Diet, Digestion, and Autoimmune Disease
ARE ALL CONNECTED

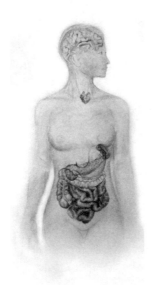

Chapter 1

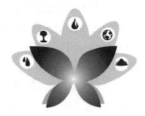

FUNCTIONAL MEDICINE AND THE FIVE PHASES OF DIGESTIVE HEALTH

*In the Western medical model, diet is not, for the most part, considered a viable treatment. And dietary recommendations are given as afterthoughts or as vague general recommendations. Instead pharmaceutical drugs are prescribed, and these tend to disrupt physiological function(s) and can lead to other health issues that, in turn, must be treated with **more** medication.*

Functional medicine, on the other hand, views diet as not only a legitimate treatment, but also as something foundational for helping restore the body to proper physiological function. And diet can play an important role as both the foundation for other treatment and as a primary modality.

As I have written in the past, Chinese medicine is the original functional medicine. And Chinese dietary therapy has been used for centuries and is extremely refined and sophisticated. Furthermore, diet has always been thought to be important as a causative factor of diseases and as a legitimate treatment modality.

Ancient Chinese doctors recognized that the different systems of the body were not static machine parts, and they recognized them to be living ecosystems that were constantly in flux and constantly interacting with, influencing, and affecting one another.

The five elements are a very clever template for understanding these complex interactions.

In my first book, I introduced the theories of yin and yang and the Five Elements System, and we looked at the five elements in relation to Hashimoto's and hypothyroidism and discovered how the thyroid influenced all the systems of the body.

This time around I want to take you to the next level and to explore these five interacting systems not as static entities but as constantly moving parts, much like a solar system with all the planets moving in their various orbits.

In order to understand this better, we're going to change the terminology a little bit too and refer to them as the *five phases*. I will explain more in a moment, but first let's review yin and yang, and then we'll explore all of this in the context of diet and digestive issues.

YIN AND YANG IN NATURE

The theory of yin and yang is prescient because it comes from nature. All one has to do is to be in the natural world to see it play out. Night and day, darkness and light, winter and summer, hot and cold, wet and dry, the sun and the moon . . . these are all examples of the interplay of yin and yang in daily life.

Yin and yang perfectly describes the interaction of opposites and the ways in which each, ultimately, leads to the other. For example, night becomes day and the darkest (most yin aspect) point of night is right before the dawn (which is the beginning of yang).

In the body, yin and yang are very useful concepts for describing biological and physiological functions.

All the processes of the body can be divided into yin and yang.

These yin and yang types of relationships become significant when they impact the body's anatomy and physiology, and it is precisely these designations that are used in the diagnosis of imbalances in Traditional Chinese Medicine (TCM).

When using foods and diet to heal, we look at the yin and yang properties of food and use them to nourish or counterbalance.

In addition, when we look at the way that Hashimoto's affects the body and particularly the digestive system, we see yin and yang interplay all over the place.

The hormones of the endocrine system are yang. The endocrine organs are yin. The main organs of the immune system, the lymphatic system, and the spleen, etc., are yin. In contrast, the immune responses of inflammation and defense are considered yang.

Disease and disease progression can also be viewed in terms of yin and yang.

With digestive health and digestive function, yang metabolic activity is necessary for extracting yin nutrients. And pathologies are often caused by deficiencies of this yang or qi, which leads to excesses of yin or pathogens like dampness and/or damp heat.

And it is precisely this dynamic that leads to the formation of diseases; even people with the same disease of "Hashimoto's" can have radically different things going on in their bodies. Yin substances like dampness and phlegm can be excessive, and yang substances like hormones, stomach acid, and enzymes can be deficient. And these can all result in pathology and systemic disease.

In the next section, we are going to look at the ideas of a renowned ancient doctor whose theories about disease are surprisingly accurate today and describe the process of autoimmunity amazingly well. This theory includes something called "yin fire," which is another way of describing the systemic inflammation at the root of autoimmune disease.

In this case, the metabolic balance of yin and yang are out of whack, and yang is too weak (this is what hypothyroidism causes) and unable to balance yin. Therefore, because yang is deficient over time, then yin becomes imbalanced too. This illustrates that not only do yin and yang balance each other, but they also mutually generate each other.

And diet can play a huge role in both reestablishing balance and in providing the proper nutrients and substances to give us the raw materials that enable us to heal.

This is the yin fire that we will soon explore. But first, let's review the five elements and look at them in the context of the dynamic movement that they so beautifully illustrate.

FOOD AS MEDICINE: *TANGERINE PEEL*

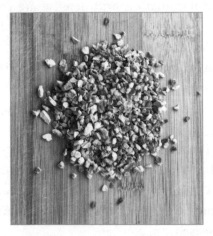

Here's a great remedy and something you'd probably throw away before you thought of using it.

But Mother Nature, in her infinite wisdom, wastes nothing!

Tangerine peel, called *chen pi* in Chinese, is considered a little sweet, spicy, and bitter. It has an affinity for the spleen and lung.

The peel supports and activates qi and dispels dampness and phlegm. And it's carminative (a fancy way of saying it relieves farting and gas).

And the rest of the tangerine is no slouch either. It's considered warm, sweet, and sour. It's also carminative; it opens the channels, strengthens the stomach, and stops coughing and gas.

It's great for nausea, vomiting, cough with an excess of white or clear mucus, chest tightness, and rib pain.

Here are a couple of simple remedies:

- For nausea, vomiting, or stomach pain, make a tea from organic tangerine peel and ginger. (It's good for hangovers too.)

- For chest fullness or rib pain, use the fruit combined with rice wine and water to make a tea.

Next time you have a tangerine, don't forget to save the peel. You can dry it and chop it up. That's what you see in the photo.

Have a great day! Unless you have other more sweet, spicy, and bitter plans.

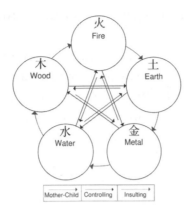

FIVE ELEMENTS INTO MOTION: THE FIVE PHASES

The ancient Chinese doctors and the Taoists, like Lao-tzu and Chuang-tzu who influenced them, studied nature. I would even argue that they were nature scientists, observing, experimenting, and learning from the natural world.

And the natural world included their own bodies. After all, where do we connect with nature more completely than inside of ourselves? Sometimes we forget that. Want to be out in nature? Go meditate for 15 minutes. There is no separation, except the one that we have created in our thinking and our behavior.

Do you want to learn how to heal? Learn how to work with the natural order of things to get your body back to balance. And how do you learn about the natural order of things? By looking inside. In my opinion, it's really that simple.

This is why I devote so much time and energy to helping you understand why things happen the way they do. I want to teach you about you. Because there is no doctor or practitioner or medical medium who knows you better than you do.

And if you can learn to listen to and work with your body as it goes through its changes, you'll be well on your way to getting better. I promise you.

The five elements, or five phases, as we are now going to refer to them, perfectly exemplify this notion.

Indigenous cultures that are sometimes called primitive observed, by necessity, the natural world. They charted the movement and cycles of the stars, the planets, and the moon.

And these celestial movements were connected to the growing seasons, the weather, and animal migration. Most cultures eventually transitioned from hunter-gatherers to agriculture societies as they grew. This required learning how to predict climate patterns and seasonal changes and how to use this information to optimize crop yields.

The ancient Chinese developed quite sophisticated systems for recording celestial movements and for forecasting the seasonal and climatic rhythms of life. For example, in 2254 B.C., legend has it that Emperor Yao ordered that the timing of the four solar seasons be charted so that farmers could know when to best plant their crops. Solstices (when the sun is at its extreme points) and equinoxes (when days and nights are equal) were both identified.[1]

Chinese doctors also sought to learn about the body's own internal rhythms. The five elements were originally written as *wu xing*. *Wu* meaning "five" and *xing* being translated as "element." But, really, the character *xing* suggests movement like walking, marching, and circulating: that is, all things that are active, movement-oriented processes.[2]

Wu xing has often been translated into the term *five elements* and I used this phrasing in my last book to keep that familiar association. However, in this book, I have chosen to use this other translation because I want you to start thinking in terms of this dynamic movement rather than just static elements.

(The reason for this change will be clearer in the second part of this book, where I will give you strategies for adapting to these movements and changes in your body.)

In addition, I will expand on an idea I introduced in my last book, and that is how to be a "gut farmer." Thinking in terms of the five phases like the seasonal changes of growing crops will give you a good sense of the direction we are going in. (More will always be revealed, my friend.)

THE FIVE PHASES DESCRIBE CYCLES OF MOVEMENT IN YOUR BODY

Another way to think about the five elements of wood, fire, earth, metal, and water is that they represent the different periods of the growth and maturation of plants grown by farmers.

What does that look like?

Well, think about planting your garden. In the spring, all is green as you plant the seeds, and the activity is the budding and sprouting of those seeds out of the ground. This is the Wood phase. Spring is thought to be the time of the liver and gallbladder. It's a great time to do a liver cleanse by using the liver diet and herbs that I share with you in Chapter 12.

Then comes the red heat of summer, and the movement is growth. The plants push up and out and go through the most dramatic period of their development. This is the Fire phase and the time of the heart and small intestine.

In some texts, the season of the earth is "Indian summer" or "long summer." This is when plants reach their final stages of growth. If we were farmers growing grain, this is where grain grows to its most mature stage and becomes ready for harvest.

However, in the *Su Wen*, or *Yellow Emperor's Classic of Medicine*, one of the most important texts in Chinese medical history, the Earth phase has no particular season.

Qi Bo, the doctor who teaches the Yellow Emperor, explains why the Earth phase has no season like this: "The spleen is earth and manages the center. It constantly promotes the growth of the other four viscera throughout the four seasons. . . . Earth engenders all the tens of thousands of things in accordance with the laws of heaven and earth. Hence [the spleen] reaches up to the head and down to the feet with no whole season for it to rule."[3]

In my opinion, this suggests the importance of the Earth phase, and we can see how all the other phases depend on it. It "manages the center" and is a kind of fulcrum or leverage point for health and disease.

For the purposes of this book, we're going to look at the five phases like this because it's consistent with the approach that we are going to take.

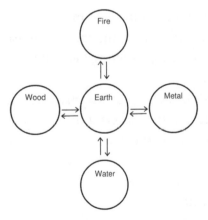

Next, green plants like rice and wheat turn yellow ochre when they are ready for harvest. Autumn is when we harvest and gather our crops. We harvest them and turn this yellow ocher into white grain. This is the Metal phase and time of the lungs and large intestines.

And finally, the black or deep, dark blue of winter comes. We store the crops that we have harvested. This is the Water phase and the time of the kidney and urinary bladder.

And then we wait for the spring and do it all over again. That's just how we accumulate another birthday in our lives. Cycles repeat and repeat.

This is not just metaphorical; the ancient Chinese doctors actually believed that the organ systems that are associated with each element also go through seasonal changes. And understanding the influences of the seasons on our internal organs was also considered an important skill for a practitioner to have.

THE FIVE PHASES GIVE US AN ALGORITHM FOR COMPLEX INTERACTIONS

Another amazing thing that five phase theory gives us is a way to understand interactions between the various organ systems in real time. In Western medicine, focus is almost always on a single system and because most doctors are specialists, they don't think outside their specialty.

Well, in reality, the body is interconnected and all these systems interact and affect one another all the time. And when things go wrong in one place, it impacts all the other systems in multiple ways. This can be completely overwhelming and difficult to understand.

There is nothing in the Western medical model to explain interactions between systems. Research has found that these interactions exist, but there is no overarching theory for understanding and predicting behavior between the systems. Chinese medicine gives us this tool.

The five phase interactions help us to see this, and the amazing thing about this template is that it works on multiple levels. I'll show you what I mean in upcoming chapters, but one thing I discovered is that you can use it for various individual systems as well. For example, in researching this book I discovered the five phases of the endocrine system, which is completely mind-blowing. Stay tuned—I'll be sharing some of my insights with you.

Take a look at the diagram of the five phases on page 29. What you'll see are three distinct types of interactions. The first is called the "mother-son" or promoting cycle. These are the arrows that point from one phase to the next and make the outer circle.

For example, water is considered the mother of wood, which, in turn, is the mother of fire. It's logical, as water creates life in the form of wood. Wood can be burned to create fire. Fire, in turn, is the mother of earth, as ashes become soil. Earth is the mother of metal, just as the earth creates metal ores like iron. Then metal is the mother of water, as minerals meld with water. And thus, the cycle repeats.

What is also true about these relationships is that they are mutually influential. If there is weakness or pathology in a mother, it will affect the child. And like any family if there is weakness or pathology with the child, it will have a profound impact on the mother.

And we can see this play in real-life physiology; it's not just silly old metaphors. For example, liver and cardiac disorders have been widely documented in medical literature.[4] We know heart diseases affect the liver, and liver diseases affect the heart. There are even diseases that affect both systems at the same time. The ancient Chinese gave us a way of understanding it.

If you look at the diagram again, you'll notice that there is a kind of pentagram at the center of the circle. Also notice that the arrows go in two different directions. These are called the controlling and insulting modes. And these are really interesting in that they give us clues to other forms of influence among the organ systems.

THE CONTROLLING MODE

This type of influence of one system over another is that of a controller or regulator. This has a kind of retraining or counterbalancing effect. Kind of like the negative feedback mechanisms that are common in the body.

I find this particularly helpful when we look at the five phase interactions of the endocrine system. One example of this is the relationship between insulin produced by the pancreas (earth) and cortisol produced by the adrenals (water). Insulin surges can modulate the cortisol response.[5]

We'll explore this further as we look at the Earth phase, for this has some really important implications when it comes to carbohydrate levels in your diet because these can cause surges in insulin.

THE INSULTING MODE

This type of influence involves the same two systems, just in the reverse direction. This is often a good clue about pathology or something being out of balance. In Chinese medicine, this is also where excess or deficiency in one phase affects the other.

For example, if your adrenals are depleted (deficient), then you may develop problems breaking down glycogen (stored sugar), and this can lead to hypoglycemia (low blood sugar).

And if your adrenals are overactive (excess) and you are stressed, then this can cause a faster breakdown of glycogen to glucose, which suppresses insulin and leads to too much sugar in the blood, or insulin resistance.[6] Again, we'll explore this further when we look at how to use diet more effectively.

Holy moly! My mind is blown by how much these ancient doctors understood! The more I dig into this and learn, the more I am in awe and so grateful for the insights they have provided us.

Time for a quick recap . . . we just covered a metric ton of stuff!

RECAP: **THE FIVE PHASES**

1. The five phases are the five elements in motion. They give us an algorithm or template for understanding interactions and relationships between the systems of the body.

2. Because this is a dynamic, fluid system, there are three different types of interactions:

   - **The Mother-Child Cycle:** This is where one system gives support or promotes another. This is a way of explaining how these organ systems affect one another, and it helps us identify important relationships.

   - **The Controlling Mode:** These connections help us identify feedback loops and allows us to see where nourishing or strengthening one system can have a positive effect on another.

   - **The Insulting Mode:** This is the same connection as the controlling mode but in the opposite direction, and this offers us clues about pathology and imbalances. Often when one system is "excess" or "deficient," this mode may come into play.

   Next we're going to be looking at this with earth as the center of these interactions because the digestive system is a kind of fulcrum or leverage point for all these interactions. And understanding these relationships gives us insights into using the diet to heal all kinds of dysfunction in the body.

WHAT DOES ALL THIS HAVE TO DO WITH HASHIMOTO'S AND DIET?

This information shows us where our points of leverage are. In my first book, I wrote about the 80/20 principle, which states that 80 percent of your symptoms are being caused by 20 percent of some imbalance. And the five phases show us where the 20 percent solutions are that will get us 80 percent better.

Because the Earth phase is at the center, as the *Yellow Emperor's Classic* teaches us, it is a place where we can get an 80 percent return on our 20 percent investment.

Hopefully all of this will lead us to finding simpler, more elegant solutions. It's a way for us to do less by focusing on the places that need our attention. Does that make sense?

In this book, I will use this theory to help you understand how to better navigate a diet for Hashimoto's and to help you make changes when the time comes for you to make them.

Next, let's look at the work of an ancient Chinese master named Li Dong-yuan who made healing through the digestive system his focus and life's work. In my opinion, he has some incredible insights into how we can heal Hashimoto's and other autoimmune diseases.

LI DONG-YUAN'S YIN FIRE THEORY

Li Dong-yuan, also known as Li Gao, was in contention for being MVP of the Jin-Yuan Dynasty. The Jin-Yuan period was from A.D. 1115 to 1368. This was a time of great change in China and a period that ushered in the rule of the Mongols and Genghis Khan, one of history's unparalleled leaders. It was the beginning of the height of the Mongol empire that extended all the way to Europe.

Li came from a wealthy family in the Hubei province in Central China. He began his studies under one of the most famous physicians in the region named Zhang Yuan-Su and was a diligent student of his school called the Yi Shui School. Li eventually moved on and formed his own school of medicine known as the Earth School.[7]

While they were ruthless, the Mongols were keen on medicine and imposed a strict system of medical practice, banning certain toxic medications. Li Dong-yuan was one of the most prominent physicians of this period, and he is known for his focus on how lifestyle affects the body's organs.

Li developed his own theories that most disease was formed as a result of damage to the digestive system. Li believed that damage to the Earth system (the stomach and spleen in TCM) was caused by three main factors:

1. Excessive eating and drinking (especially overconsumption of excess amounts of cold, raw, fatty, or unclean foods).

2. Overwork and exhaustion. Li identified that illness could also be caused by poverty, war, and oppression. In other words, he identified that stress caused illness.

3. Emotion. Li also believed emotion was a causative factor in disease and that excess emotions and repeated emotional drama could agitate the body and lead to poor digestion.

This was a time of great social upheaval and unrest in China as the results of the conquest of the Mongols. Li observed the toll that this conquest took on his people and he saw some of them left poor, powerless, and unable to access proper nutrition. This made them vulnerable to diseases, and it affected their health physically, emotionally, and spiritually.

There's an old saying among scholars of Chinese medicine: "For external diseases, Zhang Zhong-jing, for internal diseases, Li Dong-yuan."[8] (Zhang Zhong-jing is a famous Chinese doctor and also an undisputed genius in my mind; but we have much to cover in this book, and I can't get to him too.)

Hashimoto's is an internal disease. What that means is the problem is not from an external source. It is caused internally by our immune system attacking itself. (Zhang Zhong-jing lost a large percentage of his family to smallpox; he understood how to treat external pathogens. And it could be argued that the pathogens, like Epstein-Barr, that are known to be causative factors also make Hashimoto's an external disease, but for now our focus is on the internal nature of the disease.)

Autoimmune disease is a problem that comes from the inside. What is autoimmunity, after all? It's the loss of self-tolerance. You can't get much more internal than that. We're being attacked from the inside by our own immune systems.

Li is remembered, historically, as being the founder of the *Bu Tu Pai*, the School of Supplementing the Spleen and Stomach, and his masterpiece is the *Pi Wei Lun (Treatise on the Spleen and Stomach)*.

Let's take a look at his revolutionary theory.

YIN FIRE: SYSTEMIC INFLAMMATION

Li's main theory is known as the Theory of Yin Fire. Li thought that most diseases, eventually, lead to heat patterns. Heat in Chinese medicine is another way of saying, in my opinion, systemic inflammation. Li thought with chronic diseases, "heat" was also mixed with deficiency or compromise and, especially, deficiency of the Earth phase.

The term *yin fire* can also have more than one meaning.

First, it develops in the lower burner, the yin part of the body. The lower burner is part of the triple burner in TCM. This is a concept that is unique to Chinese medicine and has no direct correlation to Western medicine. The lower burner is located below the belly button; and it includes the liver, kidneys, large intestine, small intestine, and bladder.

You can think of it as the peritoneum, or you can also think of it simply as space, essentially, like a room or a part of your house. And this part of the house is in your lower torso. An important feature of the triple burner is that it controls the flow of water or fluids in the body. It's like part of the river and delta that flows to the ocean.

Second, yin fire is commonly associated with *yin evils*. This is another way of saying "disease symptoms." Disease is yin, as opposed to health and "righteous qi," which is yang. And autoimmunity is a "yin evil" disease.

And lastly, this heat or "fire" is pathological; it is intimately linked with the disease process. I'm fond of saying inflammation is the root of all evil. Yin fire is also the root of all evil.

To summarize, yin fire is pathological change, it is destructively hyperactive, and it is the upward movement of "ministerial fire."

(Good Lord, how many terms do we have to define? Stay with me, we're getting to the good stuff now . . .)

Okay, *ministerial fire* is SUPER IMPORTANT!

In my opinion, it's really a metaphor for a kind of root of metabolic activity. And what is responsible for that? Yup, the thyroid! This is the movement of thyroid hormone, manifest in the body. Or perhaps, more accurately, it is the totality of metabolic activity, which is really endocrine-immune-neurological activity.

Because, for all intents and purposes, this metabolic activity is intertwined; when you think of the body as a whole, it's all interconnected. The entire endocrine system is a five-phase constellation. And it and the immune system and neurological system are all talking to one another and impacting each other. The sum is exponentially bigger than the parts.

The idea that these glands (or systems, for that matter) are separate is nonsense. The endocrine system is like the solar system. You need to step back and see the bigger picture. And the ministerial fire is like the sun or, if you think about the earth, the hot molten core at the center of our bodies.

Furthermore, when you look at all the symptoms of deficiency of ministerial fire, it looks an awful lot like hypothyroidism or, in a larger sense, deficiency or weakness of this foundational energy.

It's like the heat in the earth's core is getting too weak.

And according to Chinese medicine, this ministerial fire is only healthy when it is anchored in the lower burner. So it's as though this fire must be contained, for when it spreads throughout the body, trouble ensues and trouble is yin fire.

THE FIVE MECHANISMS OF YIN FIRE

According to Li, there are five basic mechanisms for yin fire. And because everything is connected in the body, each of these mechanisms can give rise to any other.[9]

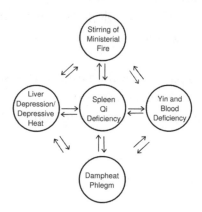

They are as follows:

1. Spleen qi deficiency

2. Damp heat/phlegm

3. Liver depression/depressive heat

4. Yin and blood deficiency

5. Stirring of ministerial fire

Notice in the diagram that the earth (the spleen) is in the center. I adjusted the five phase diagram so that we could see both together. Let's start there. Spleen qi deficiency has a number of potential causes and when you look at the symptoms, it sounds an awful lot like hypothyroidism and Hashimoto's.

These include fatigue, cold hands and feet, pale complexion, obesity, puffy edema (myxedema), and a tendency toward loose stools and/or constipation.

Sometimes this is accompanied by kidney qi deficiency, and this has all the above symptoms plus low libido, dizziness, tinnitus, infertility, menstrual irregularities, and low back and knee pain.

And, of course, not everyone has every symptom. But these are exactly the same symptoms I see in my Hashimoto's patients every day.

Li attributed this spleen qi deficiency to overthinking, anxiety, worry, too little exercise, poor diet, improper medical treatment (that's a cause that never gets enough attention), etc.; and all of these were thought to damage spleen qi.

Once damaged, the spleen can't properly do its job, and this can lead to a host of other issues. One function of the spleen in the body is to take yang energy and bring it up into the lungs and upper part of the body.

When the spleen is weak, this can result in this yang energy becoming depressed, and when depressed it can transform into pathological heat (inflammation). And this inflammation mixes with the ministerial fire, which if you recall is this totality of endocrine-immune-neurological metabolic activity.

So, essentially, this pathological heat, or inflammation, ends up affecting other organs like the stomach, the liver, the lungs, the heart, and eventually the kidneys. And it can even lead to psychological problems by affecting the spirit of the heart.

What does this process describe? Well, in my opinion, it perfectly describes autoimmunity affecting various tissues in the body. This is the destructive systemic inflammation of autoimmune disease.

Another problem that arises when the spleen qi becomes weak is that it can't properly move and transform water and liquids in the body (another way of saying properly digest and assimilate). And this can result in dampness and phlegm.

Once again, because the yang energy is trapped and can't go anywhere, it becomes pathological heat and mixes with the dampness. This damp heat affects the lower body and can also manifest in all the organs.

Issues that are associated with damp heat include nodules, edema with redness and pain, bacterial and viral infections, Candida, urinary tract infections, yeast infections, and more.

Holy crap! Once again, lots of issues we commonly see in our community.

Another function of the spleen in Chinese medicine is that it makes and transforms blood. If the qi of the spleen is weak, it may not properly make blood. This then leads to blood deficiency, and this can lead to yin deficiency.

What are symptoms of blood and yin deficiency?

Blood deficiency symptoms include anemia, hair loss, weak and brittle nails, pale complexion, infertility, etc.

Yin deficient symptoms include neurotransmitter and hormone deficiencies, neurological weakness, brain-related problems, etc.

Once again, these are many common issues that confront Hashimoto's patients!

One consequence of this blood and yin deficiency is that it also affects the yin organs, especially the liver. If blood fails to nourish the liver and yin fails to moisten the liver, then it becomes compromised.

And when the liver becomes compromised, it is thought to become depressed and its qi stagnates. And this stagnation can also lead to pathological heat. Liver qi stagnation can result in (and also be caused by) anger and unfulfilled desires, and this can result in pathological heat that can damage other organs like the spleen, the stomach, the heart, and the lungs.

Symptoms of liver depression and depressive heat include nodules, emotional depression, anger and irritability, joint pain, gallbladder issues and gallstones, problems with liver detoxification, poor bile flow, poor thyroid hormone conversion, etc.

These are also very common issues with Hashimoto's and hypothyroidism.

So, as you can see in the previous diagram and from all these symptoms and interactions, Li Dong-yuan is clearly articulating five common mechanisms of Hashimoto's. This book was written in the 12th century, about 800 years ago.

Amazing, right? What's truly incredible to me is that we now have a way to wrap our minds around a bunch of symptoms common to Hashimoto's that most Western doctors and most practitioners, really, would never see as related.

And we can see that not only are they related, they actually lead to each other. In combination, this theory of yin fire and the five phase theory give us a map of the disease process in Hashimoto's.

What are maps good for? They help us find our way.

And Li Dong-yuan's masterpiece, the *Pi Wei Lun*, is loaded with formulas and treatment strategies.

Basically, they can be broken down into protocols that address the five mechanisms we just discussed.

He shows us how to:

1. Fortify the spleen and boost qi in cases of spleen qi deficiency

2. Clear damp heat and resolve phlegm in cases of damp heat and phlegm

3. Resolve liver depression and clear heat from the liver in cases of liver depression and depressive heat

4. Nourish blood and yin in cases of blood and yin deficiency

5. Restore the balance of ministerial fire when it has become pathological

He even explains how to prioritize when you have a combination of issues!

I'm feeling some gratitude right about now.

Let's recap, because we just tore through one of the greatest works of Chinese medicine in about seven pages. Don't worry. In the next several chapters, we will unpack this and look at how to apply what Li Dong-yuan teaches us to specific issues. We'll also look at how we can use diet (and some herbs) to heal.

RECAP: **YIN FIRE**

Yin fire is master Li Dong-yuan's theory of the process of internal diseases, of which Hashimoto's is definitely one.

1. **Spleen qi deficiency**, which is at the root of it all and is the earth element that controls the digestion system and can be healed through diet, etc. Symptoms include things like fatigue, cold hands and feet, pale complexion, obesity, puffy edema (myxedema), and a tendency toward loose stools and/ or constipation. In other words, what we see every day in Hashimoto's and hypothyroidism.

2. **Damp heat and phlegm**, which are associated with things like nodules, edema with redness and pain, Candida, urinary tract infections, yeast infections, and more.

3. **Liver depression and depressive heat**, which is associated with nodules, emotional depression, anger, joint pain, gallbladder issues and gallstones, problems with liver detoxification, poor bile flow, poor thyroid hormone conversion, etc.

4. **Blood and yin deficiency**, which includes issues like anemia, hair loss, weak and brittle nails, pale complexion, infertility, neurotransmitter and hormone deficiencies, neurological weakness, brain-related problems, etc.

5. **Abnormal behavior of ministerial fire**, which is another way of saying the endocrine-immune-nervous system is out of whack.

Okay, time-out! All of that being said, it's still important to put this in perspective and to understand that figuring out which changes to make and making those changes may not always be easy. This is a map, but it doesn't tell you where you need to go. And some of us need to go to some *radically* different places.

So, that's where you come in. You have to participate in this process, and you have to get to know your body well enough to be able to identify what's going on. And you have to be willing to try some different things and be open and willing to make changes.

And that takes time and commitment and dedication. In my opinion, you should be meditating daily, you should be doing some sort of rejuvenating exercise (like yoga or qi gong) regularly, and you should be keeping at least one journal of your diet, activities, and symptoms.

And remember back to what I wrote about conducting experiments. We're going to be conducting some diet- and herb-related experiments, and you're going to need to keep track so that we can learn from them and build healing momentum.

THE EARTH IS THE CENTER BUT NOT NECESSARILY THE ONLY PRIORITY

According to Li, a strong, healthy spleen and Earth phase is important for keeping yin fire at bay. And because spleen deficiency plays a role in all the yin fire scenarios, one will always have to, in some measure, work to strengthen and fortify the spleen and stomach.

Often this means also treating the liver to ensure that it works harmoniously with the spleen. It will often also involve treating the stomach and intestines because they are key to nutrient absorption, microbial balance, and autoimmune flare-ups.

In many cases, there will be "evil heat," destructive inflammation that will have to be cleared. And there may be a damp element to this heat, as in damp heat or phlegm that may have to be addressed.

In addition, many of these things are interrelated: qi and blood, qi and body fluids, blood and body fluids, qi and yang, blood and yin, and all the organs and bowels . . . holy crap! My head is exploding.

Remember back to the beginning of the book? When faced with overwhelming challenges, ask yourself, *Where can I do less?*

In these many scenarios, we have to be in touch with our bodies enough to find the top priority. If "heat evil" and inflammation are most prominent, that's where we start. If liver depression is most prominent, then that's where we start. If it's phlegm, then that's where we start.

And we always keep in mind that Earth is at the center, so we add a little something for that.

Whew! Let's take a breather. You've earned it! We've covered some amazing stuff.

Next, before we actually get further into the five phases and yin fire, let's dive a little deeper into our digestive tract and really get to know the Earth phase.

And hopefully, you get a sense of where your starting point(s) may be. Then in the second part of the book, we'll look at actual diets and larger dietary approaches that you can use as a foundation for this more specific work.

HASHIMOMENT:
The Importance of Self-Forgiveness

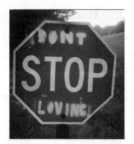

Sometimes the temptation with Hashimoto's is to feel that your body has betrayed you. That it has let you down. Try not to give into that temptation.

First of all, there are so many factors that go into the formation of something like Hashimoto's. There are genetics, environmental toxins, exposure to some kind of virus or pathogen, stress, leaky gut, etc.

What do most of these have in common? They weren't choices you made. And even autoimmunity is the result of your body trying to heal itself and balance. For some reason(s), that system went haywire.

The physical body is closely connected to the subconscious mind. The best way to overcome these feelings is to forgive your body and yourself. Healing begins with forgiveness.

We must forgive our immune systems for attacking our body, forgive those who don't understand what we are going through, and forgive ourselves for not being perfect.

Recently, I stumbled upon some interesting research on how being compassionate toward yourself can actually help reduce inflammation in your body.

In an article in the journal *Brain, Behavior, and Immunity* published in 2014, researchers concluded that:[10]

"Taken together, these findings suggest that individuals who are higher in self-compassion may be buffered from increased inflammation following unfamiliar psychosocial stress, whereas individuals who are lower in self-compassion may be especially vulnerable to the adverse effects of this form of stress.

"Efforts to help people cope more effectively with acute stress and reduce disease risk should seek not only to relieve negative emotions and appraisals but also to foster positive emotional states such as self-compassion."

Inflammation is the root of all evil when it comes to chronic diseases like Hashimoto's. Self-compassion is anti-inflammatory.

And self-compassion begins with self-forgiveness.

Take a moment today to sincerely forgive yourself for whatever you are holding on to. You might be surprised by how you feel.

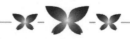

Chapter 2

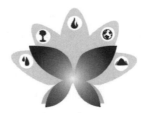

UNDERSTANDING THE TERRAIN:
Exploring the Many Ecosystems
of the Earth Phase

If we really want to heal the Earth phase, it will help if we get a better sense of it physically and geographically. And I think it's important to understand that while it is one system, it contains diverse ecosystems that all perform important functions. And all of these ecosystems can be impacted by Hashimoto's, hypothyroidism, and autoimmunity.

Since the Earth phase is the center, it deserves to be the center of our attention for the next few pages. And keep in mind that this tour of the geography and physiology of the digestive tract is also a narrative of how Hashimoto's is formed and how it proliferates.

Ultimately, this terrain is also where we have a tremendous opportunity to heal.

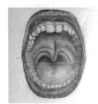

The Mouth: As we all learned in grade school, digestion begins in your mouth when you take your first bite. Chewing makes food easier to digest (a good reason to really take time to chew your food well), and saliva mixes with food to begin breaking it down so that you can absorb nutrients from it.

Enzymes and other substances are a critical part of this process. One such example is lysozyme, which offers an antiseptic function as defense against bacteria and viruses. The mouth is rich in bacteria, and some of these bacteria have been linked to both Hashimoto's and rheumatoid arthritis. They induce an inflammatory response in our bodies that cause an immune protein called IL-6 to increase.

Because the tissues of the gums are so similar to tissue of the throat and, yup, you guessed it, the thyroid, the immune system sometimes confuses the two and attacks both this bacteria and the thyroid. This is a phenomenon known as "molecular mimicry."[1]

Molecular mimicry is a theory that says the amino acid sequences of proteins of things like bacteria or viruses are similar enough to some tissue in our own body that this can result in an autoimmune attack on our tissue.

So, Hashimoto's and autoimmunity can actually begin in your mouth.

In the back of your mouth are your tonsils, and while not involved in digestion, they are certainly involved in protecting you from food-borne pathogens like bacteria and viruses. The tonsils contain up to a billion lymphoid cells about 50 percent of which are T cells.[2]

Cytokines such as gamma interferon and natural killer cells are also present in the tonsils, and these can kill viruses and tumor cells. One study from Sweden noted a higher prevalence of autoimmune disease in people who had tonsillectomies (surgical removal of their tonsils).[3]

I had my tonsils removed at age four, as many people in my generation did. At that time the tonsils were thought of as unnecessary, and removing them was often recommended whenever they became infected. It turns out, however, that this could be yet another factor in the formation of autoimmune thyroid disease.

The Esophagus: Next, food travels into the esophagus. It runs from the top of your throat all the way down to your stomach.

This area of the throat is also where the Epstein-Barr virus (EBV) attacks. EBV is a form of herpes virus (also known as human herpesvirus 4) that affects an estimated 95 percent of the population; it is transmitted in saliva and initially affects epithelial cells in the oropharynx and nasopharynx, just above the pharyngeal sphincter. EBV then enters the underlying tissues and infects B cells (and can infect T cells, as well).[4]

And essentially, the virus becomes part of these cells. It's a hybrid of virus and our own cells. After the initial infection, EBV becomes "immortalized" in memory B cells for the rest of a person's life. And the virus can shift between an active and latent state.

EBV has also been linked to Hashimoto's and is thought to be one of the potential causative factors.[5] It can become active and cause debilitating fatigue and a number of gastrointestinal symptoms. I've added a whole section on dietary treatment for EBV in Part II of this book because it's so common.

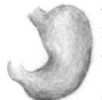 **The Stomach:** Next food enters the stomach. The stomach plays a hugely important role in digestion. It mixes and crushes food, mechanically, and it also releases some enzymes that are vital for digestion.

Pepsin is the main gastric enzyme. It is activated by stomach acid, and it works to break down protein. Lipid and carbohydrate digestion starts in the mouth, but protein digestion does not begin until the stomach. This matters to us because food sensitivities are directly related to proteins, and if proteins are not broken down sufficiently, they can cause an immune reaction.

Hydrochloric acid (HCL) is stomach acid, which is made of positively charged hydrogen atoms produced by parietal cells. HCL mainly functions to denature proteins, and this makes them biologically inactive. It also helps to destroy any bacteria or viruses that may remain in food, and it activates pepsin.

It is this process of denaturing and breaking down of proteins that is critically important in minimizing food reactions. Another common problem for people with Hashimoto's is sensitivities to various foods (for example, gluten and other grains, dairy, nightshades, and lectin-containing foods). And hypothyroidism can cause the stomach to produce less of a hormone called gastrin.

Gastrin, which is actually an endocrine hormone, enters the bloodstream and eventually returns to the stomach where it stimulates the parietal cells in the stomach wall to produce HCL and intrinsic factor.

With Hashimoto's and hypothyroidism, another common problem that may result from this is acid reflux. And this is where the discomfort is experienced. One of the reasons for this acid reflux is hypochlorhydria, or too little stomach acid.

This can be caused by hypothyroidism because the thyroid hormone affects the amount of gastrin that is released.[6] And when there is too little stomach acid, you don't break your food down properly and you wind up with what is basically a traffic jam. And this can lead to these stomach fluids leaking into the lower esophagus.

Another common problem caused by too little stomach acid is the bacteria *Helicobacter pylori*, or *H. pylori*. *H. pylori* is also very common, and it attacks the lining of your stomach. With Hashimoto's and hypothyroidism, one theory is that the lower levels of stomach acid can make people more vulnerable to *H. pylori* infection. It can also lead to ulcers in the stomach.

And *H. pylori* can also lower stomach acid itself, thereby compounding the problem. This can be a double whammy and it may be difficult to figure out which came first. Low stomach acid caused by hypothyroidism or low stomach acid caused by *H. pylori*?

CLINICAL PEARL:

Sometimes, it doesn't matter what the root cause is. More importantly, what is the problem NOW and how do we resolve it? This is a perfect example. It could be H. pylori, it could be hypothyroidism, it could be both. We need to evaluate and treat both if necessary.

Another important protein produced by the parietal cells of the stomach is intrinsic factor (IF). This is essential in the absorption and utilization of vitamin B12. As I mentioned, the saliva initially produces haptocorrin, which binds to B12 and carries it safely through the stomach into the duodenum.

In the duodenum, pancreatic enzymes liberate (or "cleave") B12 from haptocorrin. Then this freed B12 binds with intrinsic factor released by the parietal cells in the stomach and creates vitamin B12-IF complex. This is then transported to the next section of the small intestine, the ileum, where it is absorbed into the bloodstream so that it can be used by the body.

Some people have autoimmune antibodies to parietal cells and/or intrinsic factor, and this can make getting proper levels of B12 really difficult. Low stomach acid and hypothyroidism can also impact this process.

Do you see why it's important to know this information?

Chances are, most endocrinologists won't be looking for this. But now that you are learning how all of this is connected, you will be. And if you have problems with B12 levels, we've now identified a few really common reasons. (MTHFR mutations are another potential cause.)

FOOD AS MEDICINE: *GINGERROOT*

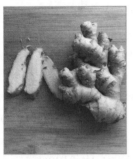

Ginger is one of my favorite herbs. I use it in cooking, and it has phenomenal healing properties as well.

Traditionally in Chinese medicine, it is considered warm and pungent. It promotes sweating, it is an anti-toxin, it is a good antidote for seafood poisoning (one reason why it's served with sushi), it benefits the lungs and stomach, and it expels pathogens.

It is traditionally used to treat common colds, cough (with clear white mucus), nausea, vomiting, diarrhea, and certain types of arthritis (cold type).

One common problem for people with Hashimoto's is low stomach acid. This can cause numerous related issues such as poor absorption and assimilation of important vitamins and minerals, and it can also cause downstream problems such as sluggish bile flow.

Ginger is the perfect remedy for both problems since it promotes the release of gastrin, which is responsible for the release of stomach acid and helps promote bile flow. An awesome one-two punch!

Recent studies may confirm that ginger directly affects the gastrointestinal tract, helping to improve muscle tone and to prevent abnormally rapid and strong intestinal contractions.

Research has shown some promise for supplemental ginger in the treatment of both osteoarthritis and rheumatoid arthritis.

Due to its tremendous circulation-increasing qualities, ginger is thought to improve the complexion. It has reduced nervousness, eased tendonitis, and helped sore throats return to normal. Studies demonstrate that ginger can lower cholesterol levels by reducing cholesterol absorption in the blood and liver. It may also aid in preventing internal blood clots.

Gingerroot was recently the subject of a startling new research report presented at The American Association for Cancer Research conference in Phoenix. In the study, ginger actually suppressed cancer cells suggesting that the herb was able to fuel apoptosis, or the death of the cancer cells. Ginger has been shown to work against skin, ovarian, colon, and breast cancer.

Some common applications are:

- For colds, cough, or vomiting: Simply make ginger tea.

- For diarrhea: Apply a plaster to the belly.

- For arthritis: Rub fresh ginger directly on the painful areas, and drink tea (contraindicating in hot, red types of arthritis).

- Nausea: Squeeze ginger juice into some water and sip.

Tastes great, and it's good for ya!

THE SMALL INTESTINE: (DUODENUM, THE ILEUM, AND THE JEJUNUM)

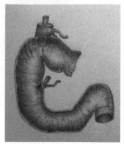

The Duodenum: After food leaves the stomach, it enters the duodenum. This is the top 12 inches of the small intestine, and it is arguably the most important 12 inches in the entire digestive tract.

This is a place of an insane amount of metabolic activity that just began in the stomach. Once the chyme (partially digested food) arrives there, bile from the gallbladder, bicarbonate, and lots of enzymes from the pancreas are released through the ampulla of Vater (named after the German anatomist who first described it in 1720, Abraham Vater. Thanks, Abe!). This is where it all comes together!

This is like the Amazon River. Have you ever seen a map of South America? There are many tributaries meeting and flowing into the Amazon. The duodenum is the Amazon of metabolic activity.

And ducts from the liver, the gall bladder, and the pancreas all converge.

BILE

Bile's role in digestion is that it helps to break down fats in food. They do this by acting like surfactants (which are common in many household cleaners). These basically weaken the surface tension between two liquids.

In the body these liquids are water and fat. Bile salts are water loving on one side (hydrophilic) and water hating on the other (hydrophobic). So they surround little droplets of fat.

What this does is create a much larger surface area for the enzyme pancreatic lipase to break it down. This allows the triglycerides to be broken down and absorbed by the villi in the small intestine. The body is so ingenious!

Hashimoto's and hypothyroidism can cause a decline in both pancreatic enzyme release and in gallbladder function. Hypothyroidism also slows cholesterol metabolism and excretion of bilirubin though the bile is diminished. One theory is that increased cholesterol levels found in patients with myxedema is caused by too much cholesterol in the bile, and this can result in a higher incidence of gallstones.[7]

Thus, all of this beautiful symphony of metabolic activity can be slowed and impaired, which means that you aren't going to absorb nutrients as well as you should.

This can lead to nutrient deficiencies that can cause a whole bunch of health issues, including making hypothyroidism symptoms worse.

BACK TO THE DUODENUM

The duodenum itself has hormones, peptides, and its own groovy enzymes called "brush border enzymes" that it releases in order to orchestrate all of this like some crazy genius conductor.

The small intestines are the place where leaky gut often happens. And the walls of the small intestines are lined with tiny little hairlike protrusions called microvilli. On a regular microscope, they kind of look like a tiny, fuzzy paintbrush.

This fuzzy appearance is why they came up with the term *brush border* to describe them.

WHERE ABSORPTION HAPPENS

This is the place where absorption happens. And many people with Hashimoto's suffer from deficiencies of important vitamins and nutrients (like vitamin D, vitamins B12 and B6, zinc, selenium, magnesium, iron, etc.). One of the reasons for this is the breakdown of these brush borders.

Foods high in lectins or other inflammatory substances (like gluten and other grains, beans, and nightshades) can actually cause these brush borders to get crushed and destroyed.

The microvilli (little hairs) that make up the brush border have enzymes for this final part of digestion anchored into their membrane as membrane proteins. These enzymes are found near to the transporters that will then allow absorption of digested nutrients.

BRUSH BORDER ENZYMES

Brush border enzymes amylase, cellulose, and invertase can be effective in digesting carbohydrates, proteins, and fats without causing irritation and digestion of the intestinal walls.

Brush border enzymes are safe, well tolerated, and can be a good tool in healing these tiny little paintbrushes.

CLINICAL PEARL:

One concern when supplementing with digestive enzymes is that those that contain enzymes that break down proteins can actually attack your own exposed proteins if you have leaky gut or intestinal permeability. Brush border enzymes are gentler because they are found at such close proximity to the intestinal lining. Sometimes these are a better, safer choice for supplementation.

All of these juices are slowly mixed with the chyme by the duodenum until all of this material is chemically transformed and digested. It's the ultimate in natural alchemy.

Then slow waves of peristalsis or contractions push it all through the duodenum. Each pulse moves the chyme ever so slowly down the duodenum toward the next part of the small intestine, the jejunum. This process can take up to an hour just to travel those 12 inches. Most of the water that we ingest is also absorbed in these two parts of intestines (a little is also absorbed in the stomach and in the colon).

Most absorption of important nutrients and minerals happens below the duodenum with a few important exceptions. Iron is absorbed in the duodenum. Sufficient amounts of stomach acid are required for proper iron absorption, and this can result in iron deficiency anemia.

Calcium is also partially absorbed in the duodenum. If you are low in calcium, specific cells in the duodenum will actively absorb calcium using special transport proteins. This process is partly controlled by vitamin D.

Other minerals including copper, magnesium, phosphorus, and selenium are also absorbed in the duodenum. Selenium is very important for proper thyroid function, as it used by the enzyme family of iodothyronine deodinases to convert T4 to T3, and it is also important for the glutathione peroxidase enzyme system. Glutathione is a vital antioxidant responsible for protecting the body from damage from environmental toxins.

Time-out! Let's just take a moment to appreciate the complexity and specificity of these substances. There is a great deal of metabolic activity; there is also a great deal of inherent physiological intelligence. And I don't mean that metaphorically—I mean that literally.

This part of the body has its own nervous system called the enteric nervous system. It's sometimes referred to as the body's second brain. We will explore it further when we get to the section of the book on the brain/gut connection.

But, I want you to understand that this is why an ancient Chinese master like Li Dong-yuan viewed the Earth phase as the center. It *is* the center and like the city of Rome, all roads lead to it.

JEJUNUM

Next we travel down into the jejunum. This portion of the small intestine is about two-fifths of the small intestine, or about 2.5 meters (about 8 feet) long on average. It is really the portion of the small intestine that specializes in absorbing nutrients.[8]

All of the enzymes we discussed that are excreted into the duodenum are still active in the jejunum, and carbohydrates are converted into glucose, fats into fatty acids, and proteins into amino acids.

In addition, vitamins A, B1 (thiamine), B2 (riboflavin), B3 (niacin), B5 (pantothenic acid), B6 (pyridoxine), B7 (biotin), and B9 (folate), as well as vitamins D, E, and K, are all absorbed here. Minerals such as calcium, chromium, iron, magnesium, manganese, molybdenum, phosphorous, potassium, and zinc are also absorbed. And most of this, about 90 percent, happens in the first 100 to 150 centimeters.[9]

As you may know, many of these minerals are important for thyroid function:

Selenium—Acts as a catalyst to convert T4 to T3 and helps protect the body from oxidative damage.

Magnesium—Proper thyroid function depends on a fine balance between calcium and magnesium. Magnesium is also used by the body in more than 300 enzyme reactions.

Zinc—Needed to form TSH and too little can impair T4 to T3 conversion.

Another interesting thing to note about this section of the small intestine is that because all the villi (or brush-like projections) are so numerous and so spread out in order to have more surface area for absorption, this is also an area where the development of leaky gut or intestinal permeability can take place.

When the lining of the digestive tract is inflamed, the connections between the pieces of lining known as "tight junctions" break down and allow large, undigested compounds—toxins and bacteria—to leak into the bloodstream.

These substances all react with the intestine's immune system and cause an exaggerated immune response. This overreaction by the immune system becomes a vicious cycle that leads to more intestinal damage.

And as this problem grows, diet, lifestyle, medications, and infections can cause further intestinal inflammation that can ultimately lead to more serious problems.

This damage can lead to malnutrition, further intestinal inflammation, further permeability challenges, the development of food sensitivities, bacteria and yeast overgrowths, and an impaired immune system leading to irritable bowel syndrome, Crohn's disease, and other autoimmune diseases like Hashimoto's.

These self-destructive patterns can be very difficult to unwind. This is exactly why it's so important for us to address healing through diet.

A couple other common issues that can be associated with this part of the bowel are abdominal bloating and distention. These can have many different causes, and it's really important to do a proper assessment to determine which of them may lead to this symptom in your body. (I will address the various causes in Part III of the book.)

ILEUM

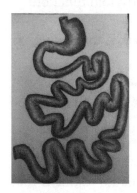

The ileum is the final section of the small intestine and connects to the large intestine via the ileocecal valve.

Here vitamin B12 is absorbed, and bile salts are reabsorbed by the body so that they can be recycled and reused.

The chyme released by the stomach is held here so that it can be carefully analyzed by the immune system for pathogens and if found they can be attacked and eliminated. And this is all controlled by the ileocecal valve, which seals off the first part of the large intestine called the cecum and the terminal ileum.

In addition, because it connects to the large intestine, which has large quantities of microbial life (bacteria), the ileum is also lined with Peyer's patches. These are rough egg-shaped lymph nodules that are similar in structure to the tonsils and the appendix in that they are not encapsulated like normal lymph glands.

Peyer's patches are thought to be there in order to analyze and respond to pathogens in the ileum. Antigens (foreign substances or toxins that cause an immune response) from microbes in the gut are absorbed by cells on the surface of each Peyer's patch. These antigens are then passed onto the lymph tissue where the immune system triggers a response that attacks them locally, and this also triggers a body-wide immune reaction.

Another interesting thing to note about this part of the intestines is that there is a very fine balance that is constantly being negotiated between an aggressive immune response to food-borne pathogens (like bacteria, viruses, fungi and parasites) and a tolerance (or calming of the immune response) to food-borne proteins (at this point most of these are broken down into protein fragments—amino acid sequences).

And this delicate balance is also what can lead to autoimmune disease because if this balance is lost and the immune system gets locked into attack mode, then attacks on our own tissue can become collateral damage. Because here's the thing: our tissues are also made of proteins, and sometimes they have the same sequences as these protein fragments.

If you just think about it for a second, it's a really difficult tight rope to walk, and it's not hard to see that things can go sideways in a hurry. This balance that stops the attack on food-borne proteins is called oral tolerance.

Oral tolerance is defined as your immune system NOT REACTING locally and systemically to antigens such as food proteins. In other words, oral tolerance is when you eat a certain protein and you become tolerant to that protein.

When this tolerance breaks down, chronic diseases follow, such as celiac disease, Crohn's, and ulcerative colitis (these all occur locally in the intestines), as well as other systemic autoimmune disease like multiple sclerosis and even Hashimoto's.

In other words, oral tolerance is a kind of dimmer switch—it turns down the attack both in the intestines and in the rest of the body.

When you have oral tolerance, your immune system doesn't attack as aggressively. When you lose oral tolerance, you wind up with things like celiac disease (which is an autoimmune disease, not just a food intolerance).

This is such an important concept that I have devoted an entire chapter to it later in the book. It is the reason, in my opinion, why some people develop more food sensitivities on restrictive diets like the autoimmune paleo diet.

ILEOCECAL VALVE

From the terminal ileum, chyme is slowly released into the first part of the large intestine called the cecum, via the ileocecal valve. This is another area where a lot can happen. Weakness or a prolapsed ileocecal valve can result in bacteria leaking out of the large intestine into that part of the ileum. (Hypothyroidism is actually a potential cause of ileocecal valve dysfunction.)

Issues like SIBO (small intestinal bacterial overgrowth) and FODMAP (Fermentable Oligo-, Di-, Mono-saccharides and Polyols—a group of compounds that can contribute to irritable bowel and other gastrointestinal disorders) can both develop as a result.

SIBO, as you may know, is the bacteria in the small intestine mutinying. They decided that the large intestine was too restrictive for them. So they made a break for it and escaped to the small intestine (and lots of gas can result).

Once there, the bacteria can wreak havoc. The stomach and the duodenum and jejunum normally contain relatively few bacteria. As we have seen, this region of the bowel is all about absorption—it's not a bacterial playland—it's all about enzymes and HCL and juices that break things down. Bacteria have difficulty surviving there.

On the other hand, when we get to this region of the bowel (the terminal ileum and the cecum), it's the beginning of Disneyland for bacteria.

Let's put this in perspective. Normally, the stomach, duodenum, and jejunum contain about 10,000 bacteria per millimeter.[10]

But, the terminal ileum has 1,000,000,000 bacteria per millimeter and the colon has 100,000,000,000 bacteria per millimeter. It's quantum. It's like the difference between our solar system and the Milky Way.

Movement through the small bowel and sufficient stomach acid are the most important factors for preventing SIBO. Guess what inhibits both? Yup, Hashimoto's and hypothyroidism. Common symptoms are nausea, abdominal cramping, bloating, farting, and diarrhea.

If it's severe, it can impact B12 and/or vitamin D absorption. Bottom line, it must be dealt with. And we will deal with it in Part II of the book.

LARGE INTESTINE

The large intestine consists of the cecum, the appendix, the colon, the rectum, and the anal canal.

But we must press on. (We're on the back nine.) The final part of digestion is the large intestine, which has a number of dynamic ecosystems. Let's start with the cecum and appendix.

CECUM AND APPENDIX

Basically, the cecum is a pouch about two inches long; and it's a transition point, like a border guard patrolling the state of the ileum and the state of the large intestine. It absorbs digestive fluids passing out of the ileum and lets the waste material through to the rest of the colon.

At the bottom of the cecum is the appendix. For years, it was believed that the appendix was useless and could be removed, without repercussions. But the appendix is *actually a bank of good bacteria* and replenishes your intestines with the species that are beneficial.

So, it's like money in the bank. And the more we learn about this microbiome, the more valuable this bank becomes.

THE COLON: ASCENDING, TRANSVERSE, AND DESCENDING

Researchers are just beginning to understand the virtues of microbial life in the digestive tract. We now know that gut bacteria carries on a symbiotic relationship with all the systems of our body including the endocrine system, nervous system, immune system, and, of course, the digestive system.

What we are also learning is that antibiotic treatments that alter and destroy some of these populations have wide-ranging, long-term health consequences that no one had foreseen. We really need these critters for an amazing variety of metabolic functions. One important function that they perform is to convert thyroid hormone T4 into T3 so that it can be utilized by the cells of the body. And I have had firsthand experience where antibiotic treatment caused a rapid and dramatic increase in TSH levels in one of my patients. This was reversed with probiotics.

ASCENDING COLON

About 90 percent of the nutrients in digested food has already been absorbed by the time it gets here. This food is mixed with bacteria in the cecum to form poop, and waves of peristalsis move this up the length of the ascending colon.

As this waste material passes through this area, bacteria digest what the human body couldn't and liberate vitamins K, B1, B2, and B12. The walls of the colon then absorb this and most of the water that is also present.

In addition, because of all the microbial life in the large intestine, it is rich in lymph nodes and these lymph nodes have been found to be important players in oral tolerance.[11]

TRANSVERSE COLON

The transverse colon is the longest part of the colon, and it is bordered by a lot of other organs and connecting tissues. Above it are the liver, gallbladder, stomach, pancreas, and spleen. The peritoneum runs right into it, and below it contacts all three parts of the small intestine. It's a crowded neighborhood!

The transverse colon absorbs water and salts.

DESCENDING COLON

The descending colon is the final major portion of the large intestine and is a waste storage center, holding and gradually solidifying stools as they get ready to be pooped out.

A very common symptom of Hashimoto's and hypothyroidism is constipation. And the reality is transit and motility in the entire digestive tract can be compromised. It can happen in the esophagus and lead to heartburn.

It can happen in the upper duodenum and lead to nausea and vomiting. This can all lead to bacterial overgrowth, which can result in abdominal pain or discomfort, gas, and bloating. It can slow motility in the ileum and the colon, which can lead to constipation.

Hypothyroidism can also impact signaling from the vagus nerve, and this affects both hormonal activity in the gut and neuro-electrical function of nerves needed to keep the intestines moving.

Both diarrhea and constipation can have multiple causes. I will address them more specifically in Part III of the book.

Finally, colon cancer is a serious, life-threatening disease that can sometimes go undetected for years. Signs that may indicate cancer include sudden bowel changes, bleeding from the rectum, black stools, frequent constipation, and mucus in the stools.

SIGMOID COLON

This is the final area of storage for stools before they are sent out into the rectum and anus for elimination. It's also the final stage of absorption of water, nutrients, and vitamins.

Common problems here include problems of the diverticula, which are little sacs or outpockets that come off of the wall of the colon. These can bleed and be quite painful and are often exacerbated by foods like seeds and popcorn that don't get broken down in digestion. These can get lodged in the diverticula and cause pain and in some cases infection.

RECTUM AND ANUS

Finally we reach the end of the hollow organ that is the bowels. This is of course where stools are eliminated. A very common problem here for people are hemorrhoids. These are basically engorged blood vessels in the anal canal.

They can become swollen and inflamed and be quite painful. In their normal state, they actually act as cushions to help control the stool. There are both internal, which are not painful but may bleed, and external, which tend to be painful and can also bleed.

Hypothyroidism can lead to hemorrhoids because it slows transit and motility and creates more pressure in this area. Constipation is also one of the most common causes of hemorrhoids.

RECAP:

The entire digestive system is important both for the development and progression of Hashimoto's, but also as a means for healing.

Here's a quick review of the important elements we just touched on:

Mouth: Where digestion begins and where complications like gingivitis and periodontal disease develop. These tooth infections can make Hashimoto's worse.

Throat and Esophagus: Where the tonsils are found and tons of other organs and glands like the thyroid, the parathyroid, lymph glands, nerves, blood vessels, and more. Epstein-Barr virus can attack here, and it can be an important driver in the initiation and progression of Hashimoto's.

Stomach: So important for absorbing and breaking down nutrients, vitamins, and minerals. The bacteria *Helicobacter pylori* can attack here and cause major problems for people with Hashimoto's.

One major problem for many people with Hashimoto's is too little stomach acid. This can lead to *H. pylori* infections and can also be caused by them.

Duodenum: An area of a HUGE amount of metabolic activity. These 12 inches of the small intestine may be some of the most important real estate in the digestive tract. So many important nutrients, vitamins, and minerals are actually absorbed here.

Jejunum: The next region of the small intestine, where leaky gut can occur and where bacterial overgrowth can start to creep.

Illeum: This is the final region of the small intestine that connects via the ileocecal valve that connects it to the large intestine. This valve can become compromised in Hashimoto's and hypothyroidism and can lead to bacteria leaking into the small intestine that shouldn't be there.

This part of the small intestine is an area that can really be damaged by this bacteria and leaky gut. It is also rich in immune cells and Peyer's patches. This is literally ground zero for autoimmunity.

Cecum and Appendix: This area is a hugely important repository of good bacteria. This is like the central bank of the microbiome. It's like Fort Knox for good bacteria!

Ascending Colon: Water is absorbed here and fecal matter is pushed through. It's also very rich in good bacteria.

Transverse Colon: More bacterial wonderland.

Descending Colon: The final part of the colon, where the last bits of water are absorbed and where constipation and diarrhea can originate.

Sigmoid Colon: This is the last section of the descending colon, where inflammation and diverticula can form.

Rectum and Anus: The end of the digestive tract, where hemorrhoids and fissures can sometimes form.

FOOD AS MEDICINE: *WATERMELON*

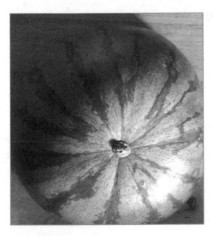

There's nothing better on a hot day than a delicious slice of watermelon.

Watermelon is considered cold and sweet in TCM.

It quenches thirst, relieves irritability, dispels summer heat problems*, promotes diuresis, and detoxifies.

It can be used to treat sores, dry mouth, summer heat irritability, bloody dysentery, jaundice, edema, and difficult urination.

It's generally contraindicated in cold conditions, for those with a week stomach and polyuria or excessive urination.

*Note: The term *summer heat* in TCM refers to overactive functioning of an organ system resulting in symptoms of thirst, aversion to heat and craving for cold, infection, inflammation, dryness, red face, sweating, irritability, dark yellow urine, restlessness, constipation, and "hyper" conditions such as hypertension.

This is different from sunstroke, which can be a life-threatening condition.

Here are some traditional remedies that use watermelon. Notice that the rind and seeds are used. Always use organic when using for these purposes.

For edema from kidney inflammation: Boil a tea made from the rind and inner portion.

For jaundice: Make a tea from the rind and red beans.

For fluid in the abdomen: Make tea from the rind and skins of watermelon, squash, and winter melon (warning: this will be very bitter).

Constipation: Boil tea from watermelon seeds, then grind the seeds into meal and take with warm water.

Next up, we will explore the microbiome or the little creatures that live in the gut. Recent research of the human genome has revealed that the organisms in the gut make up a much larger part of our DNA than we previously realized.

As I have researched and studied this topic, I also believe that we have under-estimated the importance of the microbiome and that when ancient doctors like Li Dong-yuan spoke about the qi of the Earth phase, what they were really talking about was a healthy microbiome.

Chapter 3

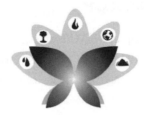

THE MICROBIOME:
We Are Bacteria

Perhaps the most important part of the digestive system is the microbiome—that is, all the tiny living organisms that co-exist in our bodies. Only recently have researchers come to realize how important this is to virtually every system of the body.

The various different species of bacteria, viruses, and fungi that live in the microbiome make up the lion's share of our DNA and are more a part of us than we previously realized.

Hashimoto's and other autoimmune diseases have multiple causes. There is no single origin and, therefore, to date there is no single solution. Instead, successful healing requires exploration into the multiple causes of the disease and healing the areas that need attention.

One such area that has recently been discovered to have a major impact on health and disease is the microbiota. In this chapter, we'll explore the role of bacteria in the formation and healing of autoimmunity and Hashimoto's.

ONE WITH OUR MICROBIOME

One of the fundamental things to understand regarding the world of microbes is that they are not separate from us. We are one. And I don't mean this in a woo-woo or philosophical sense.

I mean this in a very real, practical sense.

THE HUMAN MICROBIOME PROJECT

The Human Microbiome Project (HMP) was a United States National Institutes of Health (NIH)–sponsored project whose goal was to identify and study the microorganisms (little critters) that are found in association with both healthy and diseased humans.

Launched in 2008, it was a five-year project, with a total budget of $115 million. The ultimate goal was to test how changes in the human microbiome are associated with human health or disease.[1]

Here are some of the things that they discovered:

- "There are approximately 10 trillion bacteria in (and on) our bodies versus only 1 trillion human cells. That's right. We have 10 times more bacterial cells than we do human cells.

- There are over 1,000 species of bacteria found inside our GI tract.

- Several diseases are directly associated with a disruption to the microbiome. These include, but are not limited to Crohn's, IBS, Asthma, Allergies, and obesity.

- Pathogenic bacteria/organisms (Candida, *H. pylori*, etc.), are natural inhabitants of our gut, and are not problems in optimal conditions. Eradicating them entirely has consequences we're just beginning to understand."[2]

THE TRUTH ABOUT ANTIBIOTIC THERAPY

One thing that looking at this research makes abundantly clear is how incredibly destructive antibiotic therapy is, especially for children (for whom it is often prescribed).

Of course, these drugs have saved countless lives when they are used appropriately. But they have been abused and overused, and we are now seeing the consequences in new bacteria-resistant strains, as well as a wide variety of diseases like digestive disorders and autoimmune disease.

This is very much like the way that we treat our soil. It's time for a new paradigm. We cannot destroy ourselves to good health or good crop yields. That approach has failed us miserably.

Giving children or adults antibiotics every time they get an upper respiratory infection (most of which are caused by viruses, not bacteria) is often doing little more than setting the table for future disease and a decline in natural immunity, making them more susceptible to infections.[3]

This also has physiological consequences in our guts, and it makes us more vulnerable to pathogens because the beneficial bacteria that are killed play an important role in our immune system.[4]

It's time we stopped looking at medicine as simply a war between invading pathogens and our body. It's more nuanced than that. These microbes are not the enemy. They are spleen and stomach qi. They are metabolic energy factories, in my humble opinion.

As I have written in the past, we are a collection of interacting ecosystems, and researchers now know that these ecosystems are composed of a wide variety of friendly organisms.

Just like we need to learn to be good stewards of the earth and our external environment, we also need to view the insides of our bodies in this way and start caring for these internal ecosystems in the same way.

The lesson here is that we can't just eradicate ourselves to good health. We see this time and time again with pesticides, herbicides, and antibiotics.

Lots of doctors, practitioners, and patients still have the mind-set that says, "All we need to do is kill _____ [choose your favorite pathogen], and then you'll be healthy." And many of us have been trained to think and treat this way, whether it is with drugs or herbs and natural supplements.

Well, a lot of times this approach can result in a disruption of the ecosystem of the gut (and sometimes overgrowth of *other* pathogens). This is exactly what Li Dongyuan described as spleen and stomach qi deficiency (in my opinion, the microbiome and the organisms that populate it make up this spleen and stomach qi).

And this doesn't just happen with drugs like antibiotics; it also happens with natural products like herbs that kill pathogens in our bodies. It's time we create a new way of doing things. This is part of what this book is devoted to.

But, first let's try and figure out what a healthy microbial ecosystem is.

WHAT EXACTLY DOES A HEALTHY MICROBIOTA LOOK LIKE?

As we just explored in detail, your digestive tract is not just one ecosystem. Really, there are several distinct ecosystems that overlap and interact with one another.

The bacteria that populate each of these ecosystems are quite different.

And to complicate things, there's the intestinal mucosa and lining that houses distinctly different species than the space inside the intestine.

In addition, no two people have the same microbiota. Early research on this subject came up with the idea of "enterotypes," which are microbiota types like blood types, but they only looked at a small group of people.[5]

After looking at a lot more people from different cultures, researchers determined that it wasn't so clear-cut and there's so much variation that it's really hard to be definitive about this. (It's more nuanced. I think that's my new motto.)[6]

In the following diagram, you can get a sense of the number and diversity of bacteria that populate these various ecosystems.

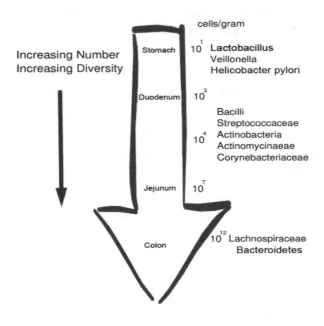

Frankly, this makes the claims and marketing of probiotics pretty ridiculous (more on that in a moment). No one or two strains of bacteria are going to properly populate your entire digestive tract. Nor does everyone need the same strains.

Furthermore, diversity is more important than overall population of certain strains. A diverse microbiome is the very definition of good health. With diversity comes proper function and more resistance to pathogens, infections, and overgrowth from other species of bacteria, yeast, etc.

HOW DO THESE BACTERIA GET HERE?

Development of a healthy and diverse microbiome is dependent on exposure to bacteria. We start with exposure to our mother's bacteria in the vaginal canal and via feces during birth. Children born by C-section are at a disadvantage because they do not get exposed to this bacteria.

After birth, we are exposed to external sources of bacteria from our mother's skin, mouth, gut, and breast milk. Breast milk is a rich and diverse source of bacteria. Spanish researchers identified over 700 species.[7]

After getting inoculated with bacteria from our mothers, additional exposure to bacteria comes from our environment and food. So, it's important to not have a completely germ-free home.

In fact, antibacterial soap, hand sanitizers, and overall germaphobia can also have a very real (and not so beneficial) impact on the development of healthy GI flora—especially related to diversity. You want your infants and kids exposed to dirt and grime. (This news will surely be liberating for some parents and horrifying for others!)

Environment also really matters when it comes to a healthy microbiome. Those who live in rural habitats generally have much greater microbiome diversity than those who live in urban settings. Working the earth is not just good for the soul, it turns out.

This also makes our widespread destruction of the soil all that more disturbing. The Earth phase is the key to good health inside and out.

FOOD AS MEDICINE: **CODONOPSIS, OR POOR MAN'S GINSENG**

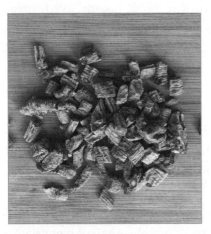

Hey, people!

I wanted to share a great herb with you that was traditionally used as both food and medicine: codonopsis.

Codonopsis can be ground into flour, cooked with rice, added to soup, and used in medicinal teas.

The roots of this herb are used and have a sweet flavor; they're thought to enter the spleen and lung channels.

Codonopsis is quite nourishing and is used to tonify qi and blood. It contains essential oils, polysaccharides, inulin, scutellarin, glycosides, alkaloids (choline and perlolyrin), and various amino acids.

Traditionally, codonopsis is used for ailments associated with weakness, fatigue, poor appetite, and anemia. It is helpful in treating diarrhea, gas, and excess stomach acid.

Laboratory testing has found that it reduces the secretion of pepsin in the stomach, and it slows down digestion. It has been used effectively to treat chronic fatigue syndrome.

Codonopsis has also been used to treat cancer patients, along with conventional cancer therapies, and may be effective in protecting cancer patients against the adverse effects of radiation therapy without reducing the effectiveness of radiation.

It also helps the body to make interferon, which can be important for people with compromised immunity. Since codonopsis is an immune stimulant (likely a Th1 stimulant), it should be used cautiously if you are Th1 dominant.

Codonopsis has anti-inflammatory effects and can be used to treat arthritis and other conditions of the muscles and joints. It has also been used traditionally to boost libido and may have aphrodisiac effects.

Pharmacologically, codonopsis has been shown to promote digestion, increase nutrient uptake, and enhance immune function. Studies have shown that it stimulates breathing and increases blood glucose levels and the production of red blood cells.

It's a pretty gentle herb and has a nice flavor. I used to cook it with oatmeal or congee (a porridge made from rice or other grains) for my kids.

As with any herb, use caution and moderation. And if you are unsure if it's right for you, consult your health-care practitioner.

HOW IS THIS CONNECTED TO AUTOIMMUNITY AND HASHIMOTO'S?

There is a good deal of evidence to support the idea that the microbiome has a profound impact on the immune system and that it is involved with the prevention as well as initiation and progression of autoimmune disease.[8]

But the idea that probiotics are always good for people with autoimmunity is not supported in the research at all. On the contrary, there is some evidence that the opposite is true and that certain strains of bacteria cause different types of immune responses and affect different autoimmune diseases differently.[9]

And there are many complicating factors here including genetics, environment, and type of disease. And mutations and changes in the microbiome can also result in different outcomes. Like most things, the reality is that there is enormous individual variation and determining whether or not probiotic therapy is beneficial and which probiotics are appropriate is not an easy thing to do.

The reality is that we are only beginning to understand this complex interaction between our immune systems and the microbiome. However, there are two theories about how the microbiota can help protect against autoimmune disease.[10]

TWO THEORIES ON HOW MICROBES PROTECT AGAINST AUTOIMMUNITY

The first is known as the "specific lineage hypothesis," and it says that in genetically predisposed animals or humans, the microbiota could provide signals that calm our body's immune responses. As a result, the microbiota stays in a homeostatic (balanced) relationship with us.

Basically, the microbes are saving themselves, and we have acquired these lineages from our mother, which have been passed down.

When a specific microbial lineage is expanded, it blocks the development of autoimmunity. It does so to improve its own odds of staying in this expanded state by suppressing our inflammatory and adaptive responses.

Our autoimmunity is calmed as a side effect of this microbial self-preservation.

The second theory is called the "balanced signal hypothesis," and this asserts that the host's interactions with microbiota are independent of the precise microbiota composition and that the host's genetics plays a critical role in the conversation with microbes.

So that your genetic profile is more important.

Whereas a balanced host response to good bacteria and this bacteria's effort to reduce this response do not affect disease development, the inability of the host to control the microbiota properly results in stronger negative signaling provided by the microbiota and a reduction of autoimmunity.

Again, the microbes are looking out for themselves and sending out signals that result in calming autoimmunity. (Both theories predict that the increase of tolerance would be lost in germ-free conditions without the microbes.)

There is also evidence that the microbiota behaves in different ways depending on the circumstances. It's not static, it adapts to changing conditions. Because it is alive and it has its own innate intelligence.

Here's the thing: the microbiota always faces two competing problems:

1. The microbiota make sure that our immune system doesn't destroy the microbes (they have to induce us into creating tolerance).

2. And our immune system must also make sure the microbiota stay under control and don't breach the barrier systems and get into the rest of the body and cause infections there.

So there's this constant balancing act that we and our microbiomes must do to keep each other healthy.

Bottom line is this: you need to be cautious when using probiotics with autoimmunity and don't just assume that any variety is going to help.

They might, in fact, not help or even make things worse. So, like everything else, you need to carefully assess your need for them and then experiment and keep track to see if they are giving you the desired result.

CHOOSING THE RIGHT PROBIOTICS

One question I frequently get is this: "Which probiotic is a good one?" As with all things Hashimoto's related, you can see that this is not a simple question. There is so much individual variability that the answer really depends.

Probiotics are big business. The global probiotics market was valued at $32.06 billion dollars in 2013.[11]

There are literally hundreds of brands, and many make outrageous health claims. I've experimented with a number of different brands, both personally and professionally. For some patients the results have been good, in others, there's been little or no noticeable effect, and for some they've actually had adverse reactions.

Some manufacturers and proponents might say these are "die-off" reactions, and they may be, but it could also be that in that particular individual with that particular genetic makeup and immune profile, they were inappropriate. (I think that sometimes practitioners use the die-off explanation to cover incompetence.)

The truth of the matter is, no one knows what probiotics are best for you. There is tremendous variability in our microbiome from person to person.

From a Chinese medicine point of view, probiotics and foods that feed them (like fermented foods) are considered warming. So, for people with damp heat or excess fire conditions, they may not always be appropriate as the first order of business.

In the next section of the book, I will show you how to determine what type of approach is correct for your unique set of circumstances.

SPORE BACTERIA: THE ANSWER?

One type of probiotic I have experimented with is called spore form bacteria. These are organisms that survive the stomach and small intestines quite well. They have evolved to be very stable in the environment and also to colonize the GI tract very effectively.

They survive digestion, they're found in the natural world, and they are of superior quality. These are not the answer for everyone, but I have known them to be effective for some people. I used them to treat the patient I mention in the case study at the end of this chapter with some compelling results.

In an upcoming chapter, I will explore oral tolerance, and these spore form bacteria have been shown to help promote oral tolerance, as well.

RECAP: **MICROBIOME**

In many ways the microbiome (the lots of tiny organisms that live in our bodies) is digestive health, immune balance, and in a Chinese medical sense, the spleen and stomach qi.

We have more bacterial DNA than we do human DNA.

Taking too many antibiotics and being too aggressive in consuming bacteria-killing herbs can wipe out the microbiome and make autoimmunity worse and long-term immune defenses weaker.

This is your body's wealth, in a very real sense. It's time we stop thinking of it as the enemy and start seeing it as the ally and close friend it really is.

CASE STUDY: Cautionary Tale of TSH and Antibiotics

Here's an interesting case study about a 60-year-old woman who had a thyroidectomy and was taking thyroid hormone replacement. What's interesting here is that she was taking levothyroxine and, as you probably know, this must be converted (by good bacteria in the colon) in order to be utilized by the body.

This case study demonstrates the effect of gut bacteria on thyroid hormone conversion and TSH levels quite clearly.

Here's her story in brief:

"Immediately after I was treated for SIBO, I began using powerful antibiotics. About one year ago, my TSH went from numbers in the teens (i.e., 17–19) all the way to the 60s and 70s, with an all-time high of 79.71. This happened despite the fact that my nutritionist was careful to add nutritional supplements to replenish gut flora.

"I'm so happy to report that your theory about increasing probiotics to three pills per day appears to be working to improve my TSH levels. I just received new lab results, which show a 20.8 point improvement. I am so excited to see and feel this improvement."

Lori C.
California

During the course of working together, this phenomenon occurred more than once. After this treatment, Lori contracted a sinus infection and was again prescribed antibiotics—and the same thing happened all over again. It's a remarkable example of the relationship between the microbiome and thyroid hormone conversion.

Chapter 4

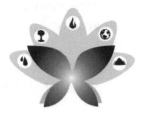

THE CHINESE MEDICINE VIEW OF THE EARTH PHASE

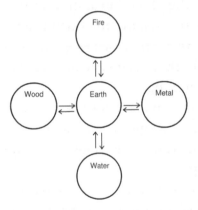

Now, given what we've just learned about all the various ecosystems of the digestive system and the microbiome, let's return to Chinese medicine and Li Dong-yuan's teachings. The genius of this way of looking at the body's physiology (and our Earth) is that it helps us understand relationships between the different parts.

Health and its antithesis, disease, never happen in a vacuum. You aren't healthy if only your muscles are healthy. You aren't healthy if only one organ system is healthy while others are compromised. You aren't healthy if your body is healthy but your mind is sick. And your mind will be affected if your body is sick.

You are not truly healthy unless the *whole* of you is healthy.

And the same is also true of our planet. We are not healthy if one group has access to good diet, nutrition, and emotional well-being while other segments of society live in abject poverty and starvation. We are not healthy when one region is pristine and clean while others are polluted with poisonous chemicals, radiation, and waste products.

We are not truly healthy unless we are all healthy. Remember, any organism that destroys its environment (and, yes, that includes our internal environment) destroys itself.

All that being said, if you have read my work and are familiar with my philosophy, you know I am not one to focus on the negative. I prefer to look for the reasons why things happen and adopt solutions. So let's dive deeper and see what we can find.

THE EARTH PHASE IS THE CENTER

As I mentioned earlier, I've chosen to shift terminology from the Earth *element* to Earth *phase,* and I've chosen to move the Earth from the outside of the five-phase constellation to the center. This is because I want you to see this as a dynamic system of constantly moving parts (like a solar system), and this book is all about using the Earth phase as leverage for healing.

Another thing to bear in mind is that these Chinese medical classics I reference are not just clinical guides. They give advice about living. One important theme I believe is that the process of healing Hashimoto's (or any disease, for that matter) is a journey of personal development.

It's an opportunity for us to take inventory of our lives, recognize where we may have erred, change our behavior where appropriate, make amends to ourselves and others, and transform and grow.

These ancient classics offer advice on living a long, healthy, and peaceful life. As mentioned earlier, *The Yellow Emperor's Classic* (a text that Li Dong-yuan quotes pretty extensively, which actually consists of two texts: the *Nan Jing* and the *Ling Shu*) is a dialogue between the Yellow Emperor (or Huang Di) and one of his doctors, Qi Bo.

Huang Di was a child prodigy. From a very early age, it was apparent to everyone around him that he was special. He possessed sincerity, wisdom, honesty, and compassion beyond his years. Huang Di became very learned and developed keen powers for observing the natural world. Like the Dalai Lama, he was chosen at a very young age to become the leader of his people.[1]

Huang Di had a voracious appetite for learning how things worked. *The Yellow Emperor's Classic* is a recorded dialogue of his ceaseless curiosity about nature and human health (and many other topics). He wanted to leave a legacy to help his people so that they could live long, happy lives. And as any of you who have struggled with your health know, being chronically ill does not a happy or healthy life make.

The Yellow Emperor's reign is said to date back to 2600 B.C. This work survived for thousands of years because it served as inspiration for many generations of physicians who did not view physical, emotional, and spiritual health as separate. They saw them as one.

In fact, the goal of physical health was to be one with the Great Tao and, thus, follow the natural order of life. And it identified that the factors that undermine our health tend to be things that separate us from heaven and its direction.

We get distracted by our five senses, lose self-control, and fall into patterns of overindulgence and emotional excesses that wind up compromising our health and shortening our life span.

In the first chapter of his masterpiece, the *Pi Wei Lun,* Li Dong-yuan looks back at the work of the masters who came before him and he quotes from a couple of different texts. First from chapter 11 of the *The Yellow Emperor's Classic*, Li quotes:

"The stomach, large intestine, small intestine, triple burner, and urinary bladder, these five are engendered by the qi of heaven and, their qi resembling heaven, they drain and do not store. Receiving the turbid qi from the five viscera, they are named bowels of conveyance and transformation. They do not keep [things] long, but transport and drain."[2]

We just spent an entire chapter looking at this in detail. The ecosystems of the digestive tract move food and water through and transform it into all the components that are vital for health and well-being (vitamins, minerals, glucose, protein, energy, etc.).

But, there's also an interesting phrase here, "receiving the turbid qi fom the five viscera," and this references the yin organs (liver, heart, spleen, lungs, and kidneys). Another role of these yang organs of the Earth phase is to help their yin counterparts stay healthy.

According to the *Nan Jing,* conditions affecting the yin organs are much harder to resolve. And certainly, if you think about it, heart, liver, kidney, lung, and spleen diseases are often much more serious and much more difficult to treat and resolve.

On the other hand, conditions of the yang organs are generally easier to treat and resolve (unless they become severe). These yin organs will naturally transfer their pathology to their yang counterparts. Transforming yin into yang. And because these yang channels have this inherent movement and transforming capacity via elimination, it is through the yang organs that the yin organs can find release.

In this first chapter of the *Pi Wei Lun*, Li reiterates several times quoting from several sources and illustrating in several different ways the rationale for the Earth phase being the center of health and well-being.

The basic crux of this is that unhealthy dietary habits and lack of moderation damage the spleen and stomach. In addition, emotion plays a key role. And the result of all of this is "fire" or systemic inflammation.

And if fire wins out, it overwhelms the Earth phase. This leads to disease.

Li continues later in the chapter:

> "In the classics, the sage concludes that the stomach qi is the root of humanity. [*The root of humanity, not just health, people!*] The sage composed these essays to bring out the meaning, throwing light [on the problem] by means of juxtaposition. He has explained all this on numerous occasions. But bad physicians read but do not understand him and make wanton use [of attacking therapy]. Much as they want to save people, the do harm to them."[3]

This is a very interesting point to me and something I have spent a good deal of time thinking about in regard to treatment. Even today, a lot of therapy of the digestive tract (and elsewhere) involves "attacking." If you think about it, antibiotic therapy, treatments for Candida, steroids, and even the newer generation of therapies (such as the TNF inhibitors like Enbrel) are all forms of attack.

I think what Li is saying is that we can't always eradicate ourselves to good health. In other words, we cannot just kill all the bacteria in our guts and hope to be healthy. The microbiome is too important and there are unintended consequences like destroying immune function and damaging the delicate balance of the microbes that live in our guts.

The underlying problem here is this imbalance and dysfunction. Once that is addressed, it will thus result in healing and the resolution of these diseases.

Furthermore, much of this dysfunction is the result of weakness and deficiency. What happens when you attack someone who is weak? Li's idea is that in some cases this fire is born out of this weakness, so we must nourish and replenish the weakness. Otherwise, we may do more harm than good.

I think this is why dietary strategies that involve concentrating on nutrient-dense foods and supplementing tonics can be so beneficial. That approach is not attacking; it's building up what has been weakened.

And people with Hashimoto's and hypothyroidism are often pretty weak constitutionally, they're exhausted all the time, they get sick a lot, and they have a hard time recovering. These are very much the signs and symptoms of deficiency in these classic texts.

Finally, Li sums it all up:

"Go by the law of yin and yang, act in conformity with the art of numbers [a reference to living in accordance with yin and yang and the five phases], keep a moderate diet, keep regular hours of life, and do not tax oneself wantonly [through sexual indulgence]. . . . From this point of view, how can diet and daily life activities be considered negligible?"[4]

Amen to that, brother! The fact that this is lost on so many physicians today is a travesty. This is the recipe for good health and longevity. (I left out the part that says this is how you live to your hundredth birthday!)

It's primitive and ignorant to just prescribe pills. Diet and lifestyle changes should be first and foremost in our treatment strategies. However, we still need to identify the problems so that we can figure out which diet and lifestyle modifications we need to make. Next, let's look at how these five-phase interactions lead to specific problems.

ACTING IN CONFORMITY WITH THE ART OF NUMBERS

If we want to live a long, active, and healthy life, then we should be in touch with yin and yang and the five phases. In order to do this, we need to understand them in our bodies. This is the key to longevity and vitality.

HOW EARTH RELATES TO ITSELF

Each of the five phases has its own character, its own season, its own flavor, its own foods, its own temperament, and its own emotion and spheres of influence.

But the Earth phase is unique in several interesting ways. First, it has no season of its own. Each of the other phases have a season (wood/spring, fire/summer, metal/

fall, water/winter), but according to Li Dong-yuan, the Earth phase adopts the last 18 days of each season in order to generate the other four yin organs.

THE SPLEEN IS DEAD YIN

He goes on to say, "The spleen is dead yin, governing no definite period, and, therefore, it too can become diseased [in any of the seasons]."[5]

Okay, time-out. DEAD YIN? What does that mean? I spent a month trying to figure it out. I read every book I could think of, and none had a satisfactory explanation. Then on the night after the solar eclipse on August 21, 2017, it came to me.

But first, let's back up. As I said at the outset of this book, I came to Arizona to get closer to the earth in hopes that I could better understand it. And it has been an extraordinary experience. I have experienced the earth in a way I have never before in my life experienced it.

And I have also experienced it in a way I did not at all expect, and this really involves understanding yin. The yang here is obvious. The sun is unrelenting. It's hot in August in Arizona. And there have been plentiful monsoon rains, so it is lush and full of abundant life. Everything is teeming with earth energy.

But the eclipse was the opposite. Think about it for a second: just conceptually, it's the moon blocking the sun. It's a very visceral injection of yin. And I was told what an opportunity it would be, and that one should meditate during the apex of the eclipse and set intentions.

My friend Stephanie sent me an e-mail in which she wrote that the eclipse was "giving us a rare chance to move forward on this earth journey we are on. . . . As the sun feeds, the moon pulls. . . . As the energies unfold and meld, it provides such an incredible time for new possibilities. During the height of the eclipse, give your attention to the unique energies that not only surround ourselves, but the planet as well."

I thought, *Marvelous! Oh, this is going to be wonderful* . . . but it wasn't, at all. As I sat and meditated during the apex of the eclipse, I felt a very cold, wet, metallic sensation. Like a samurai's sword, it was dangerous and dark. I could see that it was also death, the absolute antithesis of yang.

Yang is a hot burning sun, a mass of hydrogen and life-giving energy. In contrast, this was like a black hole, a dark place that things don't return from. I saw it like a spectator in the Colosseum sees the killing of the gladiators. It was not AT ALL what I was expecting.

But later that night, it came to me. The spleen is a graveyard. In my meditation, I had experienced the depths of yin! "Dead yin" is literal. What does the spleen do? The spleen destroys old red blood cells and platelets, in particular. It recycles iron. It metabolizes hemoglobin removed from these red blood cells.

And then it breaks them apart: the globulin is broken down into amino acids, and the heme is metabolized into bilirubin and sent to the liver where it is removed. The spleen digests red blood cells and platelets. The spleen also holds a reserve of blood, which can be valuable in cases of hemorrhagic shock. It is *so* yin!

And that's only half of what it does. The spleen is also the body's largest lymph gland; it breaks down old antibodies and antibody-coated pathogens and blood cells by way of lymph and blood circulation. And it's a huge repository of monocytes (the Pac-Man immune cells that chomp down on the bad guys).

A 2009 article in the journal *Science* reported that in a study using mice, the red pulp of the spleen forms a reservoir that contains over half the body's monocytes![6]

What they found was that these monocytes mobilize to injured tissue such as the heart after a heart attack and then turn into dendritic cells and macrophages that fend off anything that might want to invade in order to promote healing.

The spleen is a graveyard.

It is dead yin. (And by the way, this has some implications when it comes to thyroid autoimmunity.) In another study published in the *Endocrine Journal* in 1995, researchers found that hypothyroidism and higher TSH levels increase B cells and CD5-B cells in the spleens of mice.[7]

Which means higher antibodies, but the study remarked that it wasn't as pronounced in Hashimoto's patients. (It's because their Earth phase is deficient, in my opinion.)

That's what we know from modern research.

In contrast, one confusing aspect about discussing the spleen in Traditional Chinese Medicine is that is doesn't correlate well with what we know about what the spleen does in Western physiology (which we just looked at).

In TCM the spleen is linked to overthinking, the ability to hold blood in the vessels, and the "big Ds," dampness and digestion. And these links are not random; they are born out of patient studies and observation. Have no doubt; as we have seen, the ancient Chinese doctors, like Li Dong-yuan, were skilled and disciplined scientists.

Well, serotonin explains all of it.

According to Dr. Daniel Keown in his book *Spark in the Machine,* about 95 percent of the body's serotonin is found in our gut, and 99 percent of serotonin is found in platelets. What did we just learn the spleen does? It stores and destroys platelets.[8]

Therefore, the spleen is the number one organ in the body for cleaning serotonin from the blood (via platelets).

If this is true, then it is regulating all the things that serotonin regulates. For example:

It is regulating the amount of insulin receptors that transport "food" in the pancreas.

It is regulating serotonin's effect on platelets and clotting. (And the amount of serotonin that sneaks into the brain and causes overthinking.)

It is regulating the baseline amount of serotonin in the blood and gut that will lead to either constipation or diarrhea.

And it works with the pancreas (which is the endocrine gland of the earth element or spleen yang) to regulate the absorption of food and therefore our ability to form strong muscles and keep good body tone (these attributes are also linked to the spleen in TCM).

This is all done via 5HT receptors (5-hydroxytryptamine).

Holy crap!

Basically, the spleen's ability to regulate platelets and serotonin explains all of it. Boom! Mind blown. Again.

So, the spleen is the yin Earth Mother. Take a moment to feel your spleen in your body. It is literally the center of your universe. Allow yourself to experience it and give thanks.

FOOD AS MEDICINE: **SUMMER SQUASH**

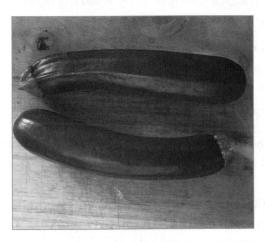

In Traditional Chinese Medicine, summer squash like yellow squash and zucchini are considered cool and sweet.

They clear heat, detoxify, promote sweating, quench thirst, and relieve restlessness. All good things during the summer!

Squash is rich in vitamin A, which is really important for gut health, and is a source of C, E, B6, niacin, and folate. It also contains magnesium, potassium, manganese, copper, phosphorous, calcium, and iron.

Squash seeds have been found to have antimicrobial and antifungal properties. They are also protective against parasites.

Some conditions they are traditionally used to treat include skin lesions, difficulty urinating, edema, summer heat, irritability, and thirst.

Note: The term *summer heat* in TCM refers to overactive functioning of an organ system resulting in symptoms of thirst, aversion to heat and craving for cold, infection, inflammation, dryness, red face, sweating, irritability, dark yellow urine, restlessness, constipation, and "hyper" conditions such as hypertension.

This is different from sunstroke, which can be a life-threatening condition.

To treat summer heat, make a salad with squash.

For jaundice, drink a tea made from squash skin (organic): 1 cup 3 times a day.

To treat edema, cook squash with vinegar until soggy and eat on an empty stomach, or make tea from squash skin.

I love grilling squash with olive oil, pressed garlic, and salt.

THE STOMACH IS THE DADDY OF EARTH'S YANG

In TCM, the stomach is said to do two main things:

1. **It controls the rotting and ripening of foods.** This is something that we've already seen from a Western physiological point of view. Breaking down food and assimilating nutrients, vitamins, and minerals.

2. **It is the origin of fluids.** This doesn't make much sense from a Western physiological perspective unless we look at the stomach as the entire gut, which is basically what it is. As we saw in the previous chapter and as I have tried to emphasize, all of these digestive organs are connected.

For all intents and purposes, the stomach is one long hollow tube of diverse and varied ecosystems. And the digestive tract is responsible for reabsorbing and redistributing water.

However, another way to view this notion of the stomach being the origin of fluids is to think about the stomach more abstractly. The Earth phase helps us establish boundaries, especially regarding the nourishment of self and others.

The quality of this balance is formed in part by our relationship to our mothers. We are connected to our mothers through the umbilical cord in the womb, and this is a graphic example of fluid nourishment from the Earth phase.

And once we are born, this connection is cut, and we are nourished by our mother's breasts with breast milk. Interestingly, the acupuncture channel for the stomach runs right through the nipple. Energetically, it is the origin of this fluid nourishment.

And really, if you think about it, it is the quality of our connection to our mother early in life that sets the stage for our relationship to the issues of need and nourishment in every aspect of our being. For people who have weakness of the Earth phase, this relationship to their mother (or a current surrogate) may have outsized importance, and they can be prone to interpreting life in terms of fulfillment of needs.

Furthermore, anyone who has weakness or deficiency of the Earth phase can struggle with the negative emotions of earth, which include worry or obsessive thinking about one's own needs or the needs of others. These are in direct conflict with the positive attributes of the Earth phase, which include proper boundaries and reciprocity or giving back appropriately.

And because Earth is the center, this can lead to selfishness and self-centered behavior. This self-centeredness may lead some to look out for their own needs regardless of others, or it may motivate them to give to others in hope of receiving validation.

This behavior often leads to resentment with the end result being that these relationships should nourish us but they have become burdensome. Symptomatically, people with weakness of the Earth phase may suffer from a lack of center or from excessive centeredness on every level of their being.

Symptoms like a prolapsed uterus, diarrhea, or even poor balance may all be an example of this. On the emotional level, losing one's center may show up as excessive thought and worry. To the other extreme, excess weight gain, digestive complaints, nodules, or selfishness could all be considered signs of excessive centeredness.

But often, with proper treatment, these behaviors of neediness and self-centeredness diminish, other symptoms improve, and the positive virtues of sincerity and reciprocity are able to find their way back again.

THE HEALTH OF THE SPLEEN AND STOMACH ARE INTERTWINED

Perhaps because of the intensity of their gravitational pull and their polar opposites, the spleen and the stomach are also unique in that their functions are often addressed together. (And interestingly, they are the only paired acupuncture channels that actually intersect and cross each other.)

If the qi of the stomach is weak, the spleen will also be weak. These two form a functional team whose job is to acquire and distribute all nourishment in life. The stomach is also the interface between the internal world and the spleen and all potential sources of nourishment outside of the self.

While the stomach is responsible for gathering and processing what comes in from the external world, the spleen must distribute the appropriate nourishment to all the other yin organs. The spleen does this through the blood, where it distributes the appropriate nutrients to every aspect of our being.

In a metaphysical sense, the spleen empowers the positive virtues of the Earth phase by incorporating what is consistent with our inner self. If the Earth phase is out of balance, other phases (such as the Fire phase) will be too. And the heart and mind can become separated and prevent the stomach from looking inward to the spleen when trying to assess the reality of our lives.

This can lead to seeking poor sources of nourishment in life that are unfulfilling. Thoughts become obsessive as we reject proper nourishment or try to consume everything and everything that might feed us.

If you can't get the proper nourishment, the boundary between fulfilling personal needs and the needs of others can become compromised. This breakdown can lead to either relying excessively on others for nourishment or attempting to be nourished by dysfunctionally taking care of others.

In the first example, people may become like a sponge, soaking up sympathy like a sponge soaks up moisture. Behaving overly sweet, trying to ingratiate themselves. Unable to meet their own needs, people with an unhealthy Earth phase may look for intimate relationships with needy or sick people who they try to nourish back to health.

This is how some dysfunctional relationships are formed. And if both partners have weakness with the Earth phase, it can create an unhealthy dynamic. This is why proper diet is so important for a healthy family dynamic.

Oftentimes the best way to heal a dysfunctional relationship or family is at the dinner table. And food choices and mealtime behavior are an important part of that healing process. Eating fast foods laden with fat and sugar while watching TV is not conducive to healing.

It's also a good way to continue to do damage to the Earth phase and may lead to metabolic syndrome and diabetes. Both involve the pancreas, which is really the yang of the spleen, which is responsible for transformation and transportation.

THE PANCREAS IS SPLEEN YANG

Oddly, the pancreas isn't mentioned at all in TCM. Its functions are just lumped together with the larger spleen. And they are intimately intertwined. They both grow out of the duodenum. In the embryo, the spleen sends signals to the pancreas to promote its growth. They share a blood supply from the splenic artery, and they also empty into the same vein.

So they share a common origin, they share a blood supply, they are literally right on top of each other. It's easy to see how they might have been combined.

The pancreas also has two functions, known as exocrine and endocrine. The exocrine includes all the enzymes or digestive fireworks (yang) that we saw when we looked at what happens in the duodenum. They literally are responsible for the *transformation* of food attributed to the spleen.

The endocrine function includes insulin and glucagon, which both regulate sugar. And this accounts for the *transportation* function attribute to the spleen. It's how sugar gets into the cells of the body.

Earlier we looked at serotonin and how, remarkably, it explained a lot of the activities associated with the spleen in TCM. As I mentioned, serotonin regulates insulin. With many other hormones, serotonin is like an on/off switch. But with insulin, their interactions are so intertwined that you basically can't separate them.

In a study from 2009, researcher Nils Paumann and his colleagues showed that serotonin plays a key role in controlling insulin secretion and that its absence can lead to diabetes. Furthermore, it does this differently than in the brain where it binds to receptors. In the pancreas it actually forms a bond with an enzyme, and it does this inside the cells.[9]

Insulin is stored in beta cells in the pancreas in what are called "secretory granules." These cells also store serotonin, and it is often released at the same time as insulin. In fact, researchers sometimes will measure serotonin levels when they want to track insulin release because serotonin is easier to monitor.

Okay, why does this matter other than being a mind-blowing geek fest for lovers of physiology like me?

Well, Hashimoto's and hypothyroidism are conditions of spleen yang deficiency. And insulin resistance and many of the emotional challenges that I mentioned previously are all common symptoms in Hashimoto's patients.

This means blood sugar balance and regulation is even more important than we previously thought. And also that serotonin balance is very important because it is intimately linked with blood sugar stability. Another study from the *Journal of Biological Chemistry* showed that SSRIs (antidepressant medications that flood the body with serotonin) cause insulin resistance.[10]

This means that serotonin is very much linked to sugar issues. Too much causes insulin resistance, too little can lead to diabetes or hypoglycemia. And, bringing us full circle, this is indisputable evidence of the role of emotion in disease. Li Dongyuan was right again!

When you think about the symptoms of serotonin deficiency, it also explains the emotional problems we discussed earlier—that is, feelings of not being adequately nurtured. A classic symptom of too little serotonin is not being able to get pleasure or enjoyment out of things. You can't enjoy hobbies, favorite activities, food, friendships, or relationships. And it can make you have feelings of dependency on others because you can't find pleasure or enjoyment in yourself.

Another way to look at all of these spleen qi deficient symptoms is that they manifest in one of the five imbalances of yin fire: dampness.

DAMPNESS IS A PATHOLOGY OF SPLEEN YANG DEFICIENCY

Dampness is a condition in the body of excessive amounts of moisture, like excess humidity. The dampness that is associated with spleen yang deficiency is a slightly different kind of fluid accumulation than those that Western doctors are familiar with and treat with diuretics.

These drugs treat fluid accumulation due to heart- or kidney-related problems. Either the heart isn't pumping properly or the kidney isn't draining fluids properly (or both). Dampness that is associated with spleen yang is really a dampness of impaired metabolic function rather than the inability to move fluids out of the body.

With heart- and kidney-related fluid accumulation, this dampness tends to accumulate in the lower extremities, and we see it as ankle swelling. In contrast, spleen yang dampness results in fluids accumulating in the gut (like a beer belly or with abdominal bloating).

And this fluid accumulation in the gut is caused by a weak and underactive pancreas, and is, essentially, the accumulation of toxins. These toxins tend to draw water through osmosis and since the body can't drain this dampness properly, both accumulate.

This can result in a sallow complexion. Another interesting fact about Earth phase–related conditions is that they manifest in the face. When stomach heat is excessive, your face may become bright red, as the stomach channel runs right through the face and ends just below the eyes.

With spleen qi dampness, the complexion can turn a pale yellow. In Chinese medicine, as we have seen with yin and yang, there are opposites in pathology. Excess conditions tend to produce brighter colors and deficient conditions produce pale, weaker colors.

This dampness can also be self-perpetuating, especially if you have an underlying hypothyroid condition, which slows all metabolic activity. And what are these "toxins"? They can be any substance that accumulates in a higher concentration than normal, and they often have a negative impact on cellular function.

One common example is sugar, which accumulates if a person eats too much of it or if the pancreas is weak and doesn't produce enough insulin. This is what diabetes is: too much sugar in the blood turning toxic.

Once blood sugar levels get too high, this excess sugar must be filtered and absorbed by the kidneys. If it remains high, your kidneys excrete excess sugar into your urine and also draw more fluids from your tissues.

This whole process has a negative effect on kidney function—and may cause you to pee more frequently, leaving you dehydrated. You become thirsty from losing all that fluid, and this gets worse and worse until the only thing that will help reverse it is insulin.

The irony here is that we have a state of dehydration caused by this dampness created by sugar. And this problem is one that normally develops gradually over time. It slowly gets worse and worse, which is characteristic of damp conditions.

They slowly and insidiously develop, often going unnoticed until they reach a tipping point and become a serious illness. That's what happens with type 2 diabetes. It's "adult onset" because it's been developing for years. And it's caused by lifestyle choices, such as eating a lot of sugary foods and carbohydrates.

Over time as this dampness develops, as we learned from Li Dong-yuan, heat can also develop with it. And when heat develops, the dampness congeals into phlegm. *Phlegm* in Chinese medicine is pathological dampness.

If you think about things in the body that contain phlegm (such as phlegm from colds and flus, mucus in the stools, and plaques that accumulate in the blood vessels), what do they all have in common? They're full of dead immune cells. These cells are drawn to the toxins and are there because they are attacking it like an invader, trying to get it out of the body.

It's an immune response, causing inflammation and eventually, it can build on itself.

This is yin fire.

Wow! We covered a ton. Let's recap some of the symptoms of spleen and stomach qi deficiency (they are so similar to hypothyroid symptoms, don't you know!).

RECAP:

These are all symptoms of spleen and stomach qi deficiency: weakness, lethargy, and/ or fatigue; decreased motivation; brain fog and dull thinking, sensing, or feeling; poor appetite; weak digestion; susceptibility to colds and flu; difficulty recovering from illness; pasty, pale complexion; poor hair growth; shortness of breath; perspire easily with exertion; low libido; muscle weakness; aversion to cold/chill easily; frequent urination; infertility; and dull, brittle nails.

Do these not sound remarkably like Hashimoto's and hypothyroid symptoms? They are one and the same!

Okay, so far we've gotten a good sense of what is involved in the entire digestive tract, which is all governed by the Earth phase. We've also met the three major actors of Earth: the spleen, the stomach, and the pancreas.

And we've also seen how deficiency in one aspect of the Earth phase can cause weakness and compromised function in other aspects of Earth and to pathology. And the brain. Of course, the Earth phase also has relationships with the other four phases. None of this happens in a vacuum.

Next, we'll take a look at how modern research confirms Li Dong-yuan's theory about the role that emotion plays in digestive health. We see this connection when we look at the relationship between the gut and the brain.

And it really emphasizes just how important emotions are in the formation and progression of autoimmune disease.

HASHIMOMENT:
Is This Your Most Important Asset?

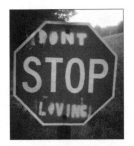

I was thinking today about something that may be the single most important asset in healing your Hashimoto's.

It's a belief that drives everything else, and it is the crucible that contains hope. I'm talking about faith. And not just in a religious sense, though that can be helpful.

I mean a basic belief, underneath it all, that you *can* be successful in overcoming this challenge.

Because here's the thing, if you lose faith, you're done.

Hope goes with it, perseverance too. Determination and optimism are also casualties.

And make no mistake: There will be times that you still have setbacks. And some of these setbacks may seem like they bring you right back to zero.

But, I can tell you from experience with working with many, many people that often:

The biggest implosions happen before the biggest insights, and the biggest defeats come before the biggest victories.

Sometimes the biggest breakdowns happen before the biggest breakthroughs.

The worst doubts come before the miracle.

So, it comes down to having faith.

My question for you today is this: Can you cultivate faith?

Is this a muscle that can be strengthened? Is this a skill that can be developed?

I think it is.

Of course, in a religious or spiritual sense, this is a belief in a power greater than yourself, however you define that, and a trust in that greater power.

Prayer and meditation and reading books that inspire this connection are vital.

And in a nonreligious sense, it's the basic belief that the solution is knowable.

That's why I spend so much time studying physiology and research, because I believe that in that data are the seeds of our solutions.

If I can figure out the mechanism, at least I can have a better idea of where the problems might be. And if I know where the problems are, I can get closer to finding the solution.

That gives me faith, or at least keeps me busy, when I'm having doubts.

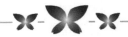

Chapter 5

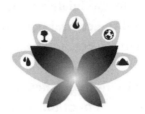

BRAIN/GUT INTERACTIONS:
Smooth Operating System

While the brain is not considered a separate system in Chinese medicine (it's part of the Water phase), I feel that it's so important that I have decided to devote a chapter to it.

In addition, in my opinion, it is an absolutely fascinating area of modern research that confirms virtually everything that ancient Chinese doctors like Li Dong-yuan were saying about the role of emotion in disease and about the importance of digestive function.

In particular, the role of the microbiome (the little critters that live in our gut) explains so much. In my opinion, the bacteria in the gut and the metabolic activity that they are responsible for is spleen and stomach qi.

Because when the microbiome is damaged or dysfunctional, it can lead to many of the symptoms that we have just been discussing in the last several chapters. Furthermore, its influence is felt body wide, and it is also one of the primary drivers of autoimmunity.

And one thing that's critically important to understand about this is that it extends far beyond what is normally thought of as basic physiology. The interactions between the gut, brain, emotions, and even things like motivation and intuitive decision-making are all connected via the gut and the microbiome.

In recent years, research in neuroscience and biopsychology has shown that the gut microbiota has direct impacts on thought and a variety of stress-related behaviors including those connected to anxiety and depression.[1]

The gut microbiome can actually modulate and influence behavior of the immune system, the endocrine system, and the central nervous system. And leaky gut is also directly impacted by the bacteria in the gut, and it can affect communication between these systems.[2]

As we have seen, the most heavily populated area of the gut by bacteria is the colon. This is important because different populations can have different physiological impacts in your body, and certain kinds of foods feed different populations.

For example, the two species Firmicutes and Bacteroidetes, which make up a large percentage of your gut bacteria, can impact your ability to lose weight effectively. It seems that some studies indicate that more Firmicutes were found in obese individuals, but there is also some disagreement in other studies, proving just how individual the composition of gut bacteria can be.[3]

ROLE IN LEAKY GUT

The main purpose of the intestinal barrier is to absorb nutrients, vitamins, minerals, and water and to keep the bad guys out of our bloodstream. This is also where tolerance to foods and autoimmunity are thought to develop. The breakdown of the gut can lead to the loss of tolerance to food (oral tolerance) and to self (this is what autoimmunity is—loss of this self-tolerance).

The bacteria that live in the gut also populate this barrier terrain and are important in keeping the integrity of the tight junctions that make up the barrier.

What's interesting about the microbiota's influence on the barrier systems is that it is not just restricted to the gut barrier. There is evidence that the blood-brain barrier is also made of the same proteins as the intestinal barrier and that when there are changes or a breakdown of one barrier system, it leads to the other breaking down as well.

In other words, if you have leaky gut, then you also may have leaky brain.

This is one of the reasons why food reactions can cause brain fog. When materials leak into the bloodstream, they can also leak from the bloodstream into the brain. The immune system then reacts and attacks them, causing inflammation in the brain.[4]

Communication between the brain and the gut occurs via the nervous, endocrine, and immune systems. And the bacteria in the gut influence this communication. This is the lifelong job of these bacteria: to keep this communication happening and to protect the barriers.

Exactly how this happens is not yet fully understood. Problems with the intestinal barrier could cause a microbiota driven pro-inflammatory response that affects the brain. An increase in gut permeability could also lead to mucosal inflammation that then leads to more barrier destruction.

This could then maintain and make worse the low-grade inflammatory response. Alternatively, systemic inflammation could increase intestinal barrier permeability and thus allow the movement of bacteria (or bacterial by-products) outside the gut and that could lead to more systemic inflammation. (This is what happens in autoimmunity and Hashimoto's.)

One theory is that damage to your microbiome early in life can set you up for problems later in life. And if you think about how common it is for young children to be prescribed antibiotics for upper respiratory and ear infections, you can see that this can have profound consequences later in life.

There are theories that a lack of diversity in bacteria in the gut can lead to chronic inflammatory disorders later in life.[5]

Furthermore, researchers have found that interactions between the immune system, the intestinal barriers, and the microbiota can lead to aging. In fact, the composition of gut bacteria is much different in frail versus healthy elderly people. Want to live to a healthy old age? Make gut-bacteria health your number one mission![6]

STRESS AND THE GUT

There is a good deal of research on the connection between stress, leaky gut, and gut bacteria. Stress has been shown to increase leaky gut.[7]

And this is true of both chronic and acute stress.

What's also interesting is that gut bacteria have been shown to affect the impact of stress-induced changes to the HPA (hypothalamic-pituitary-adrenal axis). And these probiotics also can help restore the barriers in the gut and brain.[8]

This tells us a few things. First, Li Dong-yuan was right. Emotions do have a huge impact on our health and well-being, and this extends far beyond just the gut. Research has established that there are links between childhood stress and developing depression later in life.[9]

Stress can totally alter the balance of bacteria in the gut. And this can lead to a breakdown of the barrier systems, which leads to more physiological stress and on and on. It's a vicious cycle.

IBS AND DEPRESSION

One good example of the interactions between leaky gut, the brain, and emotional health is IBS, irritable bowel syndrome. IBS is basically the medical name for leaky gut that is bad enough to cause moderate to serious symptoms.

IBS is a stress-related imbalance of the brain-gut-microbiota communication system.[10] So it's the perfect example of this process in action, and it can teach us a lot about how to heal leaky gut as well as the emotional consequences of the breakdown of this axis.

One thing that research has shown is that a significant number of IBS patients also suffer from anxiety and depression. And this is definitely not just a one-way street. Anxiety and depression also make IBS (and leaky gut) worse.[11]

What's also really interesting is that the ratio of gut bacteria (remember the Firmicutes and Bacteroidetes families that affected weight loss?) determines how severe depression symptoms are. Depression was found to be more serious in IBS patients with a high Firmicutes:Bacteroidetes ratio compared to IBS patients with a healthy microbiota signature.

So, gut bacteria actually determines psychological health! Holy crap! (Pun intended.) And there are crazy levels of granularity in some of these studies, down to specific areas of the gut that cause specific immune consequences.

This is why I wanted you to learn about all the ecosystems in the gut. They all have influence throughout our bodies.

SEROTONIN

Another interesting area of research is the influence of gut bacteria (spleen qi) on serotonin. As we have learned, serotonin is an important neurotransmitter for a variety of metabolic activities. And we saw how the spleen is a major regulator of serotonin activity via its affect on platelets.

Well, new research has shown that the serotonin system may be under the influence of gut microbes. And this plays a role in leaky gut. The largest reserve of 5-HT (serotonin) is found in the enterochromaffin cells. (These are neuroendocrine cells found in gastric glands in the mucosa, and they are responsible for producing gastric acid by the release of histamine.)[12]

This mucosal serotonin plays a direct role in leaky gut. It can decrease intestinal permeability, and in IBS patients it decreases the expression of a protein called occludin, which is like the glue that binds the intestinal cells together.[13]

So, serotonin, which is regulated by the spleen, is regulated by the gut bacteria (spleen qi)! Also, another study found that spore-forming bacteria (which I have found clinically to be superior in their healing power) increase colonic and blood 5-HT in the chromatin cells.[14]

SHORT-CHAIN FATTY ACIDS

The gut bacteria produce a number of metabolic products that are energy producing (again, in my opinion this is the metabolic building blocks of the spleen and stomach qi). These included SCFAs (short-chain fatty acids), polysaccharides, nucleic acids, structural proteins, and more.

The SCFAs are signaling molecules and are very important in maintaining a strong gut barrier. One that I particularly like to use as a supplement is butyrate. Butyrate has been demonstrated to influence expression of tight junction proteins, including claudin-2, occludin, cingulin, and zonula occludens proteins.[15]

With IBS, there is often a lesser amount of butyrate-producing bacteria.

ROLE OF DIET IN ALL OF THIS

Not surprisingly, diet plays a huge role in the health of gut bacteria. Processed food and fast food are directly linked to leaky gut and depression.[16] On the other hand, a diet rich in vegetables, fruit, and fish is associated with healthier levels of bacteria and fewer symptoms of depression.

In addition, diets high in healthy fats can influence the gut microbiota, and have been demonstrated to increase the Firmicutes:Bacteroidetes ratio and induce the growth of *Enterobacteriaceae*.[17]

PROBIOTICS, PREBIOTICS, AND "CRAZY" PSYCHOBIOTICS

Not all probiotics are created equally (and in the chapter on the microbiome, I explored which ones may be better than others), and it is clear that certain strains can help heal leaky gut. There was a term that made me laugh in the medical literature called "psychobiotics," which refers to probiotics that may actually have a beneficial effect on mood, anxiety, and cognitive function by modulating this brain-gut-microbiota axis.[18]

There have yet to be any clinical studies on this, so I think it's a bit early to know which are best, but, certainly, we have the ancient Chinese wisdom of how to use diet effectively to modulate this relationship. And we also know that the combination of certain herbs and diet can have profoundly positive impacts on mood, the brain, and the gut.

RECAP: **GUT/BRAIN INTERACTIONS**

I think the biggest takeaway here is that Li Dong-yuan was right! There is now so much research connecting emotions to profound states of physiological dysfunction and illness.

This is not a minor connection. This is a point of leverage, and ignoring it will undermine your health. For some of you, it is already undermining your health in very powerful ways. TAKE THIS SERIOUSLY! I'm not playing.

And what's also remarkable is that the microbiome has intelligence. It dictates our emotions, too. So, again, taking loads of antibiotics not only has physical consequences, but it also has emotional and psychological ones.

Okay, so far we've learned about the many ecosystems in the gut, and we've seen how ancient Chinese doctors like Li Dong-yuan viewed the gut and digestive system as central to good health. In addition, we've gone over some of the Chinese medical theory regarding the Earth phase, and we've seen that the microbiome is itself very important for systemic health as well as emotional and physical well-being.

Now let's bring it all together and start looking at some solutions! But before we go there, here's an inspiring case study about how grateful we can be when we are able to recover some of our lives back after losing them to Hashimoto's and autoimmune disease.

Also, we can see firsthand how committing to the right diet can yield some big rewards!

CASE STUDY

The pain and fatigue from Hashimoto's left me housebound for several months. I was even bedbound for a month. I was unable to work at my job as a solo flutist in my symphony orchestra for four months. When the new season was starting, it was SO important to me to prove to myself that I could get up and go out and do the one thing I love doing most.

I put all my energy into changing my diet into AIP, taking the supplements, resting, going on walks, and practicing in my head when physically I didn't have the strength to. The concert became my ONE focus and the proof to myself that I could get better. It became my huge motivational carrot—if I could get up onstage and play some of the hardest repertoire for the flute in my condition, then I knew I could get better. It would be the proof that I was on the way!

The rehearsals were so hard and the loss of muscle tone made me so tired too, but the concert was great and I played well!! I played like it was the last time I was ever going to play.

I cried unashamedly as the conductor got me to my feet during the standing ovation from my colleagues! Despite all those months of despair, pain, and fatigue, I could still do the thing I loved most. And I could still do it well. I had succeeded!

For me to get better, I had to have a goal, a plan, and sheer determination despite all the times that I felt totally in despair or scared and when I took three steps backward instead of going forward all the time.

I still have a way to go, but I know that I have the confidence in me to do it, and I will succeed!

Lorraine R.
France

PART II

The Hashimoto's
HEALING DIET

Chapter 6

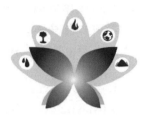

THE HASHIMOTO'S
Healing Diet Quiz

Hopefully, by now you've gotten a sense of the issues that affect the digestive system with Hashimoto's and hypothyroidism. Maybe you've started to get a sense of the mechanisms involved and you're curious about what you should do.

Next I'd like to share a simple questionnaire to help you identify your issues and show you how to pinpoint what your priorities are. As I mentioned previously, I recommend that you use the A.P.A.R.T. System as a basic tool for achieving your health goals.

As you may recall, the first *A* stands for asking the right questions, and this quiz will help you do just that. Then I'll show you how to identify which areas are priorities for you.

To begin, you need to figure out if your challenges are deficient or excess in nature (or some combination of the two—usually one predominates, however). Then you need to choose the appropriate dietary strategy to treat those issues.

Conditions that are deficient in nature are characterized by marked weakness, fatigue, and depletion. If you have trouble mustering enough energy to get out of bed and you get exhausted quickly, then chances are that you are deficient. This, then, becomes your priority because, obviously, you can't get better if you don't have the energy to take the action steps necessary to get better.

In contrast, conditions that are excess in nature are characterized by "too much." Too much heat (inflammation), too much damp and/or phlegm (fungal and bacterial infections), too much stress and emotional drama, etc., are the hallmarks of these issues.

The following quiz will help you discover your number one priority, helping you establish an action plan for dealing with whatever challenges you have. As you answer the questions, notice there are numerical values for your answers. At the end of the quiz, tally these up and that total will reflect your priorities.

TAKE THE QUIZ

1. Gender

A. Female	0
B. Male	1

2. Age

A. 0–25	0
B. 25–35	1
C. 35–45	1
D. 45 and up	0

3. I experience weakness, lethargy, and/or fatigue.

A. Never	3
B. Sometimes	2
C. Often	1
D. All the Time	0

4. I have brain fog and/or dull thinking, sensing, or feeling.

A. Never	3
B. Sometimes	2
C. Often	1
D. All the Time	0

5. I have a poor appetite and/or weak digestion.

A. Never	3
B. Sometimes	2
C. Often	1
D. All the Time	0

6. I have low libido or weak sex drive.

A. Never	3
B. Sometimes	2
C. Often	1
D. All the Time	0

7. I have infertility and/or a history of miscarriages.

A. Never	3
B. Sometimes	2
C. Often	1
D. All the Time	0

8. I have poor hair growth, hair loss, and/or dry, brittle nails.

A. Never	3
B. Sometimes	2
C. Often	1
D. All the Time	0

9. I have slow digestion and/or sluggish movement through my bowels.

A. Never	3
B. Sometimes	2
C. Often	1
D. All the Time	0

10. I am constipated.

A. Never	3
B. Sometimes	2
C. Often	1
D. All the Time	0

11. I have cold hands, feet, and/or nose.

A. Never	3
B. Sometimes	2
C. Often	1
D. All the Time	0

12. I have insomnia or difficulty sleeping.

A. Never	3
B. Sometimes	2
C. Often	1
D. All the Time	0

13. I have dry skin, hair, and/or eyes.

A. Never	3
B. Sometimes	2
C. Often	1
D. All the Time	0

14. I am slow to heal or recover from illnesses.

A. Never	3
B. Sometimes	2
C. Often	1
D. All the Time	0

15. I am easily irritated and experience rage.

A. Never	0
B. Sometimes	1
C. Often	2
D. All the Time	3

16. I have muscle tension and/or cramps.

A. Never	0
B. Sometimes	1
C. Often	2
D. All the Time	3

17. I feel bloated and experience distention or fullness in my abdomen.

A. Never	0
B. Sometimes	1
C. Often	2
D. All the Time	3

18. I have PMS and/or menstrual issues.

A. Never   0

B. Sometimes   1

C. Often   2

D. All the Time   3

19. I have lumps, nodules, and/or cysts.

A. Never   0

B. Sometimes   1

C. Often   2

D. All the Time   3

20. I have edema and/or water retention.

A. Never   0

B. Sometimes   1

C. Often   2

D. All the Time   3

21. I have myxedema (swelling of the face above or below the eyes or jawline).

A. Never   0

B. Sometimes   1

C. Often   2

D. All the Time   3

22. I have a fungal (yeast), bacterial, and/or viral infection.

A. Never   0

B. Sometimes   1

C. Often   2

D. All the Time   3

23. I have heartburn and/or acid reflux.

A. Never   0

B. Sometimes   1

C. Often   2

D. All the Time   3

24. I have bad breath.

A. Never   0

B. Sometimes   1

C. Often   2

D. All the Time   3

25. I have foul-smelling diarrhea or stools.

A. Never   0

B. Sometimes   1

C. Often   2

D. All the Time   3

26. I have hemorrhoids.

A. Never   0

B. Sometimes   1

C. Often   2

D. All the Time   3

27. I have sinus congestion.

A. Never   0

B. Sometimes   1

C. Often   2

D. All the Time   3

28. I have nausea.

A. Never 0

B. Sometimes 1

C. Often 2

D. All the Time 3

29. I am nervous and easily distracted.

A. Never 3

B. Sometimes 2

C. Often 1

D. All the Time 0

30. I am swollen with a heavy head, limbs, and/or abdomen.

A. Never 0

B. Sometimes 1

C. Often 2

D. All the Time 3

Scoring: The following scores represent zones of possibility and are not exact measurements. They're meant to help you to develop awareness of your own body so that you can make adjustments when needed.

0–25: If you scored in this zone, then you may be predominantly deficient. Read the chapter on deficient diets, and determine which deficient condition most corresponds to your symptoms.

If you aren't sure after reading, then simply follow the qi deficient diet.

Generally speaking, this diet should be everyone's default because it is the gentlest and most supportive for healing.

26–40: If you scored in this zone, you are predominantly deficient, but you have some excess issues that may need to be addressed. Our bodies don't always follow a rulebook, and sometimes we may have a mixed presentation. These types of conditions tend to be more complicated and consulting a trained physician who is familiar with these apparent contradictions may be advisable.

With this type of mixed presentation, the underlying deficiency condition may be leading to symptoms that resemble excess. For example, yin deficiency can lead to heat in the body. In other words, the underlying weakness is causing a kind of metabolic stasis that leads to stagnation.

The best approach for healing this type of presentation is to address the under-lying deficiency and to use foods and herbs to clear the underlying stagnation and excess symptoms. The qi deficient diet is your foundational diet though some tweak-ing may be needed to address the excess symptoms.

41–60: If you scored in this zone, you may have a mixed presentation that is excess in nature with this excess depleting the body and leading to deficiency. In this case it is important to address the excess condition in the short term and then return to the foundational qi deficient diet.

An example of this type of condition might be SIBO. In this case the underlying excess condition of the bacterial imbalance can lead to compromises in the intestinal lining and may cause leaky gut. The same may true of a condition like Candida, where the underlying fungal (yeast) infection may lead to damage to the intestinal lining.

In both cases you must treat the condition and then move to the default healing of the qi deficient diet. Herbal treatment or medication may also be advisable.

61–81: If you scored in this zone, you may have a predominantly excess condition. This can lead to deficiency pretty quickly, so it's important that it is addressed. For this type of presentation, review Chapter 12 on excess diets and find the symptoms that most suit your condition.

If you aren't sure, this may be a good time to test for underlying pathogens. Cyrex Laboratories offers a terrific panel called Array 12: Pathogen Associated Immune Reac-tivity Screen. This panel tests for antibodies for 29 different pathogens, including all the pathogens that I discuss in this book.

This must be ordered by a licensed medical professional. It can be quite helpful because you can quickly and easily rule out many different pathogens in one simple blood test.

Once you have addressed the pathogen or other cause of the excess condition, return to the default qi deficient diet to help restore balance and equilibrium to the digestive tract.

Chapter 7

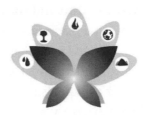

INTRODUCTION TO DIET PRINCIPLES

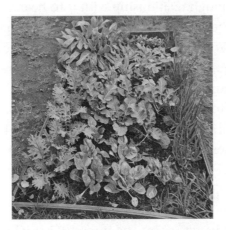

Hashimoto's is one of the most common autoimmune diseases in the United States. As you know, it is a thyroid disorder and an autoimmune disease. The autoimmune part of the equation makes virtually everything a challenge, and this is particularly true when it comes to trying to figure out what to eat.

One of the absolute truths about Hashimoto's is that no two people have the same version of the disease. There are so many variables. Some individuals are at different stages of progression and may have additional autoimmune, endocrine, digestive, or other systemic problems.

In writing this book and in working with and speaking to over 2,000 people with Hashimoto's, I have come to believe that *diet and emotions are the two most important factors in achieving long-term health goals and remission.*

In addition, I have also come to understand that a simplistic approach, which tells you to follow one diet and never deviate, is a recipe for failure. Things are going to change in your body and particularly in your gut. You need to be able to adapt when they do.

And because, as we have seen, the gut is composed of so many ecosystems and so many other things can influence the Earth phase, we have to be able to assess where the problems are and come up with the appropriate remedies for them.

I have done that for you and have made it as simple as possible. But part of what is required by you is a willingness to get to know your body. It has all the answers, but you must have a close enough relationship with it to hear them.

Therefore, you can't be a passive participant and just expect to be told what to do. You must get involved. You need to keep a journal, and you need to conduct some experiments. This is a long-term project that will yield remarkable returns if you invest the time, energy, and effort.

But before we get into the particulars, let's take a look at the big picture. With Hashimoto's and autoimmunity, generalizing about what kind of diet is the best is kind of like asking, "Where do I build my house on this minefield?"

WHERE DO I BUILD MY HOUSE ON THIS MINEFIELD?

You build it where it won't set off the mines. Researchers estimate that 70 to 80 percent of the immune system is found in the gut. Whatever the actual percentage, there is no doubt that what goes through your digestive system has a huge impact on your immune system.

Huge. This concept is just common sense, but many doctors and health-care practitioners ignore it. Why? As I mentioned earlier, one doctor friend of mine put it like this: "I don't bother trying to change people's diets. It's easier to get an alcoholic to stop drinking than to get people to change the way they eat."

People are attached to food. It has cultural, emotional, and psychological roots that run deep. And it is the playground of physical addictions to things like sugar and alcohol (which is also sugar). However, if you have Hashimoto's and you want to learn to manage it properly, you need to be prepared to abandon all of that.

Instead you must find a way to have a relationship to food and eating so that it serves you. Just as many people eat themselves to death you can use it to achieve remarkable healing and longevity. The choice is yours.

LEAKY GUT: ADDING GASOLINE TO THE FIRE

Many people with Hashimoto's also have intestinal permeability, also known as leaky gut. A healthy GI tract is one that one has a lush forest of villi, all held tightly together.

This keeps bad guys like bacteria, chemicals, environmental toxins, and undigested food out of the bloodstream. Unfortunately, the chronic inflammation of yin fire can turn this lush forest into a desert; and poor diet, blood sugar imbalances, and chronic stress can open up wide chasms that a molecular 18-wheeler could drive through.

Alessio Fasano, M.D., one of the world's leading experts on the origins of autoimmunity, has found the cause of autoimmune disease in the intestines. In a paper published in 2012 in the journal *Clinical Reviews of Allergy & Immunology*, he noted that:

> Together with the gut-associated lymphoid tissue and the neuroendocrine network, the intestinal epithelial barrier, with its intercellular tight junctions, controls the equilibrium between tolerance and immunity to non-self antigens. Zonulin is the only physiologic modulator of intercellular tight junctions described so far that is involved in trafficking of macromolecules and, therefore, in tolerance/immune response balance. When the zonulin pathway is deregulated in genetically susceptible individuals, autoimmune disorders can occur.[1]

What that means in simple terms is that the breakdown of the barrier of the intestines is the pathway to autoimmune disease. This is what actually sets the stage for the onset of autoimmune disease when the immune system short-circuits and starts confusing other stuff with our own tissue. (The one food that is most often implicated in this is gluten.)

HEAL THE GUT, SLOW THE HASHIMOTO'S

Many people also believe that the best way to heal autoimmune disease is by healing the gut. (I am one of those people.) So this begs the question, What heals the gut?

Many things can heal, potentially, and as we have seen in the first part of this book, the gut is a complex series of ecosystems, and you can have problems in any number of areas. If you are serious about healing, you have to figure out where those problems are and heal all those areas.

This is important because what the five-phase system teaches us is that problems are never confined to one area. They affect other areas, and there is a back and forth relationship that leads to further compromise if all areas are not addressed.

That being said, there are some areas that exert leverage and have important influence on others, and focusing on them can help turn the tide of momentum. But we must look everywhere and understand that things can develop slowly and insidiously. This means that we have to develop a relationship with our body that involves checking in and taking inventory on a regular basis.

HEALING STEP-BY-STEP

The first step to healing the GI tract is to simplify in order to limit your variables and to remove all the foods that are creating chronic immune responses. Eventually, you can add them back in one at a time (hopefully). When you do, you will begin to discover your own unique set of land mines.

And rather than rummaging around in the dark, now there are diagnostic tests available to help determine which foods cause an immune response in you. However, these tests are not perfect, and the gold standard remains the simple process of elimination and reintroduction.

There is no real downside to this, other than some inconvenience. If you are like me and many of the people I've worked with, you are willing to suffer a little inconvenience in order to get better. In fact, you might even be in enough pain to go to any length to get better (I was when I started this journey).

If you are having doubts, here's an example that shows just how powerful this approach can be, even when done only partially.

Mary is a 54-year-old female who was diagnosed with Hashimoto's. Her chief complaints were feelings of sadness due to her thyroid issues, weight gain, extreme fatigue, hormonal imbalances, and weary adrenals.

If we look at her Earth phase symptoms, we learn that she had more than three bowel movements daily, unpredictable abdominal swelling, and frequent bloating and distention after meals. What is that? It is textbook spleen qi deficiency.

In addition, there was evidence of too little stomach acid: gas immediately following a meal, sense of fullness during and after meals, and feeling hungry an hour or two after eating.

Mary also had a number of blood sugar symptoms: she craved sweets during the day, was lightheaded and irritable if meals were missed, and depended on coffee to both get her day started and keep her energy up. Mary felt shaky and jittery, and was easily upset and nervous. She had poor memory retention and was forgetful. These are all symptoms of hypoglycemia.

Mary had difficulty losing weight, and her blood tests revealed high cholesterol, high LDL, low LDH, normal fasting glucose, and HA1C. So, she may have also had some insulin resistance.

In addition, Mary had trouble falling asleep and couldn't stay asleep. She craved salt, was a slow starter in the morning and experienced afternoon fatigue, felt dizzy when standing up quickly, had headaches with exertion or stress, and gained weight when under stress. What does that tell us? Adrenal issues!

All of this resulted in significant thyroid symptoms: Mary was tired/weak, she required excessive amounts of sleep to function properly, she felt depressed and lacked motivation, and she noticed mental sluggishness. She also experienced night sweats.

Her blood test results revealed the following: high TSH, high TPO antibodies (they were 2,880), and low to normal T4, T3, fT3, and fT4. These findings confirm Hashimoto's and hypothyroidism.

Here's what Mary did. Because she had a lot going on in her life, she couldn't fully commit to the autoimmune paleo diet completely (but has since). She just cut out grains and legumes 100 percent.

After two months, her TPO antibodies dropped from 2,880 to 375. She also experienced dramatic improvements in energy and mood, as well as the various blood sugar and adrenal symptoms.

Mary was absolutely shocked by how much better she felt, just from simply eliminating grains and legumes.

As you can see, simplifying and eliminating foods that cause immune reactions can have dramatic effects on both antibody levels and quality of life. If you still have doubts, try it yourself and keep reading.

In the next chapter, we'll examine these food reactions and why they can be so impactful.

Chapter 8

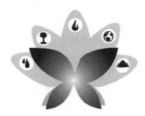

FOOD SENSITIVITIES AND DAIRY

There is no question that foods can cause immune reactions. And the unfortunate truth is that the foods that tend to be the worst are those that we, invariably, often love the most.

Foods like ice cream, cheese, bread, pasta, and alcohol are all examples. And there is a biological reason for our attachment to these foods. Both foods made from gluten and milk contain proteins that are very similar in structure to morphine. They are called casomorphin in milk and gluteomorphin or gliadorphin in wheat products. No wonder we love them; we get a very pleasant buzz from them!

In addition, sugar is a very addictive substance. Research has shown that sugar can induce reward and craving behaviors that are similar in magnitude to drugs. Experiments on laboratory rats have revealed that not only can sugar substitute for addictive drugs like cocaine, it can also actually be more rewarding and addictive.[1]

Other problematic foods include gluten, dairy, nightshades, lectin-containing foods, and more. There are plenty of books on the market with a chapter on why you shouldn't eat gluten. I'm not going to waste time writing another. If you are interested in learning more about this, visit my website and read the article titled "Celiac Disease and Hashimoto's."[2]

But before we go any further, let's take a look at the role of another problem food—dairy—and get a basic understanding of food sensitivities.

HASHIMOTO'S AND DAIRY

With Hashimoto's, as I just mentioned, sometimes the things that can cause the most problems are the things we are most attached to. Dairy certainly falls into this category.

DAIRY CAN COMPROMISE YOUR HEALTH IN TWO WAYS

There are two distinctly different problems that can be caused by dairy consumption. The first is caused by milk proteins; the second is caused by milk sugars.

Let's take a look at both.

MILK PROTEINS HAVE A SIMILAR STRUCTURE TO GLUTEN

Unless you've been living under a rock, you've probably heard about the benefits of going gluten-free for people with Hashimoto's. Well, milk-based products have a host of proteins that also can and do cause immune reactions. These include casein (alpha and beta), casomorphin (the protein that closely resembles morphine), milk butyrophilin, and whey.

These proteins are known as "cross-reactors" because they closely resemble gluten proteins and can cause a similar immune response in the body.

In a lot of cases these responses are undiagnosed, and people continue to eat these foods and/or are advised to eat these foods, and they end up damaging their intestines and robbing themselves of important nutrients.

There are different parts of the immune system that react to these dietary proteins. These are known as IgE, IgA, and IgG reactions. It's helpful to understand how they differ.

UNDERSTANDING THE DIFFERENCE BETWEEN IGE, IGA, AND IGG

Food allergies are mediated by the IgE part of the immune system. These generally cause an immediate reaction and are often what is called a "true allergy" by doctors and other medical professionals. However, this is not the only type of food reaction your body can have.

IgA and IgG systems can also lead to hypersensitivities, sometimes termed "food intolerance" or "food sensitivity." These are the antibodies that are tested when you order food-sensitivity panels. The important thing to understand about them is that they are much different in their mechanism and ability to wreak havoc in your body.

IGA FOOD REACTIONS

IgA food intolerance is the more severe reaction and happens mostly in the intestines. It is an abnormal response of the intestines to certain foods in genetically predisposed individuals. The intolerances may manifest themselves early in childhood or later in life.

IgA food intolerance results in irritation and inflammation of the intestinal tract every time that particular food is consumed. This results in damage to the intestines, and eventually it hurts your ability to absorb nutrients and can increase the risk of autoimmune diseases, cancer, and accelerate aging through increased intestinal permeability or leaky gut.

IgA food intolerances can also vary in their symptoms considerably. They may be asymptomatic or neurological, or they may present with the following symptoms: diarrhea, loose stools, constipation, acid reflux, malabsorption of nutrients from foods, and increased intestinal permeability.

They can cause IBS, gas, nausea, skin rashes (including eczema), acne, and respiratory conditions such as asthma, nasal congestion, headache, irritability, cognitive problems, and vitamin/mineral deficiencies.

The most famous IgA food reaction is celiac disease, and it is an intolerance to gluten, the protein found in wheat. Gluten's role in Hashimoto's and autoimmunity has been written about extensively, as I've mentioned.

However, dairy protein, egg, and soy protein IgA intolerances are also extremely common in people with Hashimoto's. These intolerances do not have a specific name and may be confused with other, less severe food absorption syndromes.

IGG FOOD REACTIONS

These are antibodies that provide long-term resistance to infections, called Immunoglobulin G (IgG), and they have a much longer half-life than the traditional IgE allergy. These reactions can be much more subtle, and people can live with them for years, if not their entire lives.

Symptoms range from headaches and nausea to seizures and hyperactivity, or simply just fatigue, bloating, mood changes, brain fog, memory problems, or dark circles under the eyes. They may occur hours or even days after the problem food has been ingested.

Food allergy tests like the Cyrex Labs Array #10 test both IgA and IgG reactions to foods. A positive or equivocal finding of IgG against foods may indicate that the person has been repeatedly exposed to food proteins recognized as foreign by the immune system.

CLINICAL PEARL:

IgG testing is also relevant with thyroid autoimmunity because this process of reacting to IgG antibodies can fire up the very same parts of the immune system that are already attacking our own tissue. In fact, Antithyroglobulin antibodies (TgAb) and antithyroid peroxidase antibodies (TPOAb) are predominantly of the immunoglobulin (Ig) G class, and are hallmarks of Hashimoto's.[3]

The degree and severity of symptoms vary greatly because of the genetic makeup of the individual. The complete elimination of IgG positive foods may help improve Hashimoto's symptoms because this can be a key factor in calming autoimmunity.

DAIRY ALLERGIES AND DAIRY INTOLERANCE ARE TWO DIFFERENT THINGS

Often people confuse the food immune reactions to dairy mentioned above and milk intolerance, which is caused by milk sugars known as lactose.

One thing that people don't always realize is that even tiny amounts of lactose can have a major impact on our ability to absorb thyroid medications. Worst of all, some thyroid medications actually contain lactose, defeating their own purpose!

LACTOSE CAN MAKE THYROID HORMONE NOT WORK AS WELL

A recent study published in 2014 by Mehmet Asik and colleagues found that lactose-intolerant Hashimoto's patients who were taking levothyroxine showed a decrease in TSH after lactose restriction.[4]

In other words, removing lactose improved how their levothyroxine was working.

Another study from August 2014 had a similar finding. This was published in the *Journal of Clinical Endocrinology & Metabolism* by Miriam Cellini and colleagues and found that lactose intolerance increased the need for more thyroid medications.[5]

The researchers found that the average person with Hashimoto's required an average dose of 1.31 mcg/kg/day of levothyroxine to get to an average TSH right around 1 mU/L (that would be right around 75 mcg of levothyroxine for a 125-pound person), while a person with Hashimoto's and lactose intolerance who continued to consume lactose needed a dose of 1.72 mcg/kg/day to reach the same goal (that would be like 100 mcg of levothyroxine for the same 125-pound person—that's quite a bit more).

In addition, patients who had other gut disorders in addition to lactose intolerance required an even higher dose to get to their goal TSH 2.04 mcg/kg/day, or around 116 mcg for a 125-pound person. So as you can see, the more gut-related issues, the higher the dose needed to achieve the same effect.

If your TSH levels are jumping up and down and you're having a hard time controlling them, dairy protein immune responses and lactose intolerance should be top on your list of suspects.

HOW COMMON IS LACTOSE INTOLERANCE IN HASHIMOTO'S?

Lactose-intolerance rates in Caucasians have been reported to be between 7 percent and 20 percent, and rates are much higher for those of Asian and African descents. Lactose intolerance can be secondary to other conditions and reversible, or it can be genetic and permanent.

The 2014 study by Dr. Asik and colleagues mentioned above tested 83 Hashimoto's patients for lactose intolerance and found lactose intolerance in 75.9 percent of the patients. I'd say that would qualify as pretty darn common!

Thirty-eight of those patients were instructed to start a lactose-free diet for eight weeks, and the researchers found that during that period, the patients' TSH dropped, meaning they were probably absorbing their thyroid medication better.

IF YOU ARE LACTOSE INTOLERANT, A TINY AMOUNT CAN CAUSE PROBLEMS

For some lactose-intolerant people, even tiny amounts of lactose that are found in thyroid medications can be an issue, causing impaired absorption of thyroid medications. Yes, what I'm saying is that thyroid medications could be undermining their own absorption if they contain even teeny amounts of lactose.

So if you are someone who can't get your TSH into your "Goldilocks zone" where it's just right (there is much debate about where this is, but general consensus is that TSH should be somewhere between 0.5 and 2 mU/L for people to feel best), despite taking higher and higher doses of thyroid medications, consider lactose intolerance and the possibility that the lactose in your diet or even in your thyroid medication may be hindering its absorption.

And here's the thing—the reality is that you could have lactose intolerance *and* be having an immune reaction to diary proteins. This is a potent and destructive double whammy for people with Hashimoto's, which, as you know, is an autoimmune disease of the thyroid!

So dairy can potentially wind up autoimmune tissue destruction and prevent thyroid hormone from working. The result is a rapidly accelerating decline in thyroid function.

JUST GIVE UP DAIRY 100 PERCENT

Some people will ask, "What about Lactaid?" They sometimes ask this because they can't bear the idea of living without dairy products such as cheese and ice cream. And the logic makes sense to some degree. The issue is that it doesn't really solve the long-term damage and potential problems.

It's a little bit like an alcoholic taking the drug Antabuse and continuing to drink. The real problem is alcohol. And the real problem for some people is dairy.

As far as diet, I have seen tremendous improvements in my own health and the health of my clients and readers on a dairy-free diet, so this is something that I strongly recommend for everyone with Hashimoto's (at the very least, experiment and eliminate it and see what happens).

Here's another interesting case study by someone who did her own version of the elimination diet.

CASE STUDY: Gave Up All "White Foods"

After two years of struggling with poisonous medication and an extra 60 pounds of weight that no one noticed but me, I had had enough. Enough of doctors not listening to me and wanting nothing more than to shove whatever the flavor of the month thyroid pill was. So I did my own research and finally found a doctor that was willing to believe I might know my own body better than he did. He put me on Armour Thyroid, and I also stopped eating all white foods. This included flour, rice, corn, potatoes, sugar, and dairy. I started walking every day, and just kept going farther and farther until I was up to five miles per day. I now do Beachbody workouts six days a week, and have been doing them for two years. I am down from a size 14 to a size 4 and a total loss of 65 pounds in a year and a half. I'm on the lowest dose possible of medication, and I have never felt better in my entire life, including before I was diagnosed with Hashimoto's.

Nancy C.
North Carolina

CLINICAL PEARL:

One thing that's really important to keep in mind is that when you eliminate inflammatory foods, it can improve the effectiveness of your medication. So, it's really important to monitor thyroid levels to prevent going hyperthyroid when you do an elimination diet.

BE AWARE: SOME THYROID MEDICATIONS CONTAIN LACTOSE

Here are some common medications that contain lactose as a filler and some that are lactose-free.

These medications may contain lactose:

- Synthroid

- Euthyrox

- WP Thyroid

- Nature-Throid
- Most generic brands of levothyroxine
- Some compounded medications may use lactose as a filler; check with your pharmacist

LACTOSE-FREE THYROID MEDICATIONS

These medications are lactose-free:

- Tirosint
- Armour Thyroid
- Cytomel
- Levoxyl

MEDICATION TIPS

Of all of the T4-containing medications, Tirosint has the fewest fillers that may affect absorption, and this medication was designed for people with these types of intolerance. This medication is recommended if you suspect you may have problems with dairy and lactose.

Of course some people do better with the addition of T3. Of all of the T4/T3 combination medications, WP Thyroid has the fewest fillers that can impair absorption. However, it does contain trace amounts of lactose as well.

Armour Thyroid does not contain lactose, but it does contain corn-derived ingredients that can be problematic in corn-sensitive individuals and can trigger a gluten-like reaction.

When the company that makes Armour Thyroid changed their formulation a few years ago, some people did very poorly with the new mixture, and one of the reasons was due to this corn-based filler.

OTHER FACTORS CONTRIBUTING TO MEDICATION ABSORPTION

Another really interesting research finding is that high TSH can simply be caused by absorption disorders like lactose intolerance, celiac disease, atrophic gastritis, *H. pylori* infections, inflammatory bowel disease, and/or parasites.

All of these issues commonly prevent people from getting their Hashimoto's into remission as well. These are more positive feedback loops, and they cause vicious cycles that lead to poor results in different systems of the body.

This is a perfect example of how this is not just a thyroid problem. Thyroid hormone metabolism is dependent on other systems of the body. A 2012 Polish study reported that thyroid patients who need more that 2 mcg/kg/day of levothyroxine with an increased TSH should be suspected of having an absorption disorder like the ones previously mentioned.[6]

Here's the bottom line: Get off of dairy 100 percent. What's the downside to experimenting? Treat it the same way you treat gluten, and understand that the misery it can cause is not worth the buzz of an ice-cream cone or some cheese on crackers. Also understand that having "just a little bit" is not really solving the problem at all. A tiny amount can be a tsunami to your immune system and lead to a whole cascade of problems.

Like being "sort of gluten-free," being "sort of dairy free" is like being "sort of "sort of pregnant." It's not a real thing.

FOOD AS MEDICINE: *SAGE*

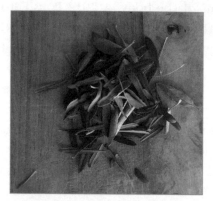

In my world, sage has few equals. The word *sage* is derived from the Latin word *salvus*, meaning well-being and, indeed, it lives up to its name and delivers on that promise.

It has a long history of use in both Chinese and Western herbalism. In fact, sage has been a primary ingredient in longevity prescriptions, and the medical verses of the 11th-century medical college in Salerno (Italy) mysteriously state that sage's supertonic effects are limited only by death.

Today, we know that sage essential oils affect the pituitary, adrenals, and gonads and enhance non-specific immunity (TH1). With its neuroendocrine restorative and immune-enhancing properties, sage reaches deeply into the core of human physiology, the higher neuroendocrine centers.

The essential oil clary sage is particularly effective in this way. I love it for whenever I'm feeling stressed or run-down.

And if you've been following me online and reading my posts, you will recall that these higher endocrine centers are core centers for connecting to spirit for the Taoists. Sage is a vehicle for this connection.

From a Chinese medical perspective, sage is considered bitter, pungent, astringent, cool, and dry.

It is restorative, astringing, stabilizing, and relaxing.

It is beneficial for the stomach, intestines, lungs, uterus, brain, nervous system, pituitary, spleen, lung, liver, and kidneys.

Sage tonifies qi, blood, and essence. It generates strength and relieves fatigue, restores neuroendocrine-immune functions, and enhances immunity. And it restores the adrenal cortex and raises blood pressure.

(Pretty phenomenal for people with Hashimoto's and autoimmunity. But, a word of caution, sage is a TH1 stimulant, so try it first before you hammer large quantities.)

It also tonifies reproductive qi, can promote and regulate menstruation, and promote labor. It increases estrogen and helps promote harmony in menopause.

Sage also promotes digestion, resolves phlegm and mucus, improves appetite, and stops discharge and secretions.

Furthermore, it's an excellent remedy for colds and flus.

Finally, sage promotes tissue repair, stimulates immunity, and benefits the skin.

Sage is basically the Swiss Army knife of the neuroendocrine-immune axis. And it's awesome with poultry. I never cook a duck or chicken without stuffing lots under the skin.

Today's mission, should you choose to accept it: go get some sage.

Chapter 9

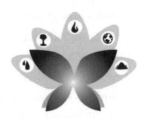

HASHIMOTO'S DIET:
Basic Principles

There is nothing more fundamental to healing the Earth phase and, indeed, healing our bodies than an appropriately designed diet. Unfortunately, for those of us with Hashimoto's and other autoimmune diseases, there is a lot of conflicting information out there about what *appropriate* means.

The genius of Chinese medicine is that it recognizes that all patients have uniquely different challenges, different constitutions and genetics, and different health issues that all require unique solutions. The design and content of the diet can be adjusted to help correct various pathological imbalances in all but the most extreme cases.

As a basic concept, the role of diet begins by focusing on treating a particular imbalance or set of imbalances and then gradually moves to a spleen and stomach qi strengthening diet. So, if you think of it as saving a burning house, first we put out the fire or fires, and then we renovate the house.

Because, fundamentally, as we have seen, healthy spleen and stomach function is the foundation of good health and necessary for all aspects of well-being, including tissue growth and repair, immune balance, healthy metabolic function, and strong reproductive and sexual activity.

As we learned from master Li Dong-yuan, maintenance of a healthy spleen and stomach (and the entire Earth phase) is central to the management of all internal disorders including Hashimoto's and other autoimmune diseases.

A detailed description of the mechanics of diet from a traditional Chinese medical point of view is beyond the scope of this book because our focus is, of course, using diet to heal Hashimoto's and Hashimoto's-related conditions. If you want to learn more about TCM diets, please see Paul Pitchford's *Healing with Whole Foods: Asian Traditions and Modern Nutrition* or Daverick Leggett's *Helping Ourselves: A Guide to Traditional Chinese Food Energetics*. Both are excellent resources in this vein.

There are two main aspects of diet to think about:

1. The kind of food you eat, and
2. The way it is eaten.

Both matter because food has properties that vary from hot to cold and dry to moist, and different foods accomplish different tasks.

Let's take a deeper look at these two aspects so that you can get a basic understanding of this.

1. The Type of Food You Eat

FOOD GROUPS AND BALANCE

Similarly to Western nutrition, TCM has three general food groups: protein, carbohydrates, and fruits and vegetables. But in contrast, each group has its own unique functions and flavors, and these also have specific nutritional and energetic activities.

For example, carbohydrates are often considered warm and sweet, and they strengthen the spleen and boost qi. Proteins (and animal protein, in particular) nourish blood, yin, qi, and jing and tend to be warmer than carbohydrates.

Fruits and vegetables tend to be more cooling, clearing, and moving in nature. They provide a kind of dietary counterpoint to the building and supplementing nature of the other two groups.[1]

So, time-out!

I want you get this. It's a conceptual shift. We can use different foods to accomplish different things. It's not just about what nutrients they contain. It's also about how we can use them to restore balance. Does that make sense?

I want you to start to think of food (and herbs) as tools for us accomplishing our goals. Food isn't just something to fill your stomach when you're hungry, you know what I'm sayin'?

There is no single diet that is appropriate for everyone. Different constitutional and genetic types require different types of food. It's primitive or naive to think that we are so similar that we should all eat exactly the same way.

So, what I'm suggesting is that even with the autoimmune paleo diet, you can accomplish different things and address particular issues by varying the proportions and focusing on how you prepare your food.

Your mission is to construct the appropriate mix of these components to suit your specific needs. Fortunately, I have done the work for you. Stick with me, and I will guide you through this.

By varying the proportions of each food group, we can achieve quite different results. For example, if you have a deficiency pattern, you will benefit from a diet based on supplementing the phases, particularly carbohydrates and proteins.

We must be particular about which carbohydrates and proteins, because the choices depend on the types of deficiency and the nature of the immune response. For example, qi deficiency needs more carbohydrates. Carbohydrates (i.e., sugar) are the fuel for our metabolic engines (spleen qi).

In the Earth phase, carbohydrates are the fuel for the reactor. The problem with autoimmunity is that some of that reactor fuel, like radiation, can be toxic. So we must be careful with which fuel we use. (And this is why the AIP diet is so helpful; it enables us to navigate which foods are safest for autoimmunity.)

In contrast, if you are blood and/or yin deficient, you want more animal protein. And organ meat like liver and heart are very effective for treating this problem.

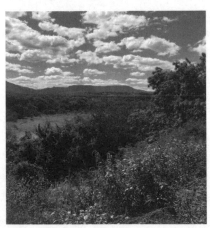

Let me tell you a story. As I mentioned, I came here to Rimrock, Arizona, just outside of Sedona, to really commune with the Earth phase. One day I went to a local farmers market to see what type of foods I could find, and I spoke with a farmer who raised his own grass-fed cattle.

His name is Zach Wolfe, and his farm is called Plowing Ahead Ranch. He and his wife, Shannon, shared with me that they were a "glass wall business," and they encouraged people to visit their farm and see how their animals are raised.

So I did. Their cows are grass-fed on land in the heart of the Verde Valley. As farmers they are fully invested in living in harmony with the earth, with their livestock, and with native wildlife. I bought a four-pound piece of liver and a beef heart because I wanted to experience the healing power of these organ meats.

The indigenous people of this region traditionally saved the organ meat from the hunt for the medicine man. It was held in that high esteem. It is in some ways the most important part of the animal and reserved for the person in the tribe who everyone depended on.

And they did so for a reason, as organ meat contains some of the most concentrated sources of just about every nutrient, including important amino acids, healthy fats, minerals, and vitamins. Compared with muscle meat, it has loads more of B vitamins including B1, B2, B6, folic acid, and the all-important vitamin B12.

Organ meat is also chock-full of minerals like phosphorous, iron, copper, magnesium, iodine, calcium, potassium, sodium, selenium, zinc, and manganese; and it provides the fat-soluble vitamins A, D, E, and K. In addition, organ meats contain high amounts of essential fatty acids, including the omega-3 fats EPA and DHA.

Do you really want to do less and accomplish more? If so, eat organ meat. It's a living multivitamin. (For some it is an acquired taste, I thought it was delicious.)

Okay, let's get back to using foods strategically. As I noted, if you are weaker or more deficient, carbohydrates and proteins should be eaten in larger proportions. But if you are tending more toward excess, then a higher proportion of fruits and vegetables is recommended.

In general, the typical American diet is high in animal protein, sugar, and fat. So, it's often overly supplementing to blood and yin. As we saw in the discussion of Earth phase pathologies, over-supplementation of this kind can lead to dampness, damp heat, and phlegm.

As we have discussed, phlegm accumulation may result in the development of deposits like plaque in the arteries, lipomas, or nodules.

It's all about balance. The correct proportions are important in designing a diet. We should seek a good overall balance, and we must also factor our underlying issues and take into account the treatment goals we have.

A meat- and protein-rich diet is appropriate for someone who is very weak and deficient. But it may not be appropriate after a period recovery and it may not be advisable long term. Diets high in animal protein and low in vegetables and fruit can lead to poor diversity of intestinal flora, declines in glutathione levels, and more inflammation. From a Chinese medicine perspective, the downside is that this diet can generate and aggravate dampness and phlegm.

Large quantities of carbohydrates act like sugar in the body and create dampness and stagnation (and blood sugar problems). Overly hot and spicy food can dry and damage the lung and stomach and further weaken qi. Too much salt can damage the kidneys and the blood (and raise blood pressure). Too much raw food can damage yin. And diets with too little protein can cause blood deficiency (anemia).

You can also further enhance or diminish the properties of foods by the way you prepare them. For example, raw is more cooling and cleansing, whereas steaming or blanching maintains some of that cooling but tempers it a bit.

INGREDIENTS MATTER

This is a no-brainer. What we put into our bodies makes a great deal of difference toward achieving or undermining our health goals. All produce should be the best quality possible and preferably organic and locally grown. Having a garden is great for many different reasons, from giving yourself healthy exposure to dirt-borne bacteria, to getting exercise, to helping you to develop a relationship with your food, and more.

Meats should be grass-fed and free of chemicals, hormones, and antibiotics. They should be locally raised, if possible. It's better to buy fresh produce a few times a week than to stockpile larger amounts that end up wilting in your fridge. You want your food to be fresh and full of qi.

FOOD COMBINING

Different food groups are digested differently. There are specific enzymes for breaking down carbohydrates, proteins, and vegetables that are released into our digestive tract during digestion. Carbohydrates and meats do not always digest well together, for instance. Carbohydrate and vegetable combinations or meat and vegetable combinations are most easily digested.

Consider rethinking your meals. In other words, you don't need to eat carbohydrates, meats, and vegetables in every meal. Experiment with these combinations, and try meals with just carbohydrates and vegetables or just meat and vegetables. Observe how you feel after eating this way.

SHOULD YOUR FOOD BE COOKED?

Raw vegan or vegetarian diets that feature raw foods and juices and avoid meat are popular in some circles. And these can be quite beneficial for those who have excess conditions. But for people with deficient conditions like Hashimoto's, cooking food may be more advisable because cooking will not further weaken the Earth phase.

Cooking partially breaks down foods and denatures proteins, making them easier to digest, less reactive and taking some of the onus off of the spleen and stomach. Cooking also begins the process of breaking down vegetables and softens cell walls, making their contents easier to assimilate and absorb. Steaming and blanching are great for this.

Digestive enzymes (spleen yang qi) tend to be temperature sensitive and don't work as effectively at colder temperatures. This is one of the reasons TCM practitioners do not recommend drinking ice water or other cold drinks at mealtime.

That being said, raw food is not prohibitive; it just needs to be used appropriately. Some people have hot, yang conditions that really need the cooling and cleansing action of raw food. Likewise, when the temperature outside is hot, raw, cooling foods can be a good counterpoint even for people who are qi deficient.

WHAT ABOUT VEGAN OR VEGETARIAN DIETS?

For some people, the choice to be vegan or vegetarian is a personal and/or philosophical one. And that's something that should be respected. However, I have worked with several individuals with Hashimoto's who were able to make dramatic progress when they switched to a paleo-style diet instead.

It may be that these people were just simply too deficient and had a compromised Earth phase, a weak spleen and stomach qi, and, therefore, couldn't withstand the common vegetarian sources of protein that are often high in inflammatory proteins like lectins.

Some may also have been deficient in yin and blood. In my opinion, this is a place where health considerations should trump all else because there's no point in rigidly clinging to a belief if it does not serve you.

That being said, I have devoted an entire chapter in the Appendix to a vegan and vegetarian approach, and in that section I give some advice for using herbs and supplements to overcome the potential downsides of these diets.

2. The Way You Eat

Chinese medicine believes that the *way* food is consumed matters as much as what is being eaten. The benefits of eating a well-balanced, nutritious diet can actually be undermined by certain factors.

THE JOY OF EATING

Flavors, colors, and textures, as well as presentation, can all make the meal more enjoyable. I think this is one area that can be a real challenge for people with Hashimoto's, digestive issues, and food sensitivities.

Dietary restrictions and fear of food reactions can make us not want to attend holiday or social gatherings, eat with friends and family, or even travel. And this, itself, can cause potential problems with the Earth phase.

Food obsessions and rigidity around food choices can feed Earth phase imbalances. On the other hand, pleasure in eating a delicious and beautifully presented meal settles the liver, calms the stomach, and facilitates the whole digestive process.

So, I think it's important to acknowledge these challenges and do our best to work within the restrictions we have and also to consciously work on healing the Earth phase so that we can move beyond the feelings of self-imposed exile.

Having good recipe books on hand and making delicious meals with the foods that we can eat is really helpful. I have included some great recipes in this book, and I've added many examples of foods and herbs that heal in the Food as Medicine sidebars scattered throughout the book. You can also get access to lots more by visiting our website: www.hashimotos-diet.com.

EATING TIMES

Because of the circadian influence of the Wood phase on the Earth phase and insulin, the spleen and stomach function best with a regular routine. Our body's natural internal rhythms are followed by the Earth phase in association with the liver to receive and process foods at certain times.

If meals are skipped or mealtimes are inconsistent, spleen and stomach functions can be compromised. Optimal eating times can vary, but there are some general rules that should be observed.

According to Chinese medicine, carbohydrate- and/or protein-rich meals should be consumed earlier in the day to supply the body with ample qi and yang for the day's activities. The optimal time to eat carbohydrates is between 7 A.M. and 11 A.M. Interestingly, this also corresponds to peak cortisol times during the day. In contrast, smaller meals are recommended later in the day as our body transitions for yang activity into yin quiet.

EATING TOO MUCH

In the U.S. and much of the developed world, people tend to eat too much for the sedentary lives that they lead. This is an important factor in the prevalence of obesity. Serving sizes have mushroomed, and many people can't think of a meal without including dessert.

Traditionally, the ancient masters like Li Dong-yuan warned of the consequences of overeating and the damage that it could do to the Earth phase. For many people with excess patterns (like damp heat, heat, and phlegm), reducing the amount of food eaten is often effective. For people who are deficient, small, regular, and frequent meals are more healing.

DIETING AND UNDEREATING

Skipping meals or severely limiting calories can damage spleen yang and qi. Moreover, quickly regaining weight with normal calorie intake after doing this is an indication of that damage.

Chinese medicine advises that we find balance, that we eat moderate amounts of nutritious foods to achieve or maintain our ideal weight.

TO FAST OR NOT TO FAST

Fasting can be useful for certain cases. People with excess conditions like dampness, damp heat, and phlegm, can find it beneficial. In contrast, for those with deficient conditions (and hypoglycemia), fasting is not recommended. In fact, it could make deficient patterns worse.

And just to clarify, fasting here is defined as no solid foods; vegetable juices and broths can both be consumed. And in terms of the length of the fast, it's generally not recommended to do multiple days. Rather, one day of fasting periodically can encourage the release of pathogens.

INTERMITTENT FASTING

A popular trend in alternative health circles is something called intermittent fasting (IF). If you aren't familiar with it, it's an approach to timing your meals that has grown in popularity. Recently a number of people have asked my opinion about doing it if you have Hashimoto's. Like all things Hashimoto's-related, this is a complicated question masquerading as a simple one.

HOW DOES IF WORK?

IF is not really a diet; it's more of an eating schedule where you cycle between your regular meal pattern and fasting (not eating at all).

The focus is not on *what* foods you should eat; it's more on *when* you should eat them. Let's take a look at the pros and cons of intermittent fasting with regard to Hashimoto's and hypothyroidism.

WHAT'S THE POINT OF IF?

The reason IF has become popular is that it has been shown in some research to have a number of health benefits.

Basically, there are three major mechanisms that have been identified as benefits of intermittent fasting:

1. **Increased insulin sensitivity and mitochondrial energy efficiency.** Fasting increases insulin sensitivity and improves energy production from mitochondria (your body's energy factories); this slows aging and disease, and helps with weight loss.

2. **Increased capacity to resist stress, disease, and aging.** Stress isn't always bad. Fasting causes a stress response inside cells (kind of like exercise). This causes genes to be expressed that help your body better cope with stress.

3. **Reduced oxidative stress.** Fasting helps reduce free radicals inside your cells and prevents damage from them.

THIS ALL HAPPENS IN PEOPLE WHO DON'T HAVE HASHIMOTO'S

Before you get all excited, it's important to understand that people with Hashimoto's are not normal subjects.

They often don't have typical insulin responses, their immune systems are hyper-vigilant, and they rarely have a normal capacity for handling additional stress. It's important to understand that intermittent fasting can help you under some circumstances but can actually do some harm in others.

PRESERVING YOUR CIRCADIAN RHYTHM TRUMPS EVERYTHING ELSE

The more I study physiology and look at the connections between systems of the body, the more I realize how incredibly important respecting your body's natural clock is.

This is one of those areas that can have a profound impact on your health and well-being and on the progression of your Hashimoto's.

Your body's natural clock regulates your hormones, affects your ability to digest food and absorb nutrients, affects immune function, eliminates toxins, and helps regulate your insulin and stress responses.

If this system is out of whack, it can result in you not sleeping properly, having digestive issues and constipation, craving sweets and carbs, having trouble losing weight, and having a really hard time handling stress. (Sound familiar? These are super common Hashimoto's symptoms.)

These chronic disruptions of your circadian rhythms are pretty much ignored by proponents of intermittent fasting.

Eating times are either random or just plain wrong. This can have huge consequences when you have Hashimoto's and autoimmunity. You cannot overlook the relationship between mealtimes and your body's internal clock, especially if you need to restore that rhythm.

WHEN ARE THE BEST TIMES TO EAT?

During the day, your sympathetic nervous system puts your body into an energy-burning mode, whereas at night your parasympathetic nervous system puts your body into an energy-replenishing, relax and sleep mode.

This is why Chinese medicine recommends eating larger, more carbohydrate- and protein-heavy meals early in the day, so you provide fuel for that energy burning.

This is also why normal cortisol peaks in the morning and gradually diminishes, and melatonin peaks at night. Unfortunately, this system is highly sensitive to getting disrupted, especially when you have autoimmunity and hypothyroidism and none of your body's systems are functioning properly.

So, if you eat a large meal at the wrong time of the day, you can cause insulin surges, and this can totally mess up your autonomic nervous system.

This can result in you inhibiting your sympathetic nervous system and turning on your parasympathetic nervous system, which makes you feel tired and fatigued during the day.

And instead of spending energy and burning fat, you'll store energy and gain more fat. This is a downward spiral and the ultimate no-win situation. The problem with many intermittent-fasting programs is that they don't pay any attention to this at all.

Another thing that is really important with Hashimoto's is blood sugar balance.

CLINICAL PEARL:

The impact of fasting on a preexisting blood sugar imbalance must be considered whenever you're doing any type of fasting. I cannot overstate how important this is. *If you are hypoglycemic and you fast, you can cause more harm than good because you may be pushing the insulin spikes and crashes, and this can have devastating physiological effects on thyroid autoimmunity.*

Let's break down some common IF programs. Here are the most common approaches that I could find:

ALTERNATE-DAY FASTING: Followers of this program eat on some days and don't eat at all on others. This is really hard to do and can result in a major surge in hunger (obviously).

If you do this and then binge eat, you are pretty much guaranteeing a massive insulin surge. This will cause a cortisol surge, which can result in LH and FSH suppression by the pituitary, problems with liver detoxification, under-conversion of T4 into T3, thyroid hormone receptor resistance and suppression of SIgA, and a breakdown of immune barriers.

If you are hypoglycemic, your blood sugar will crash dangerously, and you might wind up feeling major fatigue, having insomnia, getting irritable and/or depressed, slowing your metabolism so that losing weight will be harder, getting headaches, and experiencing hormonal imbalances. Not good.

There are reports from people who have tried this that they experience sleeping disorders, constipation, and persistent fatigue. In other words, this can be an absolute disaster for people with Hashimoto's.

ONCE A WEEK OR TWICE A WEEK FASTING: Fasting once or twice a week is a little easier to do than alternate-day fasting, but the problems mentioned above still persist. Coming off of it can generate massive insulin surges, and hypoglycemics will suffer in a big way.

FASTING EVERY OTHER WEEK OR EVERY MONTH: This is even worse than once or twice a week and, basically, it's an attempt to create an easy, fast program. Half measures almost never result in half successes; in my experience, they result in disappointment and failure.

SKIPPING DINNER: This totally goes against your body's natural rhythms. If you're hypoglycemic, you're just prolonging the punishment and the damage. If you are insulin resistant, you may once again wind up with an insulin surge when you have breakfast.

This can also make sleep problems worse. People who are in favor of this approach say that breakfast is more important than dinner and should not be skipped.

I agree, but most Americans have a breakfast that is heavily weighted toward sugar and carbohydrates. That is a recipe for insulin surges and a day filled with misery. However, a breakfast of healthy carbohydrates combined with some proteins and good fats can give you a nice bit of energy for the day.

SKIPPING BREAKFAST: Some people feel that this is better than skipping dinner, especially if you exercise in the morning. But this also can cause problems.

Again, if you are hypoglycemic, you will not have had anything for 6 to 9 hours (fasting is technically the gap between meals minus digestion time—so even though you don't eat for 12 to 16 hours, you're actually fasting for 6 to 9 hours).

No matter how you calculate it, that's just too long.

WHAT'S THE BEST APPROACH?

For hypoglycemics or people with Hashimoto's who have a mixed presentation of hypoglycemia and insulin resistance, I think it's far more important to work to balance blood sugar and to restore and preserve circadian rhythms.

In my experience, that will make you feel much better, help you to have enough energy to exercise and be active, and get you in a position to actually lose weight.

And your choice of foods is also very important. Eating foods that are high in nutrient density and avoiding inflammatory foods like gluten, dairy, and non-fermented soy is also much more important than fasting for reducing systemic inflammation.

IS THERE A FASTING APPROACH THAT CAN WORK FOR PEOPLE WITH HASHIMOTO'S?

It really depends on how bad things are and where you are in the progression of the disease. If you have major disruptions in your circadian rhythms and you have major imbalances in blood sugar, I would strongly discourage attempting the intermittent fasting programs.

I've found that most people who are being treated for their Hashimoto's are advanced enough where intermittent fasting just doesn't give them enough benefits for all the serious downsides that may result.

However, if you have healed to the point where you have restored your circadian rhythms and your blood sugar is well balanced, then perhaps the one-day-per-week juice and/or broth fast could be something that you attempt.

This is really the only viable option for keeping balance of your body's clock and maximizing the beneficial effects of intermittent fasting. If you exercise, you'll need to feed your muscles post-workout with a low glycemic index recovery meal to avoid the dangers of insulin surges.

And consuming proteins and carbs that are quickly assimilated before your workout can help load glycogen in your muscles, nourish the fast fibers in those muscles, and help boost max strength and performance.

With Hashimoto's, however, this is another potential land mine as the most commonly recommended form of protein is good-quality whey protein. And while whey is refined and filtered, it may contain trace amounts of casein, which can cause major immune flare-ups in some Hashimoto's folks.

Here's the main takeaway: In my opinion, intermittent fasting can have some health benefits for people whose Hashimoto's is very well managed and who have balanced blood sugar and well respected and preserved circadian rhythms.

Unfortunately, the reality is that most people with Hashimoto's have not achieved anything close to that in their lives and many have some degree of circadian disruption and some degree of blood sugar dysfunction.

For them, working to restore their body's natural clock and keeping their blood sugar stable throughout the day is much more important than jumping on the IF bandwagon.

Daily focus on those two goals (body clock maintenance and blood sugar balance) is a much better use of your money, time, and energy and will yield much better long- and short-term results like more energy, better sleep, improved digestion, and a happier mood and outlook on life.

Here's another example that shows an even more dramatic improvement from using this diet:

Stephanie is a 59-year-old female who was originally diagnosed with hyperthyroidism. She later tested positive for Hashimoto's. After years of supplementing with L-Tyrosine and others, she alternated between Synthroid and Armour.

She did not like taking synthetic drugs, and Armour felt "hot." Her thyroid testing showed low thyroid. When her doctor increased the dose of Armour, it resulted in a CVA (cerebrovascular accident, otherwise known as a stroke). Stephanie couldn't simply increase thyroid hormone because there was a risk that it would literally kill her.

Before contacting me, Stephanie went off levothyroxine completely for about nine months and was taking an OTC desiccated bovine thyroid supplement. Her doctor advised her to go on low-dose naltrexone (1.5 mg/1x day) and get back on Armour.

At that time, Stephanie's lab results revealed the following: TSH 42.666 and anti-TPO antibodies 6,688.

Her symptoms included serious fatigue, exhaustion, brain fog, inability to concentrate, and inability to cope well with work-related stress.

Stephanie decided to go on the autoimmune paleo diet. We also worked on a number of other things, like cleaning up her liver function, healing her adrenals, getting her sleeping again, and reducing her stress levels.

Her most recent test results (one year later) revealed: TSH 5.950 and anti-TPO antibodies 233.

In addition, her energy has increased dramatically, her brain fog has diminished, and she can now cope with work-related stress in a way she could not before.

Stephanie's antibody levels dropped 6,455 points!

Of course, I can't promise everyone will get these results. But for Stephanie, it was completely miraculous. There's still work to do, but she is inspired to keep doing it.

Chapter 10

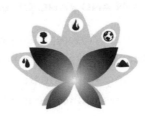

HASHIMOTO'S DIET:
Getting Started

In this chapter we will explore some of the basics of the thermal nature and flavors of foods, and we'll look at proper proportions for achieving our treatment goals.

In order to understand how to use diet effectively, we need to start thinking of food not just as something we eat for pleasure and for nutrition, but also as something that we can use to restore balance to the body.

And while herbs are medicinal, they are also foods that can be added to meals and beverages to enhance certain properties and to strengthen the effects that we are trying to achieve. The thermal nature and the flavors of foods are a way of describing how these foods affect our body.

And it's important to understand that these properties don't always correspond to how they taste and feel when we eat them. For example, beef and chicken are considered sweet, whereas lettuce and broccoli are bitter.

In Chinese medicine both herbs and foods have different temperatures, meaning they are cooling, neutral, or warming in varying degrees. In addition, both herbs and foods are thought to have an affinity for different organs and organ systems, and they have flavors that correspond to those affinities. For example, sweet foods are yang and have an affinity for the spleen.

We'll also talk about how to deal with nasty food cravings that may derail your efforts to get healthy.

FOOD TEMPERATURES: THE YIN AND YANG OF EATING

The idea that different foods have different temperatures is related to the theory of yin and yang. Cold and cooling foods tend to be more yin in nature and hot and warming foods tend to be more yang. Applying these principles to your food choices and meal preparation methods allows you to use food more strategically.

YIN OR COOLING FOODS

Foods and herbs that are cold or cooling in nature are used to slow metabolic activity and to help relieve excess heat conditions. This can be beneficial, but can also cause problems if applied inappropriately.

Heat in the body is exhibited in both healthy and unhealthy ways. Healthy forms of heat include metabolic vitality (like healthy hormone levels and natural energy) and robust movement of fluids and proteins (like healthy blood and lymph flow, which results in more rapid recovery from injury and illness).

In contrast, pathological heat is found in infections and inflammatory conditions. Examples of this include fevers induced by a viral infection and the red, painful swelling of rheumatoid arthritis.

Use cold or cooling foods to help restore balance and relieve pathological heat and inflammation. But be cautious in instances of weakness and deficiency because this can exacerbate that weakness.

For example, raw foods such as salads and juices are great if you have a robust metabolism and tend to run hot. They are also helpful if you are experiencing a lot of inflammation.

However, if you are really yang deficient and have lots of hypothyroid or adrenal fatigue types of symptoms (i.e., sensitivity to cold, fatigue, lethargy, lack of motivation, sluggish digestion, etc.), they may not be a good choice for you. Raw foods also tend to be difficult to digest, so if you already have too little stomach acid or a deficiency of digestive enzymes, they can further tax your system.

Methods of preparation and cooking like steaming, blanching, and stir-frying can preserve the cooling nature of these foods, and also make food easier to digest and assimilate.

YANG OR WARMING FOODS

Hot or warming foods and herbs stimulate yang and boost metabolic activity. They help promote circulation, can generate and boost energy, and help warm your body. They also can cause problems if used inappropriately. Warm foods are helpful for deficiency and cold conditions, but too much heat can aggravate heat conditions or excess patterns.

Use warming foods to create energy, boost fertility, help the body rebuild, and restore metabolic vitality. But be cautious when there is a lot of inflammation or heat in the body.

Methods of preparation and cooking can also increase the warm properties of food (especially when you cook for prolonged periods of time, like stewing, roasting, and deep-frying). A slow-cooked stew with tonifying herbs that boost qi and warm yang can be very beneficial for healing deficient conditions and for those who are experiencing metabolic weakness.

——Flavors Are Not Just for Savoring ——

The flavors of foods are also thought to have specific yin and yang and warming or cooling properties. Incorporating these in your meals can not only make the experience of eating more enjoyable, but can also enhance your treatment.

BITTER

Bitter flavors have a yin, cooling effect. They encourage contraction and cause the energy in the body to descend. The heart has an affinity for these and bitter flavors can be used to cleanse arteries of cholesterols and fats. Some are also helpful in reducing blood pressure (green orange peel is an herb commonly used for this purpose).

Bitter flavors are helpful with inflammation, infections, and conditions that are characterized by dampness such as Candida, parasites, excess mucus, cysts, and nodules. In small amounts they also promote digestion. This is why bitters are a popular European after-dinner drink. The bitter flavor aids digestion and promotes bile flow.

An overly bitter diet, which is pretty rare because most people can't handle lots of bitter food, can weaken the spleen, damage yin and blood, and cause dryness. Some examples of bitter foods are bitter melon (it's really bitter!), alfalfa, radish leaf, amaranth, asparagus, celery, papaya and vinegar.[1]

SWEET

Sweet flavors tend to be yang in nature and are "harmonizing," which means they assist in building synergy and they make ingredients that are less palatable taste better. In addition, they have a calming, relaxing effect (sugar releases dopamine in the brain). In moderation, they can actually benefit the digestive system and are generally helpful for healing weakness and deficiency, in general.

Sweet, warm flavors (like those found in complex carbohydrates) tend to be strengthening and help to tonify yin, qi, and blood. Sweet, cool flavors (like those found in fruit) tend to be cleansing for the body.

Too many sweet foods will cause an accumulation of dampness and phlegm, and might aggravate tissue proliferation. We see examples of this in obesity, plaques, and various types of tumors and fatty deposits.

All grains are considered sweet (rye, amaranth and quinoa are also bitter).[2] In addition, all legumes (like lentils, peas, and beans) and most meats and dairy products are also considered sweet.[3] Obviously, all fruits (including tomatoes) are sweet as well.

Some examples of sweet vegetables are sweet potato, squash, beets, cabbage, celery, and lettuce (the last three are also bitter), mushrooms, eggplant, and cucumber. Nuts and seeds like almonds, coconut, walnut, and sesame and sunflower seeds are also considered sweet. As are natural sweeteners like maple syrup, honey, molasses, barley malt, and unrefined cane sugar.

SOUR

Sour flavors are yin tend to be cooling and yin. They keep fluids in, and generally promote gathering and absorption. Sour herbs are often used in Chinese medicine to prevent the abnormal leakage of fluids like sweat, sperm, and urine, as well as to treat hemorrhaging of blood, diarrhea, and more.

Sour flavors are often derived from acids such as citric acid, tannic acid, and ascorbic acid (vitamin C). And teas like green and black teas are classified as "astringents" in Western herbalism. (Astringents cause contraction of body tissue, especially the skin.)

Because of their tendency to keep fluids in, sour flavors need to be used sparingly when dampness or chronic infections (like bacteria or Candida) are present. Too much sour food is also thought to damage the tendons in the body.

The liver has an affinity for sour flavors; they can help to break down fats and denature protein. Sour ingredients can also help digest minerals and improve absorption. This is one reason why adding a little lemon juice (which boosts stomach acid) to water can be beneficial.

Examples of sour foods include hawthorne berry, lemon, lime, rose hips, sauerkraut, and sour plum. Vinegar is also sour, as are some fruits like blackberry, raspberry, tangerine, apple, and huckleberry. Yogurt is considered sour, as well.[4]

SALTY

Salty flavors are also yin, and tend to encourage downward movement. (If you've ever had a glass of warm water mixed with Epsom salts, you know exactly what I'm talking about.)

Salt is also cooling and moistening. It is used to soften and break up lumps and nodules like enflamed lymph glands and nodules. It can be helpful for relieving swelling and pain, and is an effective home remedy for sore throats (gargle with salt water), sinus infections (use a neti pot with salt water), and periodontitis (brush your teeth with fine salt).

The kidneys have an affinity for salt. In fact, salt craving is a common symptom of adrenal issues. Salt can also benefit the spleen and pancreas.

Too much salt in the diet, however, can aggravate dampness, damage the bones and blood, and cause disruptions in fluid metabolism. As always, moderation in everything.

Foods with salty flavor include many types of seaweeds (kelp, kombu, dulse), fermented soy products, millet, miso, pickles and salt plums (umeboshi).[5]

PUNGENT

Pungent flavors are yang and often warming; they cause expansion and dispersion.

These flavors help stimulate digestion and break up mucus caused by mucus-forming foods (like dairy products), and can also promote sweating and circulation.

Diaphoretic herbs like scallion, mint, garlic, chamomile, and ginger are used to treat symptoms of the common cold, and can assist the lungs in healing.

Pungent flavors can also aid digestion, and it is a good idea to have them with grains, legumes, nuts, and seeds to reduce their mucus-forming potential.

Too many pungent foods will damage qi and yin, and can lead to dryness, especially in the lungs and stomach. People who are weak and deficient must be careful not to overdo it with these foods.

Pungent foods can be either cool or warm. Pungent cool foods include radishes, watercress, cabbage, celery, and peppermint. Pungent warming foods include foods in the onion family, chilies, ginger, pepper, cinnamon, and many other common kitchen spices.[6]

Cooking tends to diminish pungent properties, so in preparing these foods, no cooking or very light cooking (such as steaming or blanching) is recommended.

PROPORTIONS: THE SECRET SAUCE

As we have seen, no single diet is going to address all of your unique health issues. We need to first determine which type of imbalance you have, choose the right flavors and temperatures of food, and lastly, eat those particular foods in the right proportions.

The simplest way to do this is to first determine if your challenges are deficient type challenges or excess type challenges. In general, a lot of Hashimoto's and hypothyroid symptoms are deficient. Hypothyroidism can slow all the body's metabolic functions, so this is no surprise.

However, as we have seen, over time underlying deficiency can lead to other types of problems. In the third part of the book, I will focus on specific symptoms and help guide you to determine if they are of a deficient, excess, or mixed origin.

Something else to bear in mind is that following a single approach for an extended period of time can cause its own imbalances. So we must also learn how to adapt and make changes as we go.

Keeping a journal, using the A.P.A.R.T. System that I created for this purpose, and applying the appropriate flavors, temperatures, and proportions are all ingredients for success.

Let's review how to use the A.P.A.R.T. System to heal the Earth phase.

USING THE A.P.A.R.T. SYSTEM TO HEAL THE EARTH PHASE

As you may recall, the A.P.A.R.T. System is a system I devised for my first book that provides you with a simple, easy-to-follow template for solving any type of health- (or life-) related problem.

A.P.A.R.T. is an acronym, and each letter stands for a specific set of actions that you should take. Let's apply these to using diet to heal.

1. Ask and Assess

First we need to determine whether or not you are deficient or excess, and we need to determine which other underlying imbalances you have.

For example, here's a list of common qi deficiency symptoms:

- Weakness, lethargy, and/ or fatigue
- Decreased motivation
- Brain fog and dull thinking, sensing, or feeling
- Poor appetite
- Weak digestion
- Susceptibility to colds and flu
- Difficulty recovering from illness
- Pasty, pale complexion

- Poor hair growth
- Shortness of breath
- Perspire easily with exertion
- Low libido
- Muscle weakness
- Aversion to cold, chill easily
- Frequent urination
- Infertility
- Miscarriage
- Dull, brittle nails

Sound familiar? These are remarkably similar to common Hashimoto's and hypothyroid (and adrenal fatigue) symptoms. And while you may not have every single one of these symptoms, if you have the majority of them, then it's safe to say you are deficient.

2. Prioritize and Plan

This next step is pretty easy. The whole premise of this book is that Earth is the center and root cause of disease. So we know what our first priority is: heal the Earth phase. That's our focus. We have some additional issues that need addressing, and we'll get to those, but first things first.

Regarding your plan, this is also simple: use diet as a foundation. The next few chapters will show you exactly how to do that.

Furthermore, since we have established that you are deficient, then what do we about that? Build qi, tonify the Earth phase, and strengthen the spleen and stomach. In general, a diet that strengthens the spleen focuses on well-cooked, simple foods with relatively few components in each meal.

I'll get into this in more depth in upcoming chapters, but basically, the plan is to simplify and do less.

3. Act and Adapt

This next step is also pretty straightforward: Put your plan into action. Follow the dietary recommendations, keep a journal so that you have data to reflect on, and review that data once a week or so and tweak as necessary.

The rest of this book can be your lifelong guide. I have painstakingly put together my guidance on a lot of different issues, so all you need to do is look them up, do a quick evaluation, and follow the plan.

4. Reassess and Reevaluate

I hope by now you realize that you can't just put your life on autopilot, eat one diet, and sail into the sunset. Things are going to change, and unexpected things are going to happen.

There are going to be consequences to what you do—some will be "good," some may be unexpected or "bad." You need to pay attention and change course when it's warranted.

This whole process should be one in which you develop a dialogue with your body and the Earth phase in particular. And when circumstances change, you don't need to freak out. Just reevaluate, make a new plan, and execute it.

Easy peasy lemon squeazy.

5. Try and Try Again

This is a long-term journey. The good news is that once you do it for a few months, you'll get the hang of it. And more good news: you don't have to memorize everything; it's all here at your fingertips.

Just remember to play the long game. Keep doing it, stay in the game. This approach works, and it will continue to work from now until the end of your journey. Just commit to it and keep circling back periodically to reassess and tweak as necessary.

You got this!

Now, let's take some time to discuss ways to deal with—and conquer—cravings.

CRAVINGS

A common problem I have seen with many people I have worked with over the years is cravings for certain types of foods. These can be powerful and can undermine even the most disciplined and well intentioned among us.

The most common types of cravings are those for sugar, salt, and fat. The food industry understands this very well, and many types of junk food incorporate all three to take advantage of these cravings and to keep you hooked.

One of the most important things to understand about cravings is that they have a beginning, middle, and an end. And once you learn how to identify these, you can often simply ride them out and not be ruled by them.

Cravings are also often accompanied by an emotional or psychological trigger. These underlying emotional motivations may also need to be addressed. Once again, I advocate keeping a food journal and recommend logging the type of craving and the emotions and events that precede it. You may be surprised by what this reveals.

SUGAR CRAVINGS

Cravings for sugar can be linked to sugar addiction. Research has shown that sugar is a highly addictive substance on par with cocaine and heroin.[7] If you are a sugar addict, you need to come to grips with that and treat it like any other addiction. This may involve a period of abstinence and detoxification. There are many sugar detox books and programs available.

Good fats (coconut oil, avocados, olive oil, etc.) and protein are both helpful substitutions for sugar cravings. If you are trying to lose weight, substituting protein is your best bet. I recommend plant-based proteins like pea or hemp protein as well as animal proteins.

For salt cravings, first be sure that you are not deficient in minerals. Sometimes this type of craving is your body's way of telling you that you need more electrolytes. Here's my favorite electrolyte lemonade recipe. It can be used before or after workouts and can be helpful as a drink to relieve salt cravings.

FOOD AS MEDICINE:
ELECTROLYTE LEMONADE

Let's use what we just learned to analyze the nutritional benefits of this recipe. This lemonade is sour, sweet, and salty. It tonifies yin and qi. The sour flavor helps with absorption of the natural minerals from sea salt or Himalayan salt, and thereby restores electrolytes that are lost from sweating and exercise. By including the pith of the lemons, you are adding citrus pectin, which is an excellent source of fiber and can help lower cholesterol and triglycerides and aid in digestion, reducing GERD (gastroesphogeal reflux disease). It tastes good, and what's more, it's good for you!

MAKES 1 PITCHER

3 organic lemons, peeled, but leave white pith intact

3 tablespoons coconut oil, olive oil, or flax oil

1 organic pear, cored

1 tablespoon Celtic sea salt or Himalayan salt

6 cups filtered water

Blend everything well in a high-speed blender.

Drink 1 glass before your workout or when you have a salt craving.

If you have elevated blood pressure, you need to be cautious with the amount of salt you consume. However, if you have low or normal to low blood pressure, adding sea salt or Himalayan salt to your diet may actually be beneficial.

FAT CRAVINGS

Fat cravings may also be a way for your body to tell you that you need more essential fatty acids and good fats. Try incorporating them in your daily routine, and be sure to choose those that are rich in omega-3 fatty acids such as: flax seeds, walnuts, hemp seeds, sardines, salmon, mackerel, chia seeds, and cod liver oil.

Having good fats with sugar in your diet can also minimize the insulin spike caused by eating them. So it may be a good idea to have these together.

DEALING WITH CRAVINGS

As I just mentioned, cravings have a beginning, middle, and end. Mindfulness training and exercises like meditation are helpful in teaching you how to observe yourself. Sometimes it is helpful to simply acknowledge that you have the craving and not give into it. Simply observe it, and let it pass. The more you do it, the easier it becomes.

In addition, it is also a good idea to not have your house filled with junk food and other foods that feed these cravings. If you don't have them within reach, it will make it much easier to resist the temptation. Instead, keep plenty of low glycemic index fruits, healthy proteins, and good fats around the house so that you reach for them when you just have to have something.

Lastly, if you find that you just can't overcome your cravings no matter what you try, you may want to consider getting some support. Twelve-step programs like Overeaters Anonymous can be quite effective in helping you create a new way of living that will support you in overcoming your food addictions.

DIETARY PROPORTIONS FOR SPECIFIC CONDITIONS

As you may recall, Li Dong-yuan identified several different mechanisms for yin fire or systemic inflammation.

These can be divided into deficiency and excess conditions:

DEFICIENCY CONDITIONS:

- Qi deficiency (particularly of the spleen and stomach)
- Yang deficiency (this is similar, but a bit more severe)
- Blood deficiency (similar to various anemias)
- Yin deficiency (like blood deficiency but another level of seriousness)

EXCESS CONDITIONS:

- Liver qi stagnation (this often has an emotional component)
- Dampness and phlegm (heat can also be part of the equation)
- Heat, Fire (this is the ministerial fire raging)

Next, let's take a look at specific dietary strategies for each of these conditions.

Chapter 11

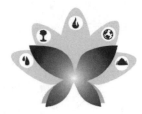

DEFICIENCY DIETS

Deficient conditions are those characterized by metabolic weakness and serious depletion. Hypothyroidism, adrenal fatigue and exhaustion, malnourishment, and weakness caused by trauma or surgery are all examples.

In some cases of deficiency, there are specific systems of the body or organs that are depleted and need to be strengthened. These different types of deficiency include blood deficiency (found in various anemias), yin deficiency (found in some organs such as the kidneys, liver, or heart), yang deficiency (very similar to endocrine disorders like hypothyroidism and adrenal fatigue), and qi deficiency (basic metabolic weakness).

Dietary treatment of deficiency conditions involves nutrient-dense foods and supplements that tonify or strengthen and help the systems and organs of the body to rebuild. A basic qi deficient type of diet can also be considered a kind of base diet that should be returned to after treating excess conditions or infections.

Here are some examples of specific diets for different types of deficiency conditions:

1. QI DEFICIENCY DIET

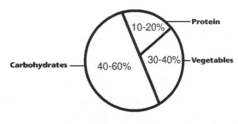

Symptoms of qi deficiency:

- Weakness, lethargy, and/ or fatigue
- Decreased motivation
- Brain fog and dull thinking, sensing, or feeling
- Poor appetite
- Weak digestion
- Susceptibility to colds and flu
- Difficulty recovering from illness
- Pasty, pale complexion
- Poor hair growth
- Shortness of breath
- Perspire easily with exertion
- Low libido
- Muscle weakness
- Aversion to cold, chill easily
- Frequent urination
- Infertility
- Miscarriage
- Dull, brittle nails

A diet that focuses on strengthening the spleen qi consists of food that is well cooked, and meals that don't have lots and lots of ingredients. This is an excellent place for us to apply the principle of "Where can I do less?"

The basis of the diet is complex carbohydrates with some high-quality protein and lightly cooked vegetables. Fresh, locally grown seasonal food is preferable, as it is most nutritious and will have the most vibrant qi.

Food should be lightly cooked, steaming or blanching vegetables just enough to preserve a light crunch. Green leafy and delicate vegetables like broccoli and beans are best cooked this way. Heavier root vegetables and grains should be cooked longer and slowly so that they retain their qi, shape, and texture.

Easily digested carbohydrates such as sweet potatoes and starchy root vegetables should make up a larger proportion of the diet (40 to 60 percent). The remainder should be cooked greens and red and yellow vegetables (30 to 40 percent), and a small proportion of high-quality animal protein (10 to 20 percent).

This is especially important in the early stages, as you are trying to rebuild. As the spleen becomes stronger, you can shift and add other elements. Salads may be added as the spleen gets stronger or if you are in a hot climate. Be aware that this larger proportion of carbohydrates can lead to dampness, and adjustments may have to be made accordingly (see the diet for dampness in Chapter 12).

Soups and stews are particularly beneficial for qi deficient conditions. You can also batch cook on weekends to last the entire week. Taking time to cook your own foods can be healing and therapeutic on its own.

From the Earth phase system, we learned about the important relationship between the Earth and Metal phase. Targeting nutrition for the spleen will also benefit the lungs and visa versa. In addition, qi gong exercises are excellent and vitally important for helping to build qi. (See my first book, *How to Heal Hashimoto's: An Integrative Road Map to Remission*, for some powerful, restorative qi gong exercises.)

Here are a few specific qi deficiency dietary recommendations:

All food cooked and warm, slow cooking of soups, stews, and broths are particularly effective. Chew your food thoroughly. Simple combinations of a few ingredients; more frequent, smaller meals, and regular mealtimes.

High proportion of complex carbohydrates and vegetables, less meat (nutrient-dense meats like organ meat are recommended).

Avoid excessive fluids during meals, overeating, missing meals, and multitasking during meals.

Beneficial foods for qi deficiency:

Neutral or sweet warm flavored foods include: artichoke, mustard greens, celery root, string beans, beets, okra, coconut milk, papaya, apricots, figs, grapes, currants, coconut, stewed fruit, chicken, beef, lamb, liver, kidney, mackerel, tuna, anchovy

Pungent flavors in small amounts help assist the natural function of dispersing and descending: onion, leek, black pepper, fresh ginger, garlic, cinnamon, and non-seed kitchen spices (sage, savory, thyme, tarragon, etc.)

Complex sweet flavors (use with caution in damp and damp heat conditions): molasses, dates, coconut sugar, cherry and date

Helpful herbs: astragalus, codonopsis, red and black dates

Optional (only to be eaten once you have eliminated and reintroduced them successfully): light grains (especially rice and rice porridge), oats, chickpeas, black beans, walnuts

Optional spices (same as above: eliminate first, then reintroduce and eat in moderation if tolerated): nutmeg, fennel

Avoid: Excessive amounts of raw vegetables. Salads, raw fruits (especially citrus), amaranth, wheat, tomato, spinach, Swiss chard, tofu, millet, seaweed, and salt. In addition, large meals and too many sweet foods and concentrated sweeteners, vitamin C (over 1–2 grams per day), beer, ice cream, and dairy products (except a little grass-fed butter), sugar, chocolate, nuts and seeds (except walnuts), nut butters.[1]

Here's a great recipe for healing the spleen:

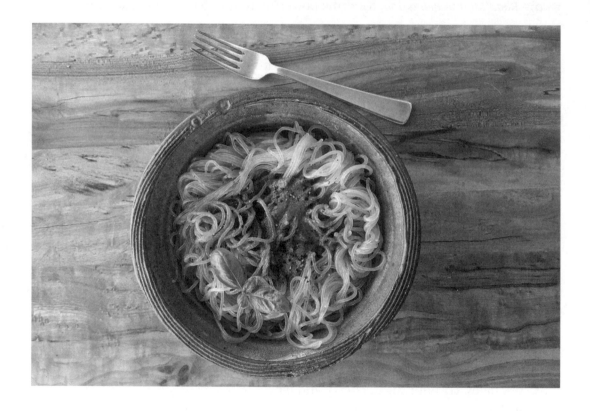

SWEET POTATO PASTA WITH PESTO

GLUTEN-FREE / DAIRY-FREE / VEGAN / SPLEEN QI TONIC / BLOOD AND YIN TONIC • *SERVES 4–6*

This is a nourishing, delicious, light, and filling dish sure to make your belly do a happy dance. Prepare pesto ahead of time, if desired. Sweet potato pasta can be found at Asian markets or ordered online.

Sweet Potato—neutral; sweet; spleen, kidney, lung, qi, blood, and yin tonic; astringes essence

Basil—warm; pungent; spleen, stomach, lung, large intestine, qi, and yang tonic; promotes circulation and harmonizes stomach

Coconut—warm; sweet; spleen, kidney tonic; produces fluids (hydrates); promotes urination; kills intestinal worms

Garlic—warm; pungent; spleen, stomach, lung, qi, and yang tonic; promotes circulation; warms middle *jiao* (tummy); kills intestinal worms

SWEET POTATO PASTA

12-ounce package of sweet potato noodles

½ teaspoon salt

1 teaspoon olive oil

PESTO

2 cups basil, packed

½ cup coconut cream

¼ cup olive oil

¼ cup fresh or frozen coconut meat (optional, for thicker pesto)

2 garlic cloves

½ lemon, juiced

½ teaspoon salt, plus more for topping

½ teaspoon pepper for topping

Bring a large pot of water to boil. Add pasta, a pinch of salt, and olive oil, and cook according to instructions (usually 7 to 8 minutes).

While pasta is cooking, place all pesto ingredients into a high-speed blender. Blend until well incorporated, about 10 to 15 seconds, or until creamy consistency is reached.

Strain pasta and cut with scissors for easier consumption. Divide pasta among bowls, and top with desired amount of pesto and salt and pepper to taste. Yum!

Store in refrigerator 3 to 4 days, or freeze in small containers for later use.

2. YANG DEFICIENCY DIET

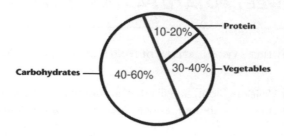

Symptoms of yang deficiency (especially spleen and kidney yang):

- Slow digestion and sluggish intestines

- Weak gums and loose teeth

- Dryness of skin and mouth

- Sore or swollen joints or muscles, especially in the face, hands, and feet

- Heaviness of head or limbs

- Weakness or soreness of the low back and knees

- Feet, legs, and back tire easily

- Diarrhea or dry small stools with bloating

- Frequent, scanty, or difficult urination

- Low libido

- Aversion to cold, easily chilled in back, legs, and arms

- Constipation and water retention following eating

- Crave salt or sweet foods

- Nervous and easily distracted

- Apathetic and insecure

(As you can see, these symptoms are very familiar for those of us with Hashimoto's and hypothyroidism. Hashimoto's is often textbook yang deficiency.)

A yang deficient diet is very similar to a qi deficient diet. Boosting spleen qi and promoting healthy spleen function is the goal. The major difference is the addition of more warming foods for the spleen and kidney and the strict avoidance of any raw food, including salads.

The proportions are the same as for the qi deficiency diet.

GENERAL RECOMMENDATIONS:

Spleen yang deficiency foods are the same as spleen qi deficiency foods plus more warming ingredients like parsnip, sweet potato, onion, leek, stocks and broths (bone broth), lamb, beef, chicken, stewed fruit, and chestnut.

In addition, more warming spices like ginger, clove, cinnamon, rosemary, and turmeric are recommended.

For kidney yang deficiency, add clove, fenugreek, black pepper, cinnamon bark, dry ginger (more warming than fresh ginger), rosemary, chestnut, lamb, salmon, onion, leek, chives, mussels, lamb and/or beef kidney.

Avoid for both: raw fruits and vegetables, sprouts and salads, tomato, spinach, tofu, soybean, millet, kelp, excessive salt and sweet foods, dairy products, nuts and seeds, soymilk, and refrigerated or iced drinks.[2]

3. BLOOD DEFICIENCY DIET

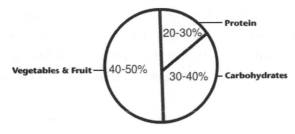

Symptoms of Blood Deficiency:

- Restless fatigue
- Irritability
- Insomnia
- Itching skin or scalp
- Dryness without thirst
- Weak or blurred vision
- Hair loss or thinning hair
- Dizziness
- Dry or hard stool
- Premature aging of skin
- Dry skin, eyes, and hair
- Anemia

- Numbness of hands and feet
- Muscle cramps
- Scanty or irregular menstruation
- Bruise easily
- Slow healing
- Palpitations
- Postpartum
- weakness or anemia
- Pale lips or eyelids
- Weak, thin, or irregular pulse
- Pale complexion

Building blood requires nutrients that build and nourish blood. In addition, the body must be able to properly absorb these nutrients. As we have learned, good absorption is dependent on a healthy Earth phase and strong spleen and stomach qi.

Building blood also requires different proportions in the diet. More animal protein is recommended. It is possible to build blood on a vegan or vegetarian diet, but the progress is slower and additional herbs are often necessary.

There's an old saying in Chinese medicine that "it takes 40 parts of qi to make 1 part of blood" and the most potent blood builders are animal proteins, particularly those rich in blood like liver.[3]

Soups and broth made with organic chicken and/or beef bones, which contain marrow, are recommended. When animal protein is not an option, choose herbs like dang gui, rehmannia, peony, foti root, ligusticum, and stinging nettle.

Green leafy vegetables, which are chlorophyll-rich, are especially helpful. Chlorophyll and hemoglobin have similar molecular structure (called a porphyrin ring). These foods are helpful in generating hemoglobin production.[4]

Food additives and excessive amounts of sugar and salt can also adversely affect blood quality. Organic and grass-fed meat is preferred. When liver is used, it should always be grass-fed. Organic is preferable, but the liver is a filter and it does not store toxins, so if you can't get organic and grass-fed, fresh is a good substitute.

GENERAL RECOMMENDATIONS:

Same basic approach as for spleen qi and yang deficiency. Why? The spleen produces blood, plus iron-rich foods, folic acid, and B12. In vegetarian or vegan diets, you may need to supplement with sublingual B12.

Beneficial foods include high-quality animal protein (especially chicken meat and soup, beef, and pork liver), abalone, rabbit, salmon, oyster, mussels, shark, eel, trout, anchovy, chicken liver, sardines, herring, stocks and bone broths, and bone marrow. Vegetables and fruits include: green leafy vegetables, wheatgrass, spinach, carrots, black dates, dark grapes, blackberries, raspberries, huckleberries, currants, cherries, black fungus, chlorella, beets, parsley, molasses, miso, tempeh, seaweed, spirulina, lychee, and coconut.

CLINICAL PEARL:

The best chicken for building blood is black-skinned chicken. I once went to Chinatown with Dr. Li, my professor from acupuncture school. She took me to a butcher who had these chickens, and I made a soup from it with Chinese dates, dang gui, and goji berries. It was very potent and delicious.

For liver blood deficiency, add blood-tonifying herbs like dang gui, he shou wu, rehmannia, chuang xiong, bai shao, and stingling nettle.

Avoid the same foods as for spleen qi deficiency, plus bitter, sour, salty, and pungent or hot foods, as well as refined sugars, chemical additives, and food coloring.[5]

4. YIN DEFICIENCY DIET:

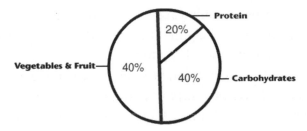

Symptoms of Yin Deficiency:

- Insomnia or restless sleep followed by deep sleep and difficulty waking up in the morning

- Nervousness and mood swings

- Fatigue

- Lumbar weakness

- Problems with temperature regulation (sensitive to heat and cold)

- Easily excited but also easily spent

- Strength tapped by hyperactivity

- Depressed or blue after prolonged mental or physical exertion

- Up for sex, but unable to sustain it

- Lack of muscle tone and joint mobility

- Anxiety

- Tension and weakness of the muscles along the spine

- Nausea, diarrhea, frequent urination (may be accompanied by anxiety)

- Craves the buzz of salty, spicy food and stimulants (nicotine, coffee, etc.)

For yin deficiency, nutrient-dense foods are critically important. If you're yin deficient, it's really important to make this diet a priority before things progress any further because this is potentially a serious condition that may affect important organs like the kidneys, liver, and brain.

Nutrient-dense foods maintain and improve tissue integrity and engender fluids and moisture. The basic diet for yin deficiency is similar to the blood deficiency diet: more animal protein, a diverse mix of green leafy and root vegetables, and more nourishing carbohydrates.

In addition, moistening and lubricating foods are helpful. For example, seed and vegetable oils and herbs can be helpful. Fish oils, oils from algae, omega-3 oils, EPA and DHA, and lecithin are all nourishing to yin.

Nutrient-rich meats like organ meat, bone broth, and bone marrow and herbs like cordyceps and American ginseng tonify yin. And just as everything else, yin must be derived from food by spleen and stomach qi. It always comes back to the center.

Regarding proportions, it's about equal carbohydrates and green leafy and watery vegetables and fruit. This is also an instance where dairy might be appropriate. Small amounts of good-quality organic cheese, cow's or goat's milk, yogurt, and grass-fed butter are all beneficial if there is dryness. (With the caveat of what we learned about the potential reactions from dairy products: If you are unsure, you can do food sensitivity testing for dairy proteins. Or simply eliminate dairy 100 percent for 30 to 60 days and reintroduce.)

GENERAL RECOMMENDATIONS:

The general focus is toward nutrient density. High-quality protein and organ meat. Use plenty of water in cooking and feature soups and stews.

Beneficial foods include: pork, chicken, duck, pigeon, bone broth and bone marrow, herring, abalone, mackerel, sardines, oyster, mussels, clams, cuttlefish, squid, octopus, kelp, spirulina, zucchini, squash, sweet potato, melon, string bean, beets, mushrooms, banana, mulberry, coconut and coconut oil, olive oil, avocado oil, and duck fat.

Helpful herbs: lily bulb, glehnia root, raw rehmannia, American ginseng.

Optional after reintroduction: adzuki beans, mung beans, tofu, tempeh, mushrooms, yogurt and cheese in small amounts.

There are also certain foods that nourish the yin of specific organs, for example:

Kidney yin: pork, beef, pork kidney, duck, string beans, blackberries, blueberries, seaweed, black fungus, tofu.

Lung yin: pears, peaches, apples, bananas, figs, strawberries, string beans, seaweed, kelp, white and black fungus (wood ears), spirulina, pork, oysters.

Stomach yin: slippery elm, white wood ear mushrooms, asparagus (root), sweet potato, oranges.

Avoid: drying, warming, bitter, and pungent foods. For example, chilies, curry, cinnamon, garlic, ginger, onion, shallots, scallion, leeks, basil, clove, wasabi, coffee, lamb, prawns, veal, game birds, vinegar, citrus, coffee, tea, alcohol, corticosteroids, recreational drugs (cocaine, amphetamines, ecstasy, etc., all damage yin), NSAIDs.[6]

Summary of Deficient Diets

Deficient Diets	Protein	Vegetables and Fruit	Complex Carbohydrates	Keys to Success
Qi Deficient	10-20%	30-40%	40-60%	Less animal protein, more complex carbs and vegetables
Yang Deficient	10-20%	30-40%	40-60%	Same as qi deficient diet with more warming foods and spices
Blood Deficient	20-30%	40-50%	30-40%	More protein and vegetables (esp. green leafy), less complex carbs
Yin Deficient	20%	40%	40%	Nutrient dense foods are critically important, i.e., organ meat

Chapter 12

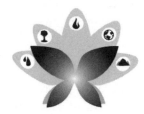

EXCESS DIETS

In contrast to deficiency diets, diets for excess conditions involve detoxification strategies and using herbs and foods that are often pungent and/or bitter and cooling to clear heat and disperse stagnation. Excess conditions can also be emotional in nature, or they can involve infections and accumulations like nodules, tumors, and growths.

These types of diets are not recommended for the long term and should just be used temporarily. Staying on an excess diet for too long can damage the flora in the gut and/or damage internal organs like the spleen, stomach, and intestines.

After treating the excess condition, it is recommended to return to a qi deficient diet to help the body recover from the harsh effects of this type of intervention.

LIVER QI STAGNATION DIET

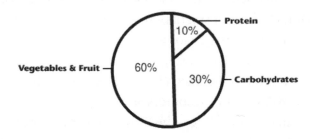

Symptoms of Liver Qi Stagnation:

- Easily irritated
- Distention or fullness in the chest or abdomen
- Mild nausea
- Muscle tension or cramps, especially in the neck, shoulders, and upper right quadrant of the abdomen
- Vague or migratory pains
- Dry eyes
- Weak or blurry vision
- Coarse, brittle, or dry nails
- Easy chilling of arms, legs, feet, and hands
- Difficult elimination; dry, tense colon
- Constipation with gas
- Irregular or scanty menstruation
- Genital hypersensitivity
- Craving sour, spicy, or fatty foods
- High-pitched ringing in the ears
- PMS
- Aggravation of symptoms by wind, heat, or drafts
- Distention or fullness of the abdomen

One of the mechanisms of yin fire, according to Li Dong-yuan is liver qi stagnation. As we have seen, the liver is the general and responsible for everything that moves through the digestive tract. Detoxification or "biotransformation" as it is known in the medical literature, is the liver's domain.

The liver processes and metabolizes, well, pretty much everything. In today's world the liver is under constant assault by artificial ingredients, chemicals, endocrine disruptors, pesticides, herbicides, and pharmaceutical drugs. It is often overburdened.

All of this adds up to liver qi stagnation. It's like you're a general and you're loyal to an insane emperor who courts chaos and craziness for sport. Every day, he stresses you out of your mind. That's liver qi stagnation.

As we have seen, although the spleen is the yin organ of digestion, the liver orchestrates timing and distribution of resources so the spleen can function efficiently. If you eat too much and/or overindulge, the liver suffers the consequences.

With liver qi stagnation, astringing or congesting foods should be avoided. Foods with a mild, pungent, dispersing nature should be featured. Here's another great opportunity to do less. Eat less, and take your last meal in the late afternoon or early evening.

Drama or conflict at mealtime is especially damaging to the liver. Meals should be calm, cool, and collected.

In contrast to the deficient diets we have seen, this diet should feature springtime foods, vegetables, fruit, and complex carbohydrates. Plenty of green, yellow, and red colors, spiced with pungent, dispersing spices. For example: curries, turmeric, ginger, and other spices used in Asian-style cuisine that move qi.

GENERAL RECOMMENDATIONS:

Eat less; main meals should be eaten earlier in the day. Focus on light and mildly spicy meals; stir-fry, poach, and steam foods. Vegetables should be featured; carbohydrates and proteins should be sparse (less than half the diet).

No eating when upset or stressed. No skipping meals, eating in a hurry, overeating, or working during mealtime.

Beneficial foods include: mild dispersing, pungent flavors. Onions, garlic, watercress, mustard greens, peas, turnips, rhubarb, endive, turmeric, basil, mint, peppermint, horseradish, pepper, dill, ginger. Be cautious with warming foods with liver qi stagnation and heat.

Small amounts of sour flavors are also beneficial. Citrus, vinegar, pickles, sour cherry, plums, blackberries, strawberries. Plenty of fresh vegetables, spouted grains, asparagus, taro root, cabbage, turnip, cauliflower, broccoli, brussels sprouts, beets, Jerusalem artichokes, olive oil, molasses, and small amounts of high-quality animal protein.[1]

Helpful herbs: fresh ginger, tangerine peel, radish seed, platycodon root.

Avoid: foods high in saturated fats and oils, cheese, eggs, ice cream, red meats, nuts, pizza, hot chips. Eliminate foods that obstruct or damage the liver. Avoid processed food, junk food, and fast food. No drugs or intoxicants. No artificial or synthetic substances, preservatives, food coloring, or drugs (unless appropriate and prescribed by your doctor). Avoid acetaminophen.[2]

DAMPNESS AND PHLEGM DIET

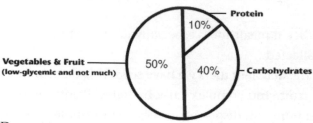

Symptoms of Dampness:

- Swollen or heavy head, limbs, or abdomen

- Tender muscles and joints

- Thick or sticky saliva or phlegm

- Sticky perspiration

- Lumps, nodules, or cysts

- Sticky or slimy stool

- Generalized water retention

- Edema of hands and feet

- Myxedema or swelling in the face (above or below the eyes and along the jawline)

- Nausea

- Sinus congestion

Symptoms of Phlegm (same as above, plus):

- Dizziness or fullness of the head with mucous congestion or nausea

- Thick, sticky discharge from the skin, mucous membranes, ears, eyes, nose, throat, vagina, urethra, or anus

- Soft, mobile lumps and enlarged lymph nodes

- Feel worse in a humid environment

- Feel worse after eating dairy products, sugar, eggs, or greasy or fatty foods

- Nausea and difficulty breathing with a feeling of fullness in the upper abdomen or chest

When treating dampness and phlegm, a couple of things need to be considered. First, a diet that supports proper function of the spleen and stomach must be strictly followed. Second, foods that cause dampness and phlegm must be avoided 100 percent. These include dairy products, processed carbohydrates, sweets, and rich, fatty foods. In addition, raw, cold, and mucus-forming foods (like ice cream) should be avoided.

Bitter, pungent, or drying foods are also helpful and can be added to food in order to further prevent dampness from forming. For example, eat meats with horseradish or bitter vegetables like turnips and pumpkins. Use pungent toppings like pesto (made without parmesan cheese), garlic, and onions.

A little wine with meat (not recommended if you are deficient), green tea with fried foods, and bitters to aid digestion are all also helpful. Most meals can be modified to reduce dampness pretty easily.

Regarding proportions, carbohydrates should be used moderately, because they are often sweet and can cause or exacerbate dampness. These should be about 30 to 40 percent of the diet. The best sources of these are some of the more drying grains like rice, millet, and gluten-free oats. (These should not be avoided during the elimination stage of the diet, which we will explore in the next chapter.)

Vegetables should be the dominant food group (40 to 50 percent of the diet) and a mixture of bitter, pungent, and sweet varieties are best. The remainder should be a relatively small amount of high-quality animal protein (around 10 percent). Nuts and seeds should be avoided altogether.

GENERAL RECOMMENDATIONS:

The general principles of the qi deficiency diet that strengthens the spleen and stomach apply here as well. Emphasize bitter and pungent flavors. All food should be cooked and warm, use oils and fats sparingly, and eat less at each sitting. No late night meals; avoid deep-fried food and junk food.

Beneficial foods include: artichoke, kohlrabi, lettuce, parsley, corn silk, endive, seaweed, celery, pumpkin, onion, shallot, scallion, garlic, plantain, musk melon, turnip, watercress, radish, extra-virgin olive oil, horseradish, quail, clam, lean grass-fed meat, white and black pepper, clove, dill, cilantro, oregano, thyme, basil, fresh ginger.

Enjoy in moderation: sweet potato, yam, green tea.

Helpful herbs: skin of fresh ginger, corn silk, poria mushroom, tangerine peel.

For dampness in the lungs and sinuses: radish, daikon, turnip, onion, shallot, scallion, garlic, horseradish, mustard greens, ginger, watercress, fenugreek.

For dampness in the urinary bladder: ginger, fenugreek, peas, adzuki beans (may be added during reintroduction phase).

Avoid: ice cream and dairy products, sugar and concentrated sweeteners, fatty meats (especially pork and duck), eggs, tofu, tempeh, butter, margarine, chocolate, nuts and seeds (especially peanuts), raw and dried fruit (especially banana and tropical fruits), salt, vinegar, beer.[3]

Here's a great damp heat–clearing recipe:

CUCUMBER AND RADISH SALAD

GLUTEN FREE / VEGAN / DAMP-HEAT CLEARING / SPLEEN QI TONIC • SERVES 4–6

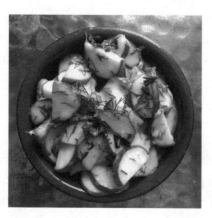

This dish is incredibly refreshing and cleansing. Traditional spring and summer salad enjoyed very much in Eastern Europe. Radish is excellent for digestion; and cucumber is loved all around for its cooling, hydrating, and detoxifying properties.

Radish—cool; pungent and sweet; stomach and lung tonic; qi and blood tonic; detoxifies; transforms phlegm and dampness; clears heat; descends rebellious stomach qi

Cucumber—cool; sweet; spleen, stomach, large intestine tonic; detoxifies; promotes urination (diuretic); hydrates and quenches thirst

Dill—warm; pungent; spleen, kidney, and qi tonic; promotes circulation

10 radishes, sliced thinly in half-moons

2 Persian cucumbers, sliced to about ½ an inch in half-moons

4 tablespoons dill, chopped

½ teaspoon salt

Combine all ingredients in a medium mixing bowl. Serve on its own, or as a side with chicken, pasta, or eggs. Let your taste buds do the deciding . . .

HEAT AND/OR FIRE DIET

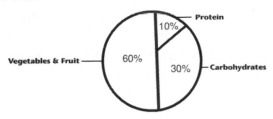

For heat and fire patterns, cooling, bitter, and pungent foods are helpful. Generally, eat less and drink plenty of fluids. And a larger quantity of raw foods (fruits and vegetables) is also helpful. This diet is also appropriate for people who tend to run hot constitutionally.

Generally, there are two types of heat patterns: acute and chronic. Acute heat patterns are often associated with a short-term attack of a cold or flu. Symptoms may involve fever, perspiration, and thirst. Lots of fluids are recommended, plenty of fruit and vegetable juices, herbal teas, and light broths and soups.

Warm or room temperature liquids are better because cold and iced beverages are thought to damage the spleen. Since these are temporary conditions, an acute heat clearing diet is only recommended for a few days, enough time to allow the condition to resolve.

In Chinese medicine, these types of conditions are known as wind heat disorders, and inducing sweating is often part of the treatment strategy. Therefore, pungent, cool, and dispersing foods and herbs are often used. For example, mint, pear, radish, watercress, and cabbage. These are often prepared in teas or soups. Warming foods like lamb, beef, chicken, shellfish, and warming spices should, obviously, be avoided in heat-related conditions.

Chronic heat patterns can be those caused by underlying deficiency. Li Dong-yuan's yin fire is a perfect example of a chronic deficiency-based heat disorder. For these types of issues, light cooking, such as steaming and stir-frying is recommended, whereas roasting, frying, and deep-frying are contraindicated.

Also, it's important to avoid heat-stimulating foods and drinks like alcohol, coffee, red meats, creamy sauces, and deep-fried foods. Foods that promote urination as a means of clearing heat from the body are recommended like celery, cucumbers, and beets.

There are other chronic heat patterns as well, such as stomach heat, and because damp and phlegm conditions can cause stagnation, damp heat, and phlegm heat.

Stomach heat is similar to acid reflux or GERD, and whole raw foods may be too fibrous and irritating to already raw tissue. In some cases, it's better to have soups and well-cooked soft or mashed foods to reduce irritation.

GENERAL RECOMMENDATIONS:

Heat/fire conditions: plenty of liquids; shorter cooking times; steam, blanch, or stir-fry. Feature soups with lots liquid and vegetables. Raw food (especially salads and sprouts). Avoid deep-frying, BBQs, roasting; avoid overeating.

Beneficial foods include: asparagus, cucumber, celery, Swiss chard, spinach, lettuce, radish, Chinese cabbage, broccoli and cauliflower, zucchini, apples, pears, watermelon, mung beans and alfalfa sprouts, kelp, spirulina, crab.

For stomach heat: foods that help form mucus to cool, moisten, and line the stomach like aloe vera juice and chia seeds. Banana, avocado, cucumber, spinach, lettuce, arugula, watercress, cabbage (cooked and juiced), tofu, yogurt made from coconut.

For liver heat: peppermint, mung beans, sprouts, celery, radish, daikon, kelp, lettuce, dandelion, cucumber, watercress, tofu.

For heat in the lungs: lemon, pear, Chinese pear, peach, radish, watercress, carrot, pumpkin, cabbage, cauliflower, Swiss chard, white fungus (wood ear).

Avoid: chilies, ginger, black pepper, garlic, horseradish, coffee, cinnamon, chocolate, heated vegetable oils, lamb, beef, chicken, alcohol, vinegar, shrimp, eggs, excessive salt, peanuts.

Damp heat conditions: eat less; light, simple foods; raw foods and juices; plenty of lightly cooked green vegetables.

Beneficial foods for damp heat include: celery, chestnuts, carrot, Swiss chard, winter squash, seaweed, spinach, Chinese cabbage, eggplant, broccoli, peas, cauliflower, plantain, asparagus, lemon, cranberry, huckleberries, watercress, arugula, lettuce, kudzu, radish, daikon, adzuki beans, mung beans, alfalfa sprouts, tofu, tempeh, green tea, water. Root vegetables and olive oil in moderation.

For liver/gallbladder damp heat: mung beans, alfalfa sprouts, celery, lettuce, leafy greens, shitake mushrooms, peppermint and chrysanthemum teas, dandelion leaf tea.

For urinary bladder damp heat: mung beans, alfalfa sprouts, celery, asparagus, diluted lemon juice, cranberry juice, blueberries, watermelon, dandelion tea, green tea.

Avoid: alcohol, greasy or fried foods, deep-fried food, fatty meats, eggs, sugar, concentrated sweeteners, chocolate, junk food, nuts and seeds, chilies, cinnamon, ginger, black pepper, garlic, horseradish, coffee, vinegar, shrimp, excessive salt.

Phlegm heat conditions: eat less and choose light, simple foods; raw foods and juices; plenty of lightly cooked green vegetables.

Beneficial foods include: bamboo shoots, watercress, radish, kelp and seaweed, turnip, persimmon, shitake mushrooms.

Avoid: all dairy products, ice cream, sugar, fatty meats, eggs, tofu, tempeh, soy sauce, nuts and seeds, bananas, avocado, pineapple, salt, coffee, alcohol, chocolate.[4]

SUMMARY OF LIVER QI STAGNATION AND DAMP HEAT DIETS

Excess Diets	Protein	Vegetables and Fruit	Complex Carbohydrates	Keys to Success
Liver Qi Stagnation	10%	60%	30%	Feature vegetables, especially leafy green
Dampness & Phlegm	10%	50%	40%	Avoid foods that cause dampness 100%: dairy, refined carbohydrates, sweets and fatty foods
Heat and/or Fire	10%	60%	30%	Feature bitter, cool, and pungent foods

Okay, so we've covered all the major permutations, and you might be saying to yourself, *Yikes! How am I going to do this?*

Don't freak out! After doing all this research and finding these various diets, I realized that this was way too complicated. So I came up with a way to simplify it all for you. Remember at the beginning of the book when I introduced the Tummy Triangle Treatment?

In case you forgot, here's a quick review of the main treatment strategies that it recommends:

- **For spleen and stomach qi deficiency:** Strengthen the spleen and stomach qi with sweet and warm foods and herbs (see the qi deficiency diet on page 151). Also include foods and herbs that are nutrient dense and tonifying. This is your default diet that can be followed long term. In addition, it should be where you return after you experiment with the diets below.

- **For liver qi stagnation:** Regulate the liver, invigorate qi, and stimulate the correct functioning of the qi mechanism with pungent, dispersing foods and herbs (see the liver qi stagnation diet on page 163). You also have to address the underlying emotional component. Ignore this, and you put up a major roadblock to healing. This diet should be used only short term, but it can be utilized regularly as a modification of the deficiency diet we just discussed.

- **For damp heat:** Clear damp heat and/or heat with bitter, cooling foods and herbs (see the dampness and damp heat diet on page 166). Many of these herbs and foods have broad-spectrum antiviral and antibacterial properties. This diet should be used only short term. Bitter, cooling foods can damage the microbiome if overused (in a similar manner to antibiotics, though these foods are much gentler).

The Tummy Triangle Treatment reminds you to think about all three of these sides of the triangle and to focus on each when appropriate. In the upcoming chapters after the discussion on the Elimination and Reintroduction/Rebuilding phases of the diet, I will guide you on how to use these with various different conditions and pathologies.

But before we get there, here's another great recipe that tonifies spleen and stomach qi and relieves liver qi stagnation. It ties these ideas together nicely and gives you a simple application of two sides of the Tummy Triangle.

ROASTED ROOT VEGGIES WITH WATERCRESS

MAKES 4–6 SERVINGS

This is one of my favorite recipes. This dish makes you feel good, like a big bear hug. It's delicious eaten alone or as a side dish. It nourishes and at the same time moves liver qi.

This dish is quite tonifying to the stomach, spleen, and lungs. It is beneficial for qi- and yin-deficient conditions. Here are the benefits of each ingredient:

Carrots—neutral; sweet; spleen, stomach, and lung tonic; dries damp and phlegm

Parsnips—sweet; nourishes spleen, lung, and yin

Sweet Potatoes—neutral; sweet; spleen, stomach, kidney, lung, qi, blood, and yin tonic; astringes essence

Beets—sweet; nourishes blood and yin

Watercress—cool; sweet and pungent; stomach and lung tonic; moves liver qi; clears heat and yang; hydrates (quenches thirst); promotes urination

Vinegar—warm; sour and bitter; moves liver and stomach qi; detoxifies; promotes circulation

4 small carrots, cut in ¼-inch slices	4 tablespoons olive oil
3 small parsnips, cut in ¼-inch slices	½ teaspoon salt
3 medium sweet potatoes, cut in ½-inch half-moons	½ teaspoon pepper
	¼ cup watercress, cut roughly
4 small beets, cut in ¼-inch half-moons	1 tablespoon balsamic vinegar

Preheat the oven to 400 degrees F.

Place the carrots, parsnips, sweet potatoes, and beets in a large baking dish; coat evenly with olive oil and salt and pepper.

Bake for about 50 minutes to 1 hour, stirring halfway through to ensure even browning. Once veggies are tender and lightly caramelized, they are done.

Remove veggies from the oven, and toss with watercress and balsamic vinegar. Serve on its own or with salad, potatoes, or a protein dish.

Chapter 13

THE HASHIMOTO'S HEALING DIET: A 90-DAY PLAN

Step One: The Elimination Phase (30 to 60 Days)

By now you should have a pretty good overview of your challenges as well as a number of different approaches to take to resolve them. You might be wondering, *What the heck do I do now?*

Of course, that depends on where you are. If you are just beginning, then this chapter will give you a good sense of how to get started. You should also still use the A.P.A.R.T. System to determine which proportions of the Tummy Triangle Treatment you need to use.

Basically, it comes down to this: Are you deficient or excess or something in between?

In my clinical experience, I have found that most people who have been recently diagnosed or are new to this approach tend to be on the deficient side. Especially if you have a lot of food sensitivities or digestive issues, that's a red flag for weakness in the Earth phase.

And remember, you're conducting an experiment with your body. A journal is an indispensible part of that. You can learn a great deal in this process if you keep notes as you try different things.

So far, I have focused on diets that include animal protein. If you are interested in a vegan or vegetarian approach, the basics still apply (that is, knowing if you are deficient or excess), but we'll need to adapt a few things and add some herbs and supplements to help you. I have devoted an entire chapter to using a vegan and/or vegetarian approach (see Appendix 2).

If you are familiar with the Autoimmune Paleo diet and have been following it for some time, then you're in a slightly different place. But the same basic strategies apply. Figure out if you are deficient or excess (and in what way) and focus on that.

The next chapter has important information that I think has been missing from the autoimmune paleo approach up until now. And that is that we must make changes when they are warranted. We can't just stay on the elimination diet forever, as there are some potentially serious health consequences to doing so.

The rest of this chapter is devoted to those who are just beginning and those who may wish to re-devote themselves to starting over. As you may recall, our theme is *Where can I do less?* And this first stage of the diet is an in-depth plan for doing so.

THE AUTOIMMUNE PALEO APPROACH

An added level of complication we have not yet addressed is that some foods can cause an immune response. The ancient Chinese had little knowledge of this because they had little knowledge of molecular biology.

They made some remarkable observations about physiology, but they did not fully understand the role of food in autoimmune disease in the way that we understand it today. The reality is many doctors are absolutely clueless about this as well.

If you have an autoimmune disease, you can't afford to be clueless. You have to understand a few basic things. First, gluten is an important trigger in all autoimmune diseases. And celiac disease is not a food sensitivity; it is an autoimmune disease.

Also, leaky gut, or intestinal permeability, the breakdown of the intestinal lining, is a necessary ingredient for autoimmune disease to develop. And there are a whole bunch of foods that resemble gluten and may cause an immune response in the digestive tract.

These include grains, legumes, and dairy products and they all can contribute to leaky gut and damage the Earth phase. In addition, nuts, seeds, and nightshades are also foods that can increase damage to the gut. They do this by either directly damaging the intestinal lining or by encouraging the growth of bacteria and yeast in the small intestine that can cause damage.

Some of the most destructive substances are lectins, digestive enzyme inhibitors, saponins, and phytic acid. Sarah Ballantyne, author of *The Paleo Approach*, has done extensive research on this topic.[1] I recommend that you read her book if you want an in-depth explanation for why these substances are so destructive to the gut and the Earth phase.

I am more concerned with providing you with dietary strategies that will get you better. So, this first phase is really designed to simplify your diet and remove all of these destructive substances so that you can heal.

BUT DOES THIS DIET *WORK*?

Who cares about anything else frankly?

Fortunately, there was recently a medical study on this approach in 2017 at Scripps Research Institute in San Diego, California. They studied the impact of the autoimmune diet on inflammatory bowel disease.

Here are the results of the study: Patients reported improved symptoms and quality of life within three weeks on the diet. By week six, disease activity markers improved significantly, and by week 11, improvements were seen on endoscopy.[2]

So not only did the people in the study feel significantly better, but there was also actual evidence of tissue repair and healing in the intestines.

Another study, published in the journal *Inflammatory Bowel Disease* in November 2017, also found that "[d]ietary elimination can improve symptoms and endoscopic inflammation in patients with IBD."[3]

Yes, it works. But I hear the skeptics among you saying, "Yeah, but . . . that's *not* Hashimoto's."

True, but we know that all autoimmune diseases have some level of damage to the gut and gut lining. And people with inflammatory bowel disease have significant damage in some cases. If it works for them, chances are good it will work for us.

And in point of fact, a 2016 study published by Italian researchers in the journal *Drug Design, Development, and Therapy* focused specifically on overweight patients with autoimmune thyroiditis (Hashimoto's) and used a diet almost identical to this.[4]

The results were pretty impressive. The dieters not only lost body weight, but also fat mass and thyroid antibodies in Hashimoto's thyroiditis.

This diet really works! And when you add the wisdom of what we have learned from Chinese medicine to tweak the diet and take it to the next level, you can really get some great results.

WHY DOES THIS DIET WORK?

The foods and substances that are avoided in the autoimmune paleo diet are the things that contribute to the destruction of the gut. By removing them from the diet, the gut lining is able to heal. And when we add insights into healing the internal organs as well, we can create significant healing momentum via the five phase relationships.

This almost always results in a lessening of symptoms and healing for those with autoimmune disease. And when we add the wisdom of Chinese medicine on top of this . . . good golly, Miss Molly! We've got a good thing going.

Let's check out the foods to avoid and the foods to include, and then review how to layer the Chinese medicine over top of that.

FOODS TO AVOID[5]

NUTS	SEEDS	EGGS	MISCELLANEOUS
almond	anise	chicken eggs	alcohol
brazil nut	canola	duck eggs	alternative sweeteners
cashew	caraway	goose eggs	emulsifiers
coffee	chia	quail eggs	food additives
cacao	coriander		food coloring
hazelnut	cumin		food chemicals
pecan	fennel seed		NSAIDs (aspirin, ibuprofen, naproxen)
pine nut	flax		Stevia
pistachio	mustard		thickeners
macadamia	nutmeg		
walnut	poppy		
	pumpkin		
	sesame		
	sunflower		
	hemp		

GRAINS	BEANS & LEGUMES	DAIRY	NIGHTSHADES
amaranth	adzuki beans	butter	ashwaganda
barley	black beans	buttermilk	cayenne pepper
buckwheat	black-eyed peas	casein	chili pepper
bulgur	broad beans	cheese	chipotle pepper
corn	fava beans	condensed milk	eggplant
faro	garbanzo beans	cottage cheese	goji berry
kamut	kidney beans	cream	ground cherry
millet	lentils	cream cheese	habanero pepper
oats	lima beans	evaporated milk	jalapeño pepper
quinoa	mung beans	frozen yogurt	paprika
rice	navy beans	goat cheese	poblano pepper
rye	pea	goat milk	potato
sorghum	peanuts	ice cream	sweet pepper
spelt	red beans	ghee	tobacco
teff	soy beans	kefir	tomatillo
tricate	white beans	milk	tomato
wheat		powdered milk	wolfberry
wild rice		sheep milk	
		sour cream	
		whey	
		whey protein	
		whipped cream	
		yogurt	

FOODS TO INCLUDE[6] AND THEIR TEMPERATURE ACCORDING TO CHINESE MEDICINE

I have also organized foods and spices in terms of their temperature so that you can continue to think of foods in this manner. This becomes important as we determine which proportions of the Tummy Triangle Treatment we will need to apply.

TEMPERATURE	VEGETABLES	FRUIT	ROOTS	MEAT
WARM	artichoke fennel kale leek mustard greens	blackberry date pineapple raspberry strawberry	onion parsnip shallot	anchovy beef bison bone broth bone marrow buffalo chicken eel lamb mussels salmon trout turkey
NEUTRAL	butternut squash celery chard collard greens mushroom	apricot blueberry clementine coconut fig grape guava kiwi marionberry papaya pomegranate plum	beet carrot celeriac jicama sweet potato taro yam yucca	duck goose herring kidney liver oysters sardines tongue venison

TEMPERATURE	VEGETABLES	FRUIT	ROOTS	MEAT
COOL	arugula asparagus bok choy broccoli brussels sprouts cabbage cauliflower cucumber lettuce pumpkin rhubarb spinach summer squash watercress winter squash zucchini	apple avocado banana cantaloupe grapefruit huckleberry honeydew melon lemon lime mango mulberry orange peach pear persimmon tangerine watermelon	daikon radish radish rutabaga turnip	abalone clams crab octopus pork rabbit squid

OTHER INGREDIENTS TO INCLUDE

TEMPERATURE	FATS	HERBS & SPICES	FERMENTED FOODS	MISCELLANEOUS
WARM	animal fat duck fat	basil chives cinnamon cloves garlic ginger oregano parsley rosemary shallots turmeric	fermented vegetables kombucha sauerkraut	apple cider vinegar coconut aminos coconut vinegar dates molasses ume plum vinegar
NEUTRAL	avocado oil coconut oil olive oil palm oil	lemongrass		coconut flakes coconut flour honey maple syrup olives
COOL		chamomile chrysanthemum cilantro dill lavender marjoram mint peppermint sage salt spearmint tarragon tea thyme	water kefir	

In general, you can organize foods as a whole on a spectrum of cool to warm.[7]

MOST COOL				NEUTRAL					MOST WARM
raw soft, juicy fruits		vegetables		grains		nuts	eggs seafood		milk cheese poultry meat
	drier, harder fruits		roots, tubers		seeds		legume		

You can also organize the manner in which you prepare food in similar terms.[8]

MOST COOL			NEUTRAL					MOST WARM
fresh raw	dried raw	steamed blanched poached	sautéed	baked	fried	dry-roasted		broiled BBQ-grilled

What this means is that you can amplify or minimize the temperature of a given food depending on the way that you prepare it.

For example, steaming or blanching will not change the nature of a food very much, but grilling will make it warmer. So if you grill vegetables, they become much warmer and lose some of their cooling properties. Whereas, poaching fish doesn't change it very much.

So, it's important to think about both the food and the manner in which you prepare it because this can give you even better results. If you are suffering from a cold condition, for instance, grilling your meat might be helpful. However, if you have damp heat, then grilling your meat is not appropriate for you.

In contrast, if you are deficient and need to tonify and warm spleen yang, then broiling or grilling could be really beneficial.

PROPORTIONS AND TEMPERATURES FOR SPECIFIC CONDITIONS

As we have already seen, the proportions and the temperature of the foods you eat can make a difference in the success of your approach. Even within the restrictions of the AIP diet, there is a whole other level of using diet that can help you get better results.

Use the A.P.A.R.T. System to determine what your overall diet should be, and be sure to keep a food journal during this process.

1. Ask and Assess

First we have to figure out whether you are predominantly deficient or excess.

Really this comes down to: Are you are exhausted, wiped out, and suffering from the common hypothyroid symptoms? And is it impacting you to such an extent that this fatigue is preventing you from doing other things? If so, this is clearly a priority and you should experiment with using the qi deficiency diet approach (see page 151).

Or are you working on clearing up some type of infection or other pathology? Or dealing with emotional issues? In these cases, you would use an excess type of dietary strategy.

Remember, the excess types of diets are temporary, so after you experiment with them for a period of time, you will return to the spleen and stomach deficiency diet. For all intents and purposes, this is your foundation and default diet.

For most, it's a good idea to begin with the basic autoimmune paleo diet for 30 to 60 days. Then the next step is to incorporate the rest of the Tummy Triangle Treatment principles (determine if the problem is primarily excess or deficient and tweak accordingly).

So, let's say (for the sake of understanding how we apply this) that you have determined that your symptoms are primarily deficient right now. Here's a quick review of deficient symptoms:

- Weakness, lethargy, and/ or fatigue
- Decreased motivation
- Brain fog and dull thinking, sensing, or feeling
- Poor appetite
- Weak digestion
- Susceptibility to colds and flu
- Difficulty recovering from illness

- Pasty, pale complexion
- Poor hair growth
- Shortness of breath
- Perspire easily with exertion
- Low libido
- Muscle weakness

- Aversion to cold, chill easily
- Frequent urination
- Infertility
- Miscarriage
- Dull, brittle nails

Write down all of your current symptoms in your journal (we will want to refer to them later to see which have improved and which remain). Now, use the proportions of the deficient diet to plan your dietary approach. Here's a quick review of proportions and temperatures for deficient types:

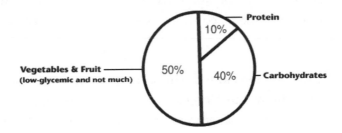

2. Prioritize and Plan

Since treating the deficiency is your priority, use the proportions of foods mentioned above and review the deficient diet (page 151). Plan your meals and decide how long you want to stay on this diet. Thirty to 60 days is a good amount of time to implement this plan and then reevaluate.

3. Act and Adapt

Follow the spleen and stomach deficiency diet for a minimum of 30 days.

4. Reassess and Reevaluate

What problem are you trying to solve? For example, if you are trying to improve antibody levels, retest after 30 to 60 days. In the study we looked at earlier, they retested after 21 days and got good results. In addition, reassess and go back over the original symptoms that you wrote in your journal and compare. Have you improved?

If yes, stay on the AIP diet for an additional 30 days and try to get more improvement. Or if you are satisfied with the results, begin to reintroduce foods.

If you have not improved, try to determine why. Review your journal and the original responses you had. Take the quiz that I created for you again. Compare your results. If your answers gave you mixed results, you may want to try treating the excess symptoms instead. If you are still confused, consult a physician who is familiar with using diet to treat Hashimoto's.

Follow your new plan for 30 days. Then, reassess and reevaluate again.

5. Try and Try Again

Keep going. After 60 to 90 days on the AIP diet, it is time to start the reintroduction process and work on improving oral tolerance.

If you have been on the AIP diet for longer than three months and are hesitant or unsure about reintroducing foods, consult a practitioner who has experience in this area for guidance.

In the next chapter, we'll explore the importance of oral tolerance and learn how to reintroduce foods while working on oral tolerance at the same time. This may be a departure from the conventional autoimmune paleo protocol that instructs you to reintroduce after a period of time (usually 30 to 60 days).

I think it's vital to reintroduce and to induce some immune responses during this period. This means that reacting to foods, especially mildly, is not necessarily bad or something to be avoided. The reason for this is simple: we want to challenge the immune system to create some level of tolerance, and sometimes we have to cause an immune response to do this.

In my opinion, a more nuanced approach should be considered. We shouldn't think in all-or-nothing terms. You may find that you can have some foods once or twice a week, or other foods once or twice a month. You may be able to tolerate a food if you don't eat it every day and give your body sufficient time to adapt to it.

HASHIMOMENT: To Heal, Go All In

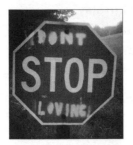

In my experience, it's really hard to heal your Hashimoto's by making a few minor changes. Remember, half measures don't lead to half results—they often lead to failure and disappointment.

This condition impacts your body in so many ways that making a half-hearted attempt at change is like blowing against a hurricane.

True healing involves transformation. True transformation often involves making real and significant changes in your life.

There's no pill or supplement that does that.

If you want real, lasting results and recovery of your energy, your mental faculties, and your old body, you need to adopt a Hashimoto's lifestyle.

WHAT IS A "HASHIMOTO'S LIFESTYLE"?

- **Follow the Right Diet:** It involves following a diet that doesn't push the progression of the autoimmune disease and make the attacks on your own tissue worse.

  For some, this can be accomplished by going gluten-, dairy-, and soy-free. For others, you may need to cut out more. The more your immune system reacts, then, usually, the more you are going to have to eliminate (at least for a period of time).

- **Manage Your Stress and Blood Sugar:** You need to make sure that you have good blood sugar balance and that you don't take on more stress than you can handle. If you are leading a very stressful life and are so busy that you don't have time for breakfast or other meals, you may be setting yourself up for failure.

- **Understand the Web:** As we have seen, Hashimoto's is much more than a thyroid problem. It's much more than an autoimmune problem. It is a complex multisystem disorder that involves every major system of the body.

You must evaluate all of them, and fix what is broken down.

- **Commit to This New Lifestyle 100 Percent:** Last, you need to stay committed. In the same way an alcoholic can't have "just one drink," you can't make these changes, feel some improvement, and then fall back to your old ways.

The stakes are too high. Slipping back can reignite the inflammation that is at the root of autoimmune disease.

Sometimes with a vengeance.

CASE STUDY: The Rewards of Going All In

Here's an e-mail I recently received from a patient whose life was transformed by committing to changing her diet. Of course, I can't promise you the exact same result, but it's a great example of what is possible when you stick with the plan.

"After using the autoimmune paleo diet approach, my doctor has lowered my Synthroid dosage a couple times now, and I've lost 30 pounds. I have a lot more energy and am enjoying the diet. There are quite a few other improvements in my overall health as well.

"My husband and I have included dairy in our list of foods to avoid, and that seems to be working well for us, although my husband is now wondering what to do with all the Lactaid pills he had stocked up on for the next year or so. I'm sure they'll get used whenever we dine out, since you can never be sure if the kitchen understands what is meant by lactose intolerance.

"I look forward to reaching my target weight, which is still 10 pounds away, but this diet doesn't really feel like a diet at all. Very easy to follow. I'm not sure what my doctor thinks about my progress, since she was not very optimistic when I first mentioned the program to her. All in all, I'd call the whole experience a success so far."

Marie G.
Vancouver

Chapter 14

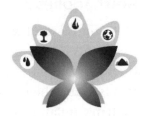

THE HASHIMOTO'S HEALING DIET: A 90-DAY PLAN

Step Two: The Reintroduction Phase and Restoring Oral Tolerance (30 to 60 Days)

As many of you know, for the last several years I have focused solely on treating people with Hashimoto's.

This has given me a tremendous opportunity to explore this health issue in considerable depth. I have had the honor and the privilege to work with over 2,000 people with Hashimoto's, and I've been privy to some cutting-edge research from colleagues like Dr. Datis Kharrazian.

Dr. Kharrazian first introduced me to the concept of oral tolerance, and I've spent a good deal of time combing through the medical literature and learning about its significance with regard to Hashimoto's and reactions to foods.

In doing so, I recently had an epiphany that has changed my way of thinking about how we can use diet to heal this disease.

In this chapter, I'm going to go deep into what I have learned about oral tolerance and its relationship to Hashimoto's, autoimmunity, and the autoimmune paleo diet.

YOU CAN'T GET BETTER WITHOUT ADDRESSING DIET

One thing I have learned (and it's the reason I wrote this book) is that diet is the foundation of success. And the reason this is true, in my opinion, is that, as we have seen, the digestive tract is ground zero for autoimmunity.

So much of the immune system is found there, and a breakdown of the gut and the intestinal lining leads to the systemic inflammation that is at the root of diseases like Hashimoto's.

GROUND ZERO FOR AUTOIMMUNITY IS THE INTESTINES

As I've mentioned, according to Alessio Fasano, M.D., an expert on the origins of autoimmunity, the cause of this disease is found in the breakdown of the tight junctions in the intestines. This is the pathway to autoimmune disease.

But this is by no means the whole story. Yes, the breakdown of the intestinal lining is a causative factor for the development of autoimmune disease; however, it's just the gateway.

This is kind of like getting a view of the door, but there is an entire landscape of immune reactions that go on beyond that door.

And what lies beyond the doorway is what we are going to explore now.

AUTOIMMUNITY IS THE LOSS OF SELF-TOLERANCE

What's happing with autoimmunity? Our immune system has lost the ability to differentiate between our own cells and foreign invaders, such as bacteria, viruses, and other proteins (like proteins found in foods).

And this confusion leads to our immune system attacking our body's own proteins. This is caused by our immune system losing the ability to have tolerance to our own tissue (made of these proteins).

The entire digestive tract is made up of multiple little ecosystems, and these ecosystems are always battling with this problem of tolerance.

Because the gut is, essentially, one long open tube; and lots of pathogens in the form of bacteria, viruses, fungi, and parasites pass through along with proteins that we need to ingest and get nourishment from.

An important part of the ebb and flow of tolerance is something called "oral tolerance."

ORAL TOLERANCE: THE HOLY GRAIL OF AUTOIMMUNITY?

Oral tolerance is defined as your immune system NOT REACTING locally and systemically to antigens such as food proteins. In other words, oral tolerance is when you eat a certain protein and you become tolerant to that protein.

We can think about this in terms of our own evolution. If you are eating something (a protein) all the time, it would be a really good thing for you to develop a tolerance to it and not attack it.

If we're only eating certain kinds of foods, we'd be more likely to survive if we could build tolerance to them.

Proteins are the things we are most often exposed to. (They're the building blocks of life, after all.)

And it turns out that tolerance to ingested proteins is also really important for the barrier function of the intestines (i.e., to prevent leaky gut).

As we saw, when this tolerance breaks down, chronic diseases follow, such as celiac disease, Crohn's, and ulcerative colitis (these all occur locally in the intestines), as well as other systemic autoimmune diseases like multiple sclerosis and even Hashimoto's.

In other words, oral tolerance is a kind of dimmer switch: it turns down the attack, both in the intestines and in the rest of the body.

When you have oral tolerance, your immune system doesn't attack as aggressively.

When you lose oral tolerance, you wind up with things like celiac disease (which is an autoimmune disease, not just a food intolerance).

HOW DOES ORAL TOLERANCE WORK?

We don't fully understand this yet.

However, what we do know is that oral tolerance works by deactivating T and B cells that target our tissues—either by clearing them out and getting rid of them or by making them not respond to proteins anymore with something know as "anergy."

Anergy is the lack of a normal immune response to a particular antigen or allergen.

Oral tolerance also works by Tregs directly suppressing these cells.

Tregs is another name for regulatory T cells (also called suppressor T cells). They are T cells that modulate the immune system, maintain tolerance to self-antigens, and discourage the development of autoimmune disease.

CAN WE IMPROVE ORAL TOLERANCE?

Of course, with autoimmune disease this may be a really important thing to achieve, if possible.

The question is this: If you can establish or reestablish or at the very least improve oral tolerance, can you remove or at least diminish the autoimmune attack?

Some researchers believe the answer is yes.[1] There is some evidence that this may be an achievable goal.

IF SO, SHOULD WE TRY TO IMPROVE TOLERANCE FOR EVERYTHING?

That's a very, very important question, because this is potentially a dangerous game. By no means is this an easy, risk-free process.

For example, should we attempt to establish oral tolerance to things like gluten and dairy (dietary proteins with tremendous destructive potential)?

In my opinion, the answer is a resounding NO!

They have been implicated in the destruction of brain tissue such as cerebellar tissue and myelin. (I'd like to keep my brain for as long as possible, wouldn't you?)

So what does that leave us with? A lot, actually.

But before we attempt to answer that, another thing research has shown us is that simply establishing tolerance alone is not enough.

We must also do other things like reduce inflammation and strengthen the regulatory part of the immune system. We must work to calm and/or eliminate stress, restore integrity and balance to the ecosystem of the gut, etc., to achieve the best results.

So first, let's look at the big picture.

What are the steps to first calming the immune system and then trying to improve oral tolerance?

STEPS FOR CALMING THE IMMUNE SYSTEM AND IMPROVING ORAL TOLERANCE

First off, if you're looking for a quick and easy solution, you might be disappointed. This isn't quick, and it isn't easy. This is a long-term project that may take several months, and it may be riddled with unexpected outcomes (welcome to the immune system).

That being said, it can also yield profoundly positive long-term results.

STEP 1: THE ELIMINATION DIET

We looked at this in the previous chapter. If you are just starting out, this is the place to begin. As we have seen, this is a very effective approach for reducing systemic inflammation and for calming the immune system. In addition, in many cases with Hashimoto's this will yield improvements in virtually all important thyroid markers, including antibody levels, TSH, etc.

And it often results in a (sometimes dramatic) improvement in weight loss, brain fog, mood, and energy. While my patients are on this diet, I also assess all the other systems of the body, and when it is called for we work on healing the gut (almost always called for), detoxifying the liver, healing the adrenals, and reducing inflammation in the brain.

That is what the approaches I have given you allow you to do on your own. The diet for liver qi stagnation will detoxify the liver; the spleen and stomach qi deficiency diet will help heal the adrenals; and all variations will reduce inflammation.

CLINICAL PEARL:

One thing I have observed with some people who tried the autoimmune paleo diet (myself included) is that it can actually increase your sensitivity to foods that you are already sensitive to.

A food that you had a reaction to in the past (like gluten) will often cause a much more severe reaction once you have eliminated it for a prolonged period of time.

And in some cases, the elimination can increase sensitivity to foods across the board. (And I have observed it seems to increase and not decrease with time. Meaning the longer some people are on the strict elimination diet, the more sensitive they become.) One theory is that what may be happening here is that the elimination of these antigens can lead to a decrease in oral tolerance. This makes logical sense because oral tolerance requires exposure to the antigens (in this case, dietary proteins).

ELIMINATING FOODS CAN INCREASE FOOD REACTIONS

There is some evidence of this in the medical literature. In fact, some researchers claim that the elimination diet is a potential cause of anaphylaxis, a severe and life-threatening allergic reaction.[2]

And many researchers and health professionals are now questioning the wisdom of not exposing children to things like peanuts in early childhood because the lack of exposure can lead to a massive immune response when they do get exposed. (In fact, they are now recommending the opposite, exposing infants to food allergens like peanuts.)

The question is, why?

If this is the case, what is the mechanism that could lead to the decline of oral tolerance?

I think the simple answer is that elimination of multiple immune-stimulating antigens can alter the entire landscape of your immune system. It has a major impact. It also alters your microbiome and eliminating diversity of foods can lead to declines in certain species of bacteria in the gut.

And while some of this is really good and, arguably, absolutely necessary (especially in circumstances like autoimmunity), it may have some unintended consequences.

This is also a great illustration of the complexity of the immune system. It has multiple parts that move in multiple directions, all the time. Overly simplistic linear thinking doesn't work when trying to understand and balance the immune system.

INCREASING FOOD SENSITIVITY IS VERY STRESSFUL

Another important observation about this process is that having to worry about food all the time and having an increasingly smaller and more restricted diet is very stressful. It makes it difficult (if not impossible) to go out with friends and relatives. It can create anxiety over what to eat, and it can make you feel further alienated and frustrated.

And of course stress is a really big deal for people suffering from autoimmune diseases like Hashimoto's. The body is already under a great deal of physiological stress—to add more daily stresses regarding what to eat and where to find the right food can be really counterproductive to the process of healing.

If we can tweak this process to make it less stressful, then that is a very valuable innovation.

STEP 2: REINTRODUCTION PHASE

Once you have done the elimination phase of the autoimmune paleo diet (usually for 30 to 60 days), the next phase involves reintroducing foods, one food at a time to see if you react to them.

In some cases, people react to an awful lot of stuff, precisely because they have been so good at eliminating these foods and have accomplished some really good things with regard to calming their immune systems.

My understanding of this phase of the autoimmune paleo approach is that this is essentially a test to see what you can and cannot eat after the elimination period.

Proponents of the autoimmune paleo approach rationalize this increase in sensitivity by saying, essentially, this is part of the healing process. They assert that once you heal your gut, you'll have fewer sensitivities. But this isn't always true, as there are people who have spent several years healing their gut and still find that they are sensitive to a number of foods.

Obviously, everyone is a little different, and some people do better than others. Some find they can reintroduce all sorts of things, while others can reintroduce just a few, and still others find their diets becoming more and more restrictive.

If you're one of the latter, this process can be really demoralizing because here you have worked your butt off to be super compliant and follow the plan, yet the end result is that your diet consists of even fewer foods.

It's the living embodiment of the expression "No good deed goes unpunished."

REESTABLISHMENT OF ORAL TOLERANCE PHASE

What I have come to see is that instead of just eliminating and seeing what happens during reintroduction, what we have is an amazing opportunity. And that is to work to reestablish or improve oral tolerance and create a much more hospitable immune environment.

How do we do that? Great question!

I'm not going to pretend to have all the answers on this, but here is what the research suggests. In autoimmune disease research, the goal with oral tolerance seems to be to suppress the Th1/Th17 response (for most autoimmune diseases).

There are two ways that researchers have tried to do this.[3] The first is by giving a high dose of an offending protein once. (This, obviously, is the heavy-handed approach.) From an immune system standpoint, when it works this can result in *anergy*, complete shutdown of both Th1 and Th2 responses.

The problem is that it doesn't always work, and obviously with autoimmunity the risk here is that you can cause massive flare-ups and discomfort.

The second approach is to take the protein at a lower dosage multiple times, which has been found to increase Tregs. The multiple-dose approach is gentler and, from an immune standpoint, a lot better suited for autoimmune disease in my opinion.

BUT YOU CAN'T JUST REINTRODUCE FOODS

Here's the real difference in approach. You shouldn't think of this phase as simply a testing phase. It could and should be much more than that.

However, before we get all excited, understand that we are wading into uncharted waters and if we are going to challenge the immune system, there are bound to be some reactions.

And not all of them will be good. In addition, maybe it's time to view reactions differently. Maybe not every reaction is just simply "bad."

Maybe total elimination of reactions isn't totally "good." It may be a bit more nuanced than that. Maybe some level of reaction is actually a good thing because it means that we're testing and provoking the immune system.

That being said, there are two things to consider during this process:

1. What helps induce or improve oral tolerance? (This would include supplements, lifestyle changes, etc.)

2. Which proteins do you want to create oral tolerance for? (This would include the approach to diet and reactions.)

Both are important because we want to do everything we can to make this a successful experiment.

Actually, there is also a third thing to consider, which is asking what we can do to minimize the discomfort and immune system flare-ups during this process.

I don't know about you, but I prefer to suffer as little as possible.

FOOD AS MEDICINE: **ALOE**

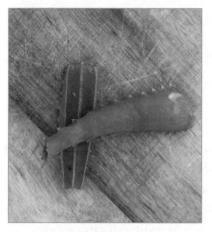

The use of aloe medicinally dates back thousands of years, and it originally comes from African medicine traditions. It was used by ancient Greek doctors and adopted by Chinese medical practitioners during the 6th century when trade routes were established with East Africa.

It was brought to the Americas during the slave trade, was used by Spanish missionaries, and adopted by Native Americans. It is truly an international herb!

Aloe is an effective remedy for a number of things and is quite gentle and minimally toxic, which means it's also great for children. It is considered bitter and cold, and is effective in heat-related conditions.

Traditionally, aloe is used as a mild laxative to treat stubborn, chronic constipation. It also kills intestinal parasites and was traditionally used to treat roundworms and ringworm in infants and children.

Aloe is also effective in promoting tissue repair and in reducing inflammation and tumors. It can be taken internally to heal leaky gut and used topically to relieve itching due to parasites or for chronic skin disorders that don't respond to other treatment.

Pharmacologically, aloe has been found to have antibiotic properties and to inhibit pathogenic fungi and dermatophytes. Alcohol extracts of aloe have also been shown to inhibit the growth of some cancer cells.

There are two forms used traditionally: aloe resin and aloe gel. The resin is used as a laxative, to reduce inflammation, and to kill parasites; the gel is used to repair damaged tissue, reduce inflammation, and treat skin conditions. This world traveler is truly an amazing herb!

Next we're going to look at how we can both introduce foods and work to increase oral tolerance at the same time. I have also created an Appendix that goes into more depth on what supplements and lifestyle changes can further enhance and improve oral tolerance (see Appendix 3). But, for now, let's focus on some general strategies that can be quite helpful.

DIETARY STRATEGIES FOR IMPROVING ORAL TOLERANCE

Understand the Importance of Proper Protein Digestion: Something that is vitally important to understand is that only dietary proteins large enough to elicit immune responses are potential food allergens.

So proper levels of stomach acid, pepsin, and digestive enzymes are critical for creating oral tolerance. This matters a great deal with Hashimoto's and hypothyroidism because low stomach acid and gastrin secretion can be caused by hypothyroidism.

In addition, make sure that you have adequate HCL, and consider experimenting with digestive enzymes that break down proteins when reintroducing foods.

A word of caution here: if you have leaky gut and exposed proteins, excessive use of digestive enzymes that degrade proteins may further damage the lining of your gut.

As always, balance is key and properly evaluating and treating leaky gut should happen prior to this stage.

The elimination phase of the diet is the ideal time to work on healing the intestinal lining. This should be done first, prior to moving to this stage of reintroduction and improvement of oral tolerance.

And that brings up an important question. How do you know if you have healed your gut enough to go to the next phase?

What if you haven't achieved 100 percent reduction in symptoms? What if you still feel like you have more work to do?

I think that the answer is a long-term project, and we need to modulate our approach periodically depending on what it is we want to accomplish.

Also, I think there is certainly some evidence that the longer people stay on strict elimination and do not attempt any reintroduction, then the more possibility there is of continued reactions, as strict elimination in some people seems to lead to more sensitivity.

So I'd say that it's a judgment call. If you haven't had any improvements, I think there's an argument for continuing with the elimination diet and applying the Tummy Triangle Treatment strategies (treating the underlying deficient or excess conditions).

If there are some improvements, but it's still not 100 percent, then you're going to have to decide when you're ready. *But at the end of the day, you have to do this at some point and the longer you put it off, the more degraded your oral tolerance can become.*

Maintain a Low-Protein Diet: This is a surprising finding because the autoimmune paleo diet features animal protein as vital to healing. And it is—there's no disputing that animal protein is nutrient rich and instrumental in healing the gut.

However, it may not be as helpful for developing oral tolerance. And one of the negatives of the AIP diet is that it can exacerbate histamine intolerance. Many of the featured foods of the AIP diet (like bone broth) are quite high in histamine. Once again, balance is critically important.

Perhaps after the period of gut healing and emphasizing meat and animal proteins, it makes sense to let the pendulum swing back and to focus on more vegetables and more variety.

Research suggests a diet of approximately 20 percent protein, but I'd push it down to 10 percent in some cases. Use the Tummy Triangle Treatment, shift, and adapt.

Think of the balance of yin and yang. You can't stay in either one for too long without consequences and an inevitable return to the other.

Incorporate Resistant Starches: Resistant starches are really interesting and have become popular in Paleo circles. They are called resistant starches because they resist digestion. There are two types of resistant starches (RS) that are helpful in the process of restoring oral tolerance.

The first is starch that isn't well digested or absorbed in the small intestines. It has a large amount of amylose, and is found in potatoes, unripe bananas, and plantains. Since it doesn't get broken down and absorbed in the small intestine, this starch continues on to the large intestine where bacteria ferment it. This fermentation process results in the formation of short-chain fatty acids (SCFAs).

SCFAs (like butyrate, propionate, and acetate) are very beneficial for the health and well-being of the large intestine. They help stimulate blood flow, help regulate and release mucus, help prevent colitis, and are important for recovery from injury or surgery. They also are generally helpful with mineral and nutrient absorption and they bind to toxins to help get them out of the body.[4]

The second kind of resistant starch is also known as "retrograde" because this starch forms after it is cooked and then cooled. It can be reheated at low temperatures to maintain its benefits as a resistant starch. Some common examples of this resistant starch are various kinds of beans, raw oats, peas, yams, muesli, corn tortillas, rice pasta, and cooked millet.

Obviously, there are a few issues here that need to be addressed. If you are on a low-carbohydrate diet or don't tolerate the above foods well, or are coming off the elimination phase of the diet and you want to take it slow, you can add resistant starches to your diet in other ways.

Bob's Red Mill Unmodified Potato Starch has roughly eight grams of RS in one tablespoon. According to Chris Kresser, L.Ac., potato starch is "generally well tolerated even by those who react adversely to nightshades."[5]

Plantains and green unripe bananas are also relatively well tolerated, I have found, and these can be added early on in the reintroduction process. These are relatively bland in flavor and can be added to cold or room temperature water, coconut milk, or mixed into smoothies. Just remember: to maintain the benefits of RS, they should not be heated above 130 degrees.

WHAT IS THE PROCESS FOR IMPROVING ORAL TOLERANCE WHEN REINTRODUCING FOODS?

I think in terms of strategy, this is another area that is highly individualized. Variations in genetic makeup and immune profiles can make a difference in your outcome. It is impossible to predict every variation.

So, understand that you are going to have to try some things. Use my A.P.A.R.T. System. Do it in a scientific and systematic way, and remember to apply the Tummy Triangle Treatment principles.

The question of whether your current issue is deficient, excess, or a mixture of the two still applies. Before we go any further, let's take a look at the energetics of foods that may be reintroduced.

TEMPERATURE	GRAINS	BEANS & LEGUMES	DAIRY	NIGHTSHADES
Warm	sweet rice		butter condensed milk whey whey protein	cayenne pepper chili pepper chipotle pepper habanero pepper jalapeño pepper paprika poblano pepper
Neutral	amaranth oats pearl barley rice	adzuki beans black beans carob chickpeas fava beans kidney beans lentils lima beans navy beans peanuts pinto beans red beans soy beans vanilla beans white beans	buttermilk cheese cream cream cheese evaporated milk ghee goat cheese goat milk kefir milk powdered milk sheep milk sour cream	ashwaganda potatoes
Cool	barley buckwheat corn millet wheat berries	bean sprouts mung beans	cottage cheese frozen yogurt yogurt	eggplant pepper tomato

TEMPERATURE	NUTS	SEEDS	EGGS	MISC.
Warm	chestnuts coffee pine nuts walnuts	anise caraway coriander cumin fennel seed mustard sunflower		alcohol
Neutral	almond cacao carob cashew hazelnut macadamia nutmeg pecan pistachio	canola chia flax hemp poppy pumpkin seeds sesame seeds	chicken eggs duck eggs egg yolk goose eggs quail eggs	
Cool			egg white	alternative sweeteners antibiotics emulsifiers food additives food chemicals food coloring NSAIDs (aspirin, ibuprofen, naproxen) Stevia thickeners

In her book *Reintroducing Foods on the Paleo Autoimmune Protocol,* Eileen Laird gives an excellent five-step method for reintroducing foods. This follows the more effective, gradual induction approach to creating tolerance I mentioned earlier in the chapter.[6]

I'd like to go over some of these and add my own suggestions for using this approach to establish or improve oral tolerance. And bear in mind, this is highly individualized and will require experimentation—not all of which will be pretty or free of unexpected results.

First, what foods should we add?

Basically, there are four stages of reintroduction recommended. Eileen's stated goal is to increase your nutrition as fast as possible with foods your body is likely to accept sooner than others. In my opinion, I don't think the order in which you introduce foods matters (there is no research data on this that I could find). There is a logic to this recommendation, however, and that is that this approach keeps inflammation to a minimum. What really matters is that you do it in a careful, systematic way, and that you focus on boosting oral tolerance.

From a conceptual point of view, lots of food reactions are an indication of deficiency in some measure. So you can also think of this reintroduction process as a rebuilding process. And it is another opportunity to apply the deficiency diet principles that we have learned.

According to the recommendations that are attributed to Sara Ballantyne, Ph.D., in the book, in Stage 1, it is suggested to reintroduce spices that come from seeds (like cumin, coriander, fennel, etc.), some oils, peas and beans, ghee, and egg yolks.[7] Of these, ghee makes the most sense for our purposes because it is a rich source of butyrate. Egg yolks are also nutritionally dense and also seem to be a food that some people really miss during the elimination phase (I know I missed them).

Stage 2 adds grass-fed butter (also an excellent source of butyrate); other seeds like chia, flax, hemp, and sesame; cacao; alcohol; and egg whites. Regarding alcohol, this is something that some people really miss during the elimination phase. However, if you are really serious about healing your gut, there is ample evidence that alcohol can be destructive to every part of the digestive tract.

Alcohol has been found to impair the muscles that separate the esophagus from the stomach. It interferes with gastric secretion in the stomach. It can impair peristalsis and can cause diarrhea. It can also damage the mucosa and inhibit the absorption of nutrients in the small intestine and can increase the transport of toxins across the intestinal walls. And, of course, it can be destructive to the liver.[8]

Even moderate alcohol use also has been linked to certain types of cancers.[9] I recommend giving it up entirely if you want to do everything you can to heal your gut (and prevent cancer).

Stage 3 adds coffee, paprika, some nightshades, and fermented dairy. While fermentation aids in the breakdown of dietary proteins and lactose that may be problematic and therefore could ease the reintroduction of dairy, given what we have learned about dairy products, I would still recommend caution.

Stage 4 adds more alcohol, nightshade spices (like various chili peppers), cheese and milk products, potatoes, white rice, soaked and sprouted beans and grains, and tomatoes. (I suspect tomatoes are problematic because they are more acidic than other nightshades.)

In addition, as I already indicated, I don't think even moderate amounts of alcohol are a good idea if your gut is compromised, let alone larger quantities. Milk products that are not fermented have all the offending proteins and lactose. I would not recommend reintroducing these foods; and I know for myself, I still to this day cannot tolerate them at all.

Many grains are considered cross-reactors to gluten (meaning that they are similar enough in protein structure to cause a similar reaction). In addition, some people develop sensitivities to the grains that replace gluten when they are on a gluten-free diet.

So be aware that you may react to these foods, and emphasize variety. Don't always eat the same thing every day. In addition, it is important to note that these grains and beans should be soaked and/or sprouted, thereby reducing the problematic antinutrients, such as lectins, tannins, and some polyphenols.

This final stage also includes adding any foods you have reacted strongly to in the past, with the exception of gluten, dairy, and unfermented soy. As I mentioned, in my own experience, I have not been able to reintroduce any type of unfermented dairy product, but I seem to be able to tolerate fermented soy products.

When should you start reintroducing foods? I recommend doing the elimination a minimum of 30 days and you can remain up to 60 days if you feel a lot better and want to continue.

As we have seen, there are consequences to *not* reintroducing. So I think we need to make some attempts and keep track to see where we are. Some foods may be okay, others may not.

In addition, I don't believe in an all-or-nothing approach, as real life is nuanced. There's nothing preventing you from doing some reintroducing and then returning to more restrictions. You may find you can have some things once or twice a month or once a week and be okay, but if you exceed that you have a reaction.

Something to consider is to score food in different categories: daily, once a week, twice a month, once a month, and so on. Find the foods in each group for you and eat them accordingly (and keep track of everything in your journal).

Okay, now let's talk about the actual reintroduction process.

The first thing to do is to decide which food you want to reintroduce. And do only one food at a time so that you minimize your variables. If you reintroduce five different things in a recipe, you won't know what you reacted to and what you didn't.

And consider the best ways to prepare those foods to minimize reactions and create tolerance. For grains and beans, soaking and/or sprouting is recommended. Cooking and cooling before eating and reheating is also an excellent way to make starches like rice more resistant and less reactive.

In addition, it's important to understand that raw proteins are different from heated, cooked proteins, and even the type of cooking can make a difference. As we have seen, the way you prepare foods can make a difference as to how they impact you.[10]

For example, some people cannot tolerate raw eggs or fried eggs or those cooked in an omelet, but they can tolerate eggs cooked in baked goods. In this case the temperature and the length of time cooked result in the proteins becoming denatured.

Next, as we learned from looking at the research regarding establishing oral tolerance, small amounts gradually introduced and increased is a good approach. So start with a small amount, a few bites. Then wait a few minutes; if there is no reaction, have a little more.

Then wait a few hours. If you still have no reaction, continue to increase the amount you eat. If at any point you experience a negative reaction, stop the reintroduction—note what happened in your journal. And remember, having a reaction doesn't mean never try it again.

When working to establish tolerance, the goal is a diminished response over time. Incorporate the many strategies I've outlined below and try again after a period of time. At first continue with foods that elicit no reaction or a relatively minor response.

A reaction is a flare-up of your symptoms. This might be digestive, such as gas, bloating, discomfort, diarrhea, or constipation. Or it could be neurological, such as pain, brain fog, memory loss, dizziness, or insomnia. Or it could be a typical allergic reaction, such as itching, rashes, or hives.

Don't rush it; give your body time. If you are experiencing negative symptoms, try these interventions to see if they can decrease or eliminate the reaction. There are two strategies that can be helpful for reducing the severity of reactions to foods:

1. Reduce inflammation. Food reactions often result in an inflammatory response. Dampening that response and calming inflammation can help minimize the adverse symptoms you experience. Turmeric, aloe vera, ginger, chrysanthemum flowers, chamomile and glutathione can all be helpful in calming inflammation in the digestive tract. Also, try to reduce stress and get plenty of sleep and support during this process.

2. Breakdown the proteins as much as possible. Dietary proteins are not as reactive if they are broken down. Boosting stomach acid with apple cider vinegar, ginger, or a betaine HCL supplement can be helpful. Taking digestive enzymes—especially gentler ones such as brush border enzymes like amylase, lactase, papain, bromelain, and lipase—can help to break down the proteins and resolve the flare-up more quickly.

If you do have a negative reaction, avoid that food for the time being. Wait for the symptoms to pass before reintroducing another food so that you have a clear baseline for each reintroduction. And work on implementing the deficiency diet and adding strategies for increasing oral tolerance. (Appendix 3 has a number of suggestions for supplements and foods that help to boost oral tolerance.)

Next, evaluate the destructive potential of the food and see if any of the interventions mentioned above help minimize the reaction. If the reaction is minor, consider additional testing to see if you can establish tolerance.

Once you have established that you can eat the food, take a break. Stop eating the food completely and watch your body for symptoms over the next two or three days. Some reactions can be gradual and may not appear right away.

If you have no reaction, that food is potentially safe for you to eat and you can eat it like a normal person. Just be careful not to go crazy and binge. Eating a large quantity is another strategy for inducing oral tolerance—it kind of shocks your system—but you also run the risk of having a massive reaction and feeling lousy for several days. The key is moderation in everything (including moderation).

There is no definitive guide to reactions to foods. Some reactions are moderate to severe and are obvious. Other reactions are more subtle and may take time to develop. And still others may be somewhere in-between. An important part of this process is keeping track in your journal and learning to read the signals that come from your body.

To establish tolerance, the safest approach may be to attempt a more subtle food reaction. Try to find a happy medium where you can consume the food without noticeable reactions. This may mean eating it a couple of times a week or a couple of times a month, but not daily.

If after eating the food for a week, your body still feels good, then you know that food is not a problem, and you can reintroduce the next one.

This is how you achieve tolerance. Little by little your immune system adapts to these dietary proteins. One thing to consider is that the foods you have a lesser reaction to may in fact help you achieve tolerance.

What other foods should you try to increase tolerance for?

I don't have a definitive answer except that we must seek to do as little harm as possible.

The best way to approach this is to look at a few different foods that you may want to try to establish tolerance for.

TOLERANCE TO LECTINS

Should we attempt to induce oral tolerance to lectins?

There's little doubt that lectins are an immune stimulant. This is precisely why removing them is the focus of elimination diets like the autoimmune paleo diet.

In addition, many researchers use them to induce an immune response (ConA and PHA are commonly used). So this is not just an issue of a reaction to a dietary protein. Lectins produce an inflammatory immune response on their own.

However, some people can eat them without a problem.

This is also a question of destructive potential. How badly do you react to them? They may be something you can eat occasionally. Remember to trust what your body tells you.

Why lectins affect different people in different ways probably has to do with multiple factors like other health issues, genetic profile, and the health of the person's intestines.

There are some things that may help reduce the impact of lectins:

1. **Soaking Them:** What this does, essentially, is ferment them, which helps break down the proteins.

2. **HCL with Pepsin:** Helps partially, but does not completely break down the proteins.

3. **Digestive Enzymes:** Helps partially, but does not completely break down the proteins.

The last thing to consider is this: Should we try to reduce reactions?

I think we should. I think there is benefit to doing a test alone and seeing what happens, then doing a similar test and try taking things that I mentioned above that may improve this process.

As you can see there's a good deal of experimentation to be done here. But I think this information should give you a good frame of reference and starting point.

FOOD AS MEDICINE: *ALBIZZIA FLOWER*

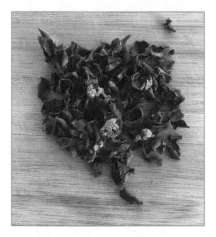

Here's a cool herb. Called *He Huan Hua* in Chinese, the albizzia is also known as the "happiness flower."

This herb comes from the albizzia tree, and both the bark and the flowers are used medicinally.

The flower is considered sweet and neutral and is associated with the liver and heart channels. Its main function is to calm the spirit, invigorate the blood, alleviate pain, and dissipate swelling.

The albizzia flower gets its nickname because it is revered as a powerful tonic for treating depression, melancholy, insomnia, anxiety, and irritability. It has the reputation of being an herbal Prozac. It is effective in my experience and rivals some of the other more common Western herbs (such as St. John's wort) for treating mild to moderate depression.

Albizzia is thought to enhance all aspects of neurotransmitter secretion and regulation. It's quite gentle, and when made as a tea has no contraindications. Because of its ability to move blood, it is not recommended in pregnancy, however.

And the bark of the plant, which has some similar properties to the flowers, is rumored to be part of the secret ingredients of Coca-Cola. Coca-Cola used to be made with real cocaine, but eventually the developers had to find an alternative ingredient that wasn't illegal. Supposedly, He Huan Hua, or the bark from the tree He Huan Pi was substituted. Maybe that's why people love Coke so much!

Pharmacologically, the active constituents of albizzia are saponins and tannins, while specifically, it contains albitocin, b-sitosterol, amyrin, 3,4,7-trihydroxyflavone, spinasteryl-glucoside, machaerinic acid, lactone, methyl ester, acaci acid, and lactone.[11]

It also contains quercetin and isoquercetin, and studies found that both of these increased pentobarbital sleeping time in mice. So, this herb should be used cautiously if you are taking sedative medication. (I have never experienced a sedative effect from taking it alone.)

It makes a nice tea. I like mixing it with chrysanthemum flowers (which I have written about in a previous sidebar) for a summertime tea that makes you feel good. And who doesn't want to feel good?

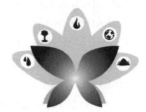

Chapter 15

SYSTEMIC INFECTIONS:
SIBO, Epstein–Barr, Candidiasis, Blastocystis, and More

Chronic systemic infections like Epstein-Barr virus, yersiniosis, and others have been implicated in both the initiation and formation of Hashimoto's. These pathogens can infect tissue in our bodies and can become permanently embedded resulting in confusion from our immune system. This confusion can lead to attacks on our own tissue and autoimmunity.

Other infections like SIBO, *Helicobacter pylori*, candidiasis, and Blastocystis can also undermine our progress by creating a state of physiological and immune stress that can result in our adrenal glands becoming fatigued or exhausted and in constant immune stimulation.

Consequently, it is really important to evaluate and rule out these infections and to provide a natural approach for dealing with them. One negative consequence of attacking these pathogens is that there can be collateral damage to our microbiome, and we have already seen how important the microbiome is for thyroid hormone conversion and absorption as well as for general health and well-being.

In Chinese medicine, there is a term known as *Gu syndrome,* which dates back to prehistoric times. *Gu* is a word that can be applied to worms, parasites, fungal infections, bacteria, or viruses. Essentially, it's a systemic infection. The origin of the term is thought to go back to ancient times and shamanic traditions.

Gu syndrome has evolved with the times, and one of the modern-day proponents of the theory is Heiner Fruehauf, founding professor of the College of Classical Chinese Medicine at the National University of Natural Medicine in Portland, Oregon, who published an influential article on this topic in 1998.[1]

The basic treatment approach used to treat Gu syndrome can be helpful in a host of digestive issues that impact people with Hashimoto's, including parasite infections, Blastocystis, and candidiasis. I discuss Gu syndrome in more detail here, and the remaining chapters in Part II are devoted to a specific chronic system infection.

As I mentioned, Gu syndrome has ancient origins and the philosophy behind it straddles conventional biomedical ideas and more esoteric ideas. According to Dr. Fruehauf, Gu syndrome actually means that your body is "hollowed out from the inside out by dark yin forces that your body cannot see."[2]

Gu syndrome originally referred to black magic, and for those suffering from it, it can certainly feel like someone put a hex on them. One explanation for this is that sometimes these types of infections are hard to identify, and sometimes tests can come back negative even though something is going on.

According to Dr. Fruehauf's 1998 article, Gu syndrome is much like what I described in my experience of dangerous yin during the solar eclipse. It is the ancient Chinese symbol for "extreme pathological yin—the dark side of life, the worst nightmare of any human being. It represents darkness, rottenness, slithering vermin, poisonous snakes, betrayal, black magic, backstabbing murder and in medical terms, progressive organ decay accompanied by tortuous pain and insanity."

However, the reality is that it isn't always so extreme and dramatic. There are a number of gradations of it. And the conditions that I mentioned also fall under the category of a more modern understanding of Gu syndrome disorders.

Here are some of the signs and symptoms associated with Gu syndrome pathologies, according to Dr. Fruehauf:[3]

DIGESTIVE SYMPTOMS

Chronic diarrhea, loose stools or alternating diarrhea and constipation, explosive bowel movements, abdominal bloating, abdominal cramping and/or pain, nausea, intestinal bleeding and/or pus, poor or ravenous appetite, peculiar food cravings.

NEUROMUSCULAR SYMPTOMS

Muscle soreness, muscle heaviness, muscle weakness, wandering body pains, physical heat sensations, cold night sweats, aversion to bright light.

PSYCHOLOGICAL SYMPTOMS

Depression, suicidal thoughts, glaring anger, fits of rage, unpredictable onset of strong yet volatile emotions, inner restlessness, insomnia, general sense of feeling muddled and confusion, chaotic thought patterns, visual and/or auditory hallucinations, epileptic seizures, sensation of "feeling possessed."

CONSTITUTIONAL SYMPTOMS

Progressing state of mental and physical exhaustion, indications of source qi damage, dark circles underneath the eyes, mystery symptoms that evade clear diagnosis, history of acute protozoan infection, history of travel to tropical regions.

So basically, if we boil it down to its basic symptoms, Gu syndrome includes digestive complaints and some neurological distress (such as body pain and/or psychological symptoms, which could be like brain fog or more severe such as hallucinations or paranoia) that aren't always easily explained by Western medical or conventional Chinese medicine diagnostics.

I think for our purposes, we can think of this as chronic, systemic inflammatory conditions, which are very common for people with Hashimoto's. And this includes infections like giardia, chronic Blastocystis, protozoa, and candidiasis.

And even Lyme disease fits this pattern perfectly. As you probably know, Lyme disease is caused by a spirochete and testing can often be inconclusive and confusing. It can also include viral infections that are potential root cause diseases for Hashimoto's, including Epstein-Barr and Coxsackie viruses.

What's really interesting about this approach is that the primary formula and the overall treatment strategy is the same across the board. And the basic approach is the Tummy Triangle Treatment with some dietary and herbal modifications for each specific pathogen.

In the remaining chapters of this section, we will explore each of these Gu syndrome infections and look at specific dietary and herbal treatment protocols for them.

HASHIMOMENT: Are You Suffering from Secondary Gain Syndrome?

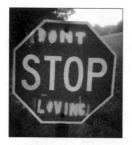

When I work with people, I'm always curious about what their challenges are and why they sought me out. And naturally, when asked, the answer is usually something negative such as, "I'm exhausted," or "I'm really sick," or "I can't lose this weight, and I can't stand looking at myself."

In my opinion, one of the keys to overcoming these struggles is to shift your focus away from what's wrong to what you want instead. This is why I encourage my patients to create a clear healing vision of exactly what they want.

I encourage them to devote some time to really feeling it in their bodies, thinking about how they will feel when they get to their goal, and considering how it will affect everyone around them. The more details and clarity you can imagine, the easier it is to get there. And the more you repeat the imaginary experience, the more possible that experience becomes.

It's very important to keep revisiting this positive visualization so that you can experience what you want rather than what is going wrong all the time. But one interesting thing I have noticed in this process is that sometimes when we make a decision to focus on what we want, fear or resistance comes up around the changes we have to make to get there.

For example: "If I'm healthy and vibrant again, I'll be expected to return to work or have to do all the housework again."

Or "If I stop eating that delicious ice cream that I love to have every night, I might have to face what's missing in my life."

And really it comes down to this question: "Who would I be without this _____ [fill in the blank with Hashimoto's, extra weight, pain, fatigue, depression, anxiety, etc.]?"

This can be a scary thought because this illness, weight, depression, anxiety, etc., may define us in some way, especially if we've been struggling with it for a long time. It's who we've become; it's our identity.

Sometimes these issues may also be connected to deeper psychological memories or traumas.

I was recently working with someone doing EFT (Emotional Freedom Techniques), and she unearthed one of these memories. (EFT, if you aren't familiar with it, is a technique that involves tapping on acupuncture points and using affirmations to release pent-up emotional issues from your body.) In the midst of our session together on letting go of her issues, she wondered out loud, "Who will I be without these memories?"

It was almost as though part of her core or essence was being removed, and some fear came up as a result. Instead of feeling fear, we decided to look at this with curiosity and start thinking of all the things she could do, think, feel, and become as a result of letting go of these memories.

The truth is that our subconscious mind sometimes wants to keep us safe and can be very resistant to change. So even if the possibility of change consciously feels exciting and new, the subconscious may do its utmost to keep us stuck where we are now, because this place is safe and familiar.

There is a payoff to staying where we are.

This is known as Secondary Gain Syndrome.

In other words, there is some benefit to staying where we are, even if we consciously want to move forward. If you aren't getting the results you had hoped for or if you continue to struggle after trying lots of different external solutions, it might not hurt to look inward and ask yourself honestly if there might be some reason why you are holding on to this struggle.

This can be its own form of Gu syndrome.

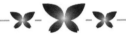

Chapter 16

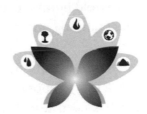

SIBO
(Small Intestinal
Bacterial Overgrowth)

WHY SIBO MATTERS TO SOMEONE WITH HASHIMOTO'S

Determining whether or not you have SIBO can be really important for people with Hashimoto's because of the role that the small intestines play in thyroid hormone conversion and absorption.

When you have Hashimoto's and hypothyroidism, this leads to problems with motor functions in the small intestine. There are thyroid hormone receptors all over the gut, and the vagus nerve fires into it.

If these parts of your body aren't getting enough thyroid hormone, things don't move through there as well, which may lead to an overgrowth of bacteria. Although this is an area that is somewhat open to debate. We don't really know what are appropriate levels of bacteria in the small intestines. Certainly, it is significantly less than in the colon, but exactly what constitutes "too much," no one really knows. What we do know is that this bacteria can interfere with thyroid hormone absorption. This may be why some people take Synthroid, Armour, Cytomel, Naturethroid, or other thyroid replacement hormones and yet it doesn't feel like it's working.

The gut is an important reservoir for thyroid hormone (especially T3) and anything that causes inflammation and malabsorption in the gut can impact the ability of thyroid hormone to do its job all over the body.

So even though you are taking thyroid hormone, it may not be effective. You still have all the symptoms like fatigue, brain fog and memory issues, weight gain, hair loss, depression, etc.

Many researchers also believe that autoimmune disease originates in the intestines.

As I mentioned in my first book, a leaky gut or damaged intestine has been found in every autoimmune disease that has been tested including rheumatoid arthritis, Crohn's disease, celiac disease, type 1 diabetes, and, yes, even Hashimoto's.

SYMPTOMS OF SIBO

SIBO has a number of possible symptoms, but mostly these involve bloating, gas, diarrhea, and/or constipation. SIBO should be considered with abdominal discomfort after eating any of the following things:

- Starches
- Sugars/fructose
- Fructans
- Prebiotics
- Probiotics
- Fiber supplements
- Rice or pea powder from metabolic powders
- Galactans

You may notice that many of the foods listed here can also aggravate Candida. And sometimes Candida is blamed for what is actually SIBO.[1]

SIBO HAS DEGREES OF SEVERITY

Just like Hashimoto's, SIBO has different degrees of severity. These are important because the more serious it is, the more work you may have to do to resolve it.

I. ASYMPTOMATIC:

Abnormal small intestine bacterial overgrowth tests and mild or no symptoms. Bloating after meals.

II. MODERATE SYMPTOMS:

Bloating with malnutrition and constipation.
Bloating with nutritional deficiencies.

III. SEVERE SYMPTOMS:

Bloating with anemia, low albumin, and low cholesterol.
Bloating with weight loss, chronic diarrhea, and malabsorption.

If you are a person who has trouble taking supplements because you just react to everything, then you may fall into the more severe symptoms category.

WHO HAS SIBO?

Here's an overview of the prevalence of SIBO in other conditions:[2]

- 15 percent of the elderly
- 33 percent of people with chronic diarrhea
- 34 percent of people with chronic pancreatitis
- 53 percent of people using antacid medication
- 66 percent of patients with celiac disease with persistent symptoms
- 78 percent of people with IBS
- 90 percent of alcoholics

What really stands out for me are two of those statistics: More than half the people on antacid medication and 9 out of 10 alcoholics suffer from SIBO.

That shows you how destructive alcohol can be to the small intestines. And, the fact is, alcohol degenerates the enteric nervous system of the gut very aggressively.

TESTING FOR SIBO

In conventional medicine, there are two types of testing for SIBO. However, both are flawed and not definitive.

1. DIRECT: ENDOSCOPIC ASPIRATION AND CULTURE

This is a direct endoscopic aspiration and culture of the small intestine. It requires a gastroenterologist, so it's costly and invasive. Another downside: many of the bacteria removed from the small intestine don't survive in culture, so they can't be analyzed.

2. INDIRECT: BREATH TESTING FOR HYDROGEN AND METHANE

This test can be inaccurate if someone has recently had antibiotics, and it may not be useful in determining all species of bacteria. You may also get false negatives due to different transit times for different people.

Another really valuable lesson I have learned from clinical experience and from Li Dong-yuan is that, often, some of the best treatments and solutions come from *subtraction*.

As we have seen, many common health problems are problems of excess. Too much sugar, too much stress, too many chemicals. An effective way of treating too much is by taking things away.

It's a simple solution, yet it's so hard to actually do. But if you have Hashimoto's, learning how to be content with less may just be the key to your healing.

ANTIBIOTIC THERAPY AND THYROID HORMONE

Another potentially serious consequence of antibiotic treatment for SIBO is its impact on thyroid hormone conversion. Bacteria in gut are (at least partially) responsible for converting T4 into T3.

Remember the story I shared earlier in the book about the woman who was treated with antibiotics for SIBO and her TSH went up to 79 points? Hers is an interesting case to look at, because she had had a thyroidectomy. So her only source of thyroid hormone was an external, controlled dose source of levothyroxine (synthetic T4).

She took spore-based probiotics, the Chinese herbal formula Si Jun Zi Tang, and some adrenal support. She was also instructed to eat a spleen qi supporting diet.

After six weeks, her TSH dropped to 44. This was a very clear example of the impact of antibiotics on thyroid hormone absorption as well as a treatment approach that followed our principles and was somewhat successful.

There are other examples in the medical research of antibiotics affecting thyroid hormone absorption. In fact, a study from the *British Medical Journal* found that the antibiotic ciprofloxacin—known more commonly by brand names Cipro, Ciproxin, or Cirpoxine—significantly decreased the absorption of the thyroid medication.[3]

In addition, some experts feel that the warning about ciprofloxacin applies also to similar quinolone antibiotics such as levofloxacin (Levaquin), lomefloxacin (Maxaquin), monifloxacin (Avelox), norfloxacin (Norox-In), and ofloxacin (Floxin).

This means that if you are taking thyroid medication and an antibiotic from the quinolone family, it could interfere with absorption, and cause you to become substantially more hypothyroid.

Most upper respiratory infections are caused by viruses. Instead of taking antibiotics for an upper respiratory infection, try antiviral herbs. I love the Chinese herbal formula Gan Mao Ling for this purpose. It's very effective and it spares the good guys in your gut.

Also, researchers have found that 80 percent of oral dosages of T4 are absorbed in the jejunum and the ileum. What this tells us is that all sorts of things that impact this part of the intestines can affect absorption.

THE SIBO DIET

The SIBO diet is a great exercise in subtraction. For the best results, it should be done for a month or so.

FOODS TO AVOID:

Fructose: sugars, artificial sweeteners, corn syrup

Grains: rice, wheat, quinoa, millet, amaranth, and some non-grains like tapioca

Legumes/galactans: beans, peas, chickpeas, soybeans, lentils

Fructan-containing vegetables: lettuce, onions, artichokes, beets, broccoli, cabbage, brussels sprouts, peas, asparagus, okra, shallots, mushrooms, green peppers, cauliflower

High-fructose fruits: grapes, apples, watermelon, cherries, kiwifruit, bananas, blueberries, mangos

Meat products: Breaded or processed meats such as hot dogs, bologna, potted meats, and most cold cuts (containing added starches). There are some experts who say to also avoid beef, pork, and lamb.

FOODS TO EAT:

Nuts: all nuts, except pistachios
Vegetables: all vegetables, except those listed above
Low-fructose fruits: apricot, avocado, cantaloupe, grapefruit, honeydew melon, nectarine, orange, peach, pineapple, raspberry, strawberry, tomato
Meats: chicken, fish, eggs; beef, lamb, and pork in moderation
Fats: animal fat, oils[4]

SIBO TREATMENT:

Generally, with SIBO there are two approaches: antibiotic therapy and diet or herbs and supplements and diet.

If you choose to go the conventional route and take antibiotics, then you will need a diet to recover and rebuild. And, for the record, the rate of recurrence of SIBO after treatment with Rifaximin (the most popular antibiotic used) is quite high. In one study, it was 12.6 percent at three months, 27.5 percent at six months, and 43.7 percent at nine months.[5]

From a Tummy Triangle Treatment perspective, this treatment will kill bacteria in your microbiome, which means you will be spleen and stomach qi (and probably yang) deficient. Antibiotics are considered to be very cold in Chinese medicine.

The best diet for treating the gut after SIBO treatment would be the spleen and stomach qi and yang deficient diets mentioned on page 156.

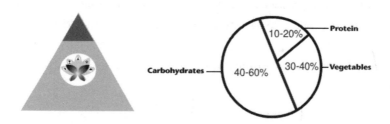

In addition, some important herbs and supplements for restoring spleen and stomach qi include the following:

A great herbal formula for helping the spleen and stomach recover from antibiotic treatment is called Bu Zhong Yi Qi Tang. This formula was invented by Li Dong-yuan, and it perfectly exemplifies the Tummy Triangle Treatment principles.

The herbs huang qi, dang shen, bai zhu, and gan cao all strengthen the spleen. Chai hu and sheng ma support these herbs in elevating qi (and also work to move liver qi); zhi shi and hou po regulate and descend qi, creating a nice balance with the other herbs; dang gui supplements blood; and chen pi regulates qi. It's a thing of beauty!

What's missing? Herbs that clear damp heat. Well, we don't need those, as we just used antibiotics to do that. Remember, antibiotics are very cold.

Other supplements to consider are probiotics (spore based) and butyrate.

NATURAL SIBO TREATMENT

If, on the other hand, you choose to treat SIBO naturally without using antibiotics, the Tummy Triangle Treatment would be a damp heat–clearing diet with a balanced herbal formula:

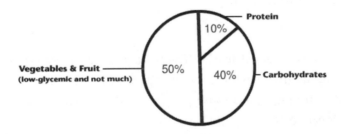

In this case, we want to first employ the damp heat diet (with the SIBO diet modifications) with an herbal antibiotic. A great formula for this is called Huang lian jie du tang.

This formula has four potent broad-spectrum antibiotic herbs: huang qin, huang lian, huang bai, and zhi zi. These are high in berberine, which is a potent antibiotic compound. Be cautious with this formula; like antibiotics it can easily damage the spleen and stomach qi. If you aren't sure how to use it, consult a trained herbalist.

This diet and this formula should only be done for a short period of time (two to three weeks). Once you have finished the treatment, return to the spleen and stomach qi deficiency diet that I mentioned previously.

If you develop diarrhea or other complications, stop the treatment and consult your physician.

USE THE A.P.A.R.T. SYSTEM TO DETERMINE YOUR STRATEGY

1. Ask and Assess

Check to see if you have the common SIBO symptoms.

Order a SIBO breath test. However, since we know that this test is hardly definitive and sometimes results in false positives, I recommend giving the spleen and stomach qi deficiency diet a chance first—especially if you don't have SIBO symptoms.

If you have SIBO symptoms and test positive, try the damp heat diet with SIBO diet modifications and the herbal formula mentioned above.

2. Prioritize and Plan

Either way, if you have it, you are going to attack the bacteria. Once you do that, you must help the gut to recover.

3. Act and Adapt

Do what you have decided to do. If you have a bad reaction, you may have to adapt and that usually involves working on healing the gut. If your approach doesn't work, your condition may be more complicated and you may need to consult a physician with experience in treating SIBO.

4. Reassess and Reevaluate

Retest and see if you accomplished what you set out to do. If you did, rebuild and work on rebuilding spleen and stomach qi.

If you didn't, I recommend consulting someone who has experience in this area.

5. Try and Try Again

Keep working on strengthening and healing the gut by keeping to a spleen and stomach qi strengthening diet.

FOOD AS MEDICINE: **WINTER SQUASH**

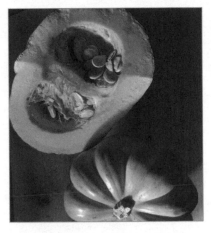

Winter squashes are those with hard skins, like acorn, butternut, spaghetti, and kabocha squash, as well as pumpkins.

These delicious squashes are considered cool and sweet. Traditionally they were thought to dispel dampness, reduce fever, relieve pain, stabilize hyperactive fetuses, stop dysentery, and benefit diabetes.

The seeds kill parasites and worms too.

Conditions they have been used to treat include diabetes, dysentery, eczema, stomachache, and yin fire symptoms such as a heat sensation in the bones.

In addition, they were used as an antidote to opium.

Traditional remedies include:

- For intestinal worms, take 1 tablespoon of ground pumpkin seeds three times a day on an empty stomach.

- For burns, apply fresh pumpkin or pumpkin mixed with aloe vera gel.

- For diabetes, eat a slice of pumpkin with every meal or better yet, bake a pie with pumpkin, yam, and potato. (Yum!)

- For vomiting, make tea from the pumpkin stem and the top cap.[6]

Chapter 17

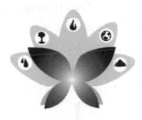

EPSTEIN-BARR VIRUS

Like most health conditions, Hashimoto's has no single cause.

It is the result of the perfect storm of factors that include a genetic predisposition, exposure to some pathogen (often a herpes virus), the breakdown of the gut and barrier systems (with or without the help of gluten), exposure to gluten, environmental toxins (like radiation, mercury, and other toxic chemicals), and often, some particularly stressful event.

Let's explore one of those causes: the herpes virus. Epstein-Barr is one form of herpes virus. In this chapter, we will explore all the herpes viruses and focus on a diet for them (and Epstein-Barr, in particular).

As many of you know, I have Hashimoto's and have made it my life's work to understand everything I can about the causes, treatment, and management of this disease.

MY OWN EXPERIENCE WITH HERPES

I also have herpes simplex 1 (along with 90 percent of the population). While this is not a life-threatening disease, it can be the cause of shame and embarrassment, especially when I get a more serious outbreak on my face or lips.

As a health-care practitioner, there are times when having an outbreak of herpes has made me feel like I'm not very good at my job because it can look much worse than it is.

But the reality is that there are few other biological entities as resilient and unstoppable as the herpes virus. All the technology at our disposal is pretty useless when it comes to trying to eradicate this infection.

And I suppose one blessing of having it is that I cannot venture too far from the things I know I need to do to stay healthy. The virus will rear its ugly head and remind me to get back in line.

In addition, one thing I have observed in my own life is that an outbreak of herpes can also affect my Hashimoto's, resulting in a debilitating double whammy that can affect me emotionally, physically, and psychologically.

So I thought I would explore this in more depth, and look at the relationship between herpes and Hashimoto's. You may be surprised by the information and the impact that these various herpes diseases can have.

HERPES VIRUSES ARE *EVERYWHERE*

There are eight different herpes viruses known to infect human beings. These include herpes simplex 1 and 2, varicella zoster (which causes chicken pox) also known as herpes 3, Epstein-Barr virus (herpes 4), cytomegalovirus (herpes 5), human herpes virus 6 and 7, and human herpes virus 8 found in people with complications due to HIV.

While the whole herpes family is believed to be linked to autoimmune disease, there is more research into the link between herpes simplex 1 and 2, Epstein-Barr, cytomegalovirus, and autoimmune thyroid disorders like Hashimoto's.

The common factors that unite them is that all of them remain in the body forever, they can remain dormant for years and then get reawakened (often by stress or stressful events), and they all have the potential to do harm to the brain because the herpes virus has an affinity for nerve tissue.

HERPES SIMPLEX 1 & 2

Herpes simplex virus (HSV) infections are very common worldwide. HSV-1 is the main cause of herpes infections on the mouth and lips, including cold sores and fever blisters. It is transmitted orally (through kissing or sharing drinking glasses and utensils). HSV-1 can also cause genital herpes, although HSV-2 is the main cause of genital herpes.

HSV-2 is spread through sexual contact. You may be infected with HSV-1 or HSV-2 but not show any symptoms. Often symptoms are triggered by exposure to the sun, fever, menstruation, emotional stress, a weakened immune system, or an illness (like Hashimoto's).

While most herpes infections do not cause serious complications, infections in infants and in people with weakened immune systems, or herpes infections that affect the eyes, can be life threatening. In addition, the herpes virus attacks nerves so it can do damage to the brain by attacking the ganglia.

EPSTEIN–BARR VIRUS (EBV)

Epstein-Barr is the virus that causes mononucleosis and is part of the herpes family. Even if you didn't come down with it in high school or college, you were very likely infected with it, as an estimated 95 percent of U.S. adults have been infected with this virus.

It can present itself without any symptoms and has been linked to both Hashimoto's and Graves' disease. In my own patient population, about 80 percent of the people I have worked with have been diagnosed with EBV.

I surveyed our Facebook group of over 40,000 members (at the time) and asked how many have also had the Epstein-Barr virus. Of the 131 (and counting) people with Hashimoto's who responded, 85 percent were aware that they had been exposed to EBV.

This is obviously not a rigorous study, but it does show you just how prevalent this infection is in this patient population.

It has also been linked to other autoimmune diseases, such as multiple sclerosis, lupus, and Sjögren's syndrome. Likewise, both fibromyalgia and chronic fatigue syndrome are linked to EBV.

Epstein-Barr can also lead to inflammation of the brain. In fact, there is a condition known as herpes simplex encephalitis (HSE). It is not known exactly how it is transmitted, but theories include transmission to the brain via major nerves (the trigeminal or olfactory nerve).

This is a serious concern with Hashimoto's because it can have a profound impact on the brain and has the potential to lead to neurodegeneration and cognitive decline.

CYTOMEGALOVIRUS (CMV)

Most people infected with CMV do not have any symptoms. Acute CMV infection can cause mono-like symptoms such as fever, enlarged lymph nodes, sore throat, muscle aches, loss of appetite, and fatigue.

In people with compromised immune function, CMV infections can attack different organs and systems in the body and can lead to blurred vision and even blindness (CMV retinitis), lung infection, diarrhea, inflammation of the liver, and inflammation of the brain (encephalitis). In more severe cases, it can lead to behavioral changes, seizures, and coma (again highlighting the impact of the virus on the brain).

HOW DO THESE VIRUSES LEAD TO AND IMPACT HASHIMOTO'S?

It is not believed that the herpes viruses directly cause autoimmune disease. But they do play a part in its initial onset and progression, and they can certainly make symptoms more intense and be a barrier to healing and feeling better.

There are many reasons for this and I will discuss them in a moment, but first let's take a look at antigens and antibodies so that you can understand how these viruses cause problems in the body.

ANTIGENS TRIGGER AN IMMUNE RESPONSE, ANTIBODIES BIND TO ANTIGENS

An antigen is a substance that produces an immune response. So, for example, foreign substances such as chemicals, bacteria, or viruses are all considered antigens. Foods can also be seen as antigens by the immune system.

However, an antigen can also be produced inside of the body, and even tissue cells can be considered to be an antigen at times, which is what happens with autoimmune conditions such as Graves' disease and Hashimoto's.

An antibody is a protein produced by the immune system that binds to a specific antigen. Once the antibody binds to the antigen, other immune system cells (i.e., macrophages) attempt to engulf and destroy the antigen.

HOW THESE ANTIBODY REACTIONS MAY LEAD TO AUTOIMMUNITY

There are a number of theories about the different mechanisms that can lead viruses to trigger autoimmune disease. A couple of examples are direct bystander activation and molecular mimicry.

Direct bystander activation: This describes an indirect or non-specific activation of autoimmune cells caused by the inflammatory environment present during infection. Think of this as being in the wrong place at the wrong time, just like being caught in a drive-by shooting.[1]

In this case, one part of the immune system becomes activated, and this turns on other parts that can kill both viral-infected cells and healthy cells as well.

So, for example, virus-specific T cells might migrate to the areas of a viral infection, and when these T cells encounter virus-infected cells, they sound the alarm and release immune proteins (called cytokines), which not only kill the infected cells, but also lead to "bystander killing" of other healthy cells nearby.

Molecular mimicry: This is a process where a foreign antigen shares an amino acid sequence or has a similar structure to self-antigens. So, for example, a certain virus can have an amino acid sequence that is very similar to the amino acid sequence of human cells.[2]

This can result not only in the production of antibodies against the virus, but can also lead to auto-antibodies against the human cells due to the similarities in the proteins.

Something else that can occur is that viral fragments can attach to human tissue and result in a hybrid that is part virus and part human, and this can also be attacked by the immune system.

HERE ARE THE POSSIBLE STEPS TO AUTOIMMUNITY

The mechanisms mentioned above are really the end of a series of potential steps that lead to autoimmunity. There are some interesting theories about how this happens, and this matters because if we can figure out how it is happening, perhaps we can find a way to treat it.

What's also interesting is that this same process takes place with all herpes viruses; it's not unique to the ones that we're looking at as examples.

IT STARTS WITH CD8+ T-CELLS

CD8+ T-cells are a kind of cell that inhibits viruses. Basically, once activated they kill bad cells.

Cells infected with the virus are used to make more virus.

Cells that viruses have infected are one example. These cells will be used by the virus to make more virus, so they must be killed by the immune system.

Having a deficiency of them is a common characteristic of virtually every chronic autoimmune disease (including multiple sclerosis, rheumatoid arthritis, systemic lupus erythematosus, Sjögren's syndrome, systemic sclerosis, dermatomyositis, primary biliary cirrhosis, primary sclerosing cholangitis, ulcerative colitis, Crohn's disease, psoriasis, vitiligo, bullous pemphigoid, alopecia areata, idiopathic dilated cardiomyopathy, type 1 diabetes mellitus, Graves' disease, Hashimoto's thyroiditis, myasthenia gravis, IgA nephropathy, membranous nephropathy, and pernicious anemia).

Some scientists believe that this CD8+ T-cell deficiency may be partially responsible for the formation of these chronic autoimmune diseases as well. And one reason is that they aren't able to control the Epstein-Barr virus or other herpes infection.

If EBV isn't controlled, it can cause all kinds of problems in the body. When EBV infects B cells, it can make them "auto-reactive," meaning that its products (antibodies) target our own tissues.

According to a paper called "CD8+ T-Cell Deficiency, Epstein-Barr Virus Infection, Vitamin D Deficiency, and Steps to Autoimmunity: A Unifying Hypothesis" by Michael P. Pender, one theory is that autoimmunity occurs in the following steps.[3]

- First you have CD8+ T-cell deficiency. This has a genetic component.

- Then EBV (or other herpes virus) infection occurs and spreads because of CD8+ T-cell deficiency (there aren't enough of these cells to kill the virus-infected cells).

- Increased antibodies against EBV (kind of like a second line of defense), your body responds and tries to bring in more help.

- EBV infects a specific organ, particularly the B cells in that organ. This corrupts the B cells to attack our own tissue. (One theory is that since viruses and bacteria have proteins similar to our own proteins, we mistakenly attack our own proteins. This confusion by our immune system is the molecular mimicry I described earlier.)

- B cells proliferate in the infected organ (your antibody numbers increase).

- T cells are drawn into the organ and also attack our tissue. Antibodies signal the attackers.

- Development of "structures" in the target organ, which causes B cells to attack our tissues. (This is dependent on Th17 cells.) This process repeats and builds on itself.

WHAT FACTORS PUSH AUTOIMMUNITY?

Some common factors that push autoimmunity are:

- Low Vitamin D

- High Estrogen

- High Chronic Stress

- Low Vitamin D

Vitamin D and sunlight are very important for CD8+ T cell production, which may explain why countries that get less sunlight have a higher occurrence of autoimmunity. People with Hashimoto's commonly have low vitamin D levels.

HIGH ESTROGEN

Estrogen also decreases CD8+ T cells, which may explain the higher incidence of autoimmunity in females. Women with estrogen dominance and/or impairment of detoxification pathways in the liver may have too much circulating estrogen, and this can cause problems with the immune system.

HIGH CHRONIC STRESS: HIGH CORTISOL/LOW PREGNENOLONE

Chronic stress can cause reactivation of EBV, probably by downgrading the TH1 immune response. (TH1 are T-helper cells that sound the alarm and also induce destruction. They are like the elite soldiers of the immune system.)

When you have chronic stress, your body keeps pumping out cortisol. Cortisol is made from cholesterol, and a hormone that helps make cortisol is known as pregnenolone.

Pregnenolone is a neurosteroid that's important in the creation of other hormones like cortisol.

When your body is under constant stress (which is the state of living with an autoimmune disease like Hashimoto's) and needs to keep producing more and more cortisol, something called the "pregnenolone steal" can happen.

This is where cortisol is "stealing" or diverting pregnenolone for cortisol production and depleting it. When pregnenolone is depleted, there will, of course, be less of it to produce more cortisol in the future.

VIRUSES HIJACK THE MEVALONATE PATHWAY

When a viral infection becomes active, it takes control over what's known as the "mevalonate pathway." Viruses use this pathway to make their protective outer coats.[4]

In answer to this, your body makes interferon, which shuts down the mevalonate pathway, which in turn suppresses the virus. However, inhibiting this pathway may also lead to a reduction in synthesis of pregnenolone and coenzyme Q10 (which also may be depleted in Hashimoto's).

One of the most common viruses that causes this pathway to be inhibited is EBV. There's also another problem.

When you're under high stress the body releases cortisol, which suppresses your immune system.

Specifically, the Th1 (or T-helper 1) part of the immune system is suppressed by chronic stress. This aspect of the immune system (Th1) protects us from viral reactivation. Cells and proteins in this family sound the alarm and kill viruses.

When this part of the immune system is suppressed, viral infections can then reactivate—including EBV, herpes, and a host of other viruses. What's really interesting about this is that Hashimoto's was originally thought to be a Th1 dominant disease, and some people with Hashimoto's do have Th1 dominance.

And here's where it gets tricky. If you stimulate Th1, then you may risk firing up the part of the immune system that is destroying your thyroid. So this requires some real skill in dealing with both Hashimoto's and EBV or other herpes viruses at the same time.

OTHER THINGS EBV CAN DISRUPT

There are some other things that EBV can cause problems with, and these are really significant because they are also common problems with Hashimoto's.

EBV can cause problems with serotonin and methylation, and can compromise the blood-brain barrier and, as we have already seen, lead to neurodegeneration.

This is really interesting because with Hashimoto's and hypothyroidism, serotonin can also become depleted. This may be one of the reasons why some people with Hashimoto's experience depression and a lack of motivation and enjoyment in things. So the combination of Hashimoto's and EBV can lead to some serious emotional issues.

Methylation issues are also quite common with Hashimoto's, and some people have MTHFR gene mutations, which can exacerbate this problem. In addition, dominance of the TH1 part of the immune system can lead to methylation problems as well.

Finally, leaky gut and intestinal permeability are the hallmark of virtually all autoimmune diseases, and this is sometimes the sign of a larger systemic problem involving all the barrier systems of the body.

The gut and the brain are very closely related; the same proteins that protect the barrier of the intestines also line the blood-brain barrier. When one area is compromised, the other can be as well.

So the combination of EBV and Hashimoto's certainly has all the ingredients of a potent, vicious cycle that can create a downward spiral of difficult to resolve physical and psychological health problems.

WHAT TO DO IF YOU HAVE EBV AND HASHIMOTO'S

Treating both EBV (and other herpes viruses) and Hashimoto's at the same time can be tricky because herbs and supplements that are known to prevent reactivation of the virus can also stimulate parts of the immune system.

And if these parts of the immune system are causing tissue destruction and flare-ups of your symptoms, then you are simply trading problems. And this approach may actually make matters worse.

So let's take a look at some obvious and less obvious treatment strategies that can keep EBV or other viruses at bay and not stoke the fires of autoimmunity.

LIFESTYLE INTERVENTIONS

One of the most important treatments for EBV (and other herpes viruses) is having stress-relieving hobbies. Many people are aware of the destructive power of stress, but it always amazes me how little they are willing to do about it.

If you have Hashimoto's and EBV and you don't do things to reduce stress daily, you are setting yourself up for failure. It's like walking into oncoming traffic and expecting not to be hit by a car or truck. You are going to be in a world of hurt if you don't have daily habits for reducing stress.

These include meditation, yoga, qi gong, music, art, relaxation, massage, acupuncture, spa days, mineral baths, etc. These are not luxuries—they are necessities for someone living with Hashimoto's and EBV.

I'm giving you permission to indulge yourself. If you need a note from your doctor for this, e-mail me and I'll be happy to write one for you.

FOODS TO AVOID WITH EBV AND HERPES VIRUSES

Another thing to be conscious of are foods and supplements that can feed and encourage the herpes virus. The most common are foods that are low in lysine and high in arginine. These include:

- Chocolate
- Coconut (coconut oil is fine since it has no amino acids)
- Seeds and nuts
- Orange juice
- Wheat products and products containing gluten
- Oats
- Lentils
- Protein supplements (casein, the protein found in milk may also increase arginine levels)
- Gelatin

What's interesting to note here is that some of these foods are ones we commonly avoid with Hashimoto's, while others are staples of the paleo and autoimmune paleo diets. (This emphasizes the importance of being flexible and of the highly individualized nature of the problem.)

Highly acidic foods and those laden with chemicals can also exacerbate viral infections and lead to outbreaks.

- Alcohol
- Caffeine
- All junk food
- Too much red meat
- Processed/white flour products
- Food additives
- Artificial sweeteners

These are all foods that can exacerbate your Hashimoto's. So there's no love lost here. Caffeine can potentiate or increase the utilization of arginine so it should be avoided or kept to a minimum.

HERBS FOR TREATING EBV AND HERPES

There are several different strategies for treating EBV and other herpes viruses. Novice herbalists will often throw lots of immune-stimulating herbs at the problem like astragalus, ashwaganda, and medicinal mushrooms like maitake and reishi.

These are great herbs, but they can be a really bad idea for some people with autoimmune disease.

Instead a more targeted approach of attacking the virus and strengthening different parts of the immune system with a more nuanced approach is a much, much better idea. The *Chinese Herbal Medicine: Materia Medica* is full of herbs that can accomplish these tasks beautifully. Here are some that specifically attack EBV and other herpes viruses:[5]

ANTI-EBV HERBS:

Angelica sinensis, chrysanthemum, citrus, lithosperum, milletia, paedria, picrorhiza

ANTI-CYTOMEGALOVIRUS HERBS:

Isatis root, baphicacanthes, cnidium, lithosperum, forsythia, gardenia, chrysanthemum, vitex, dandelion, epimedium, lonicera

ANTI-HERPES HERBS:

Belamcanda, clove, crataegous, dandelion, epimedium, houttuynia, inula, lonicera, portulaca, prunella, rhubarb, salvia, scrophularia

It's important to note that many of these herbs have multiple pharmacological properties and can therefore be used to accomplish more than one thing if combined properly.

HERBS FOR SAFELY STRENGTHENING THE IMMUNE SYSTEM

It's important to strengthen the immune system to treat these herpes viruses, but it must be done carefully.

As mentioned, vitamin D is important for strengthening CD8+ T cells, as is glutathione and superoxide dismutase, EPA, and DHA.

Turmeric is helpful because of its anti-inflammatory properties.

Also, there are a couple of essential oils that I have found are very effective for first attacking the virus and then healing the sores. Ravensara is an excellent antiviral oil that may be applied topically directly on the lesions. Heliochrysum is an oil that helps regenerate flesh and can help to heal the sores more quickly.

A colleague of mine, Olesia Farberov, makes a fantastic herbal salve with some of the Chinese herbs mentioned above, and both of these essential oils are called "The Healer." It can be purchased at www.oessencials.com.

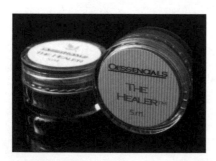

The Healer, Made with Anti-Herpes Herbs and Essential Oils: This is an absolute must for your purse, pocket, and medicine cabinet. I prescribe it to all of my patients with herpes and use it myself because it just plain works.

VITAMINS, MINERALS, AND SUPPLEMENTS:

Research has shown that a daily intake of at least 1250 mg of lysine supplements can help control herpes outbreaks.

Zinc, vitamin C, and B vitamins may also be helpful.

OTHER SUPPLEMENTS THAT CAN HELP INCREASE CB8+ CELLS INCLUDE:

N-Acetyl-Cysteine (NAC), butyrate, andrographis, and gynostemma

WESTERN MEDICATION

One area where I actually advocate using Western pharmaceutical drugs is in the treatment of these viruses. Acyclovir is a potent antiviral and for some people who have really stubborn, hard-to-treat outbreaks, it can be an effective tool in your arsenal.

Another drug to consider is low-dose naltrexone (LDN). It has the ability to modulate immune function and calm physiological stress. It can also be effective in helping the body to deal with the herpes virus.

BOTTOM LINE: IF YOU CAN'T BEAT 'EM, JOIN 'EM

At the end of the day, the reality is that these viruses are here to stay. They are remarkably adaptable and persistent, and they have their own insidious intelligence.

We cannot hope to defeat them; we have to accept them, live with them, and adapt our lives to them. The good news is that the most effective treatments for these viruses such as stress-relieving hobbies and a healthy diet are also important ingredients in our long-term health, happiness, and well-being.

USING THE A.P.A.R.T. SYSTEM TO DIAGNOSE AND TREAT EBV

1. Ask and Assess

First test for EBV.

The Centers for Disease Control and Prevention (CDC) recommends ordering several tests to help determine whether a person is susceptible to EBV or to detect a recent infection or a prior infection, or a reactivated EBV infection. These tests include:[6]

- Viral capsid antigen (VCA)-IgM

- VCA-IgG

- D early antigen (EA-D)

- Epstein-Barr nuclear antigen (EBNA)

It can be a little tricky interpreting these tests. Signs and symptoms should be taken into account. (If you are unsure, consult a health-care practitioner or a specialist in infectious diseases, specifically one who is experienced with EBV testing.)

In my experience with people with Hashimoto's and EBV, the most common symptom includes fatigue that just doesn't improve. Other common symptoms of EBV infection are fever, headache, swollen glands, etc.

Sometimes, it's just the fatigue.

If you are positive for VCA-IgM antibodies, then it is likely that you have an EBV infection, and it may be early in the course of the illness. If you also have symptoms associated with EBV (those I just mentioned), then it is most likely that you will be diagnosed with mono, even if the test for it was negative.

If you are positive for VCA-IgG and EA-D IgG tests, then it is highly likely that you have a current or recent EBV infection.

If the VCA-IgM is negative but VCA-IgG and an EBNA antibody are positive, then it is likely that you had a previous EBV infection.

If you have no symptoms and are negative for VCA-IgG, then you are likely to not have been previously exposed to EBV and are vulnerable to infection.

In general, rising VCA-IgG levels tend to indicate an active EBV infection, while falling concentrations tend to indicate a recent EBV infection that is resolving.

However, care must be taken with interpreting EBV antibody concentrations because the amount of antibody present does not correlate with the severity of the infection or with the length of time it will last. High levels of VCA-IgG may be present and may persist at that concentration for the rest of a person's life.

It's hard to know exactly what these results mean.

2. Prioritize and Plan

If you test positive or it's suspicious, you can try a course of antiviral medication like acyclovir. Consult your physician for recommendations. In my opinion, there is no real downside to a trial of this. It may not alter the test results, but it can sometimes really improve the symptoms.

If you don't want to use medication, then you can try an herbal formula. Consulting a qualified physician is recommended, but Bu Zhong Yi Qi Tang is again a good choice. You can add some of the herbs that treat EBV mentioned earlier: *Angelica sinensis,* chrysanthemum, citrus, lithosperum, milletia, paedria, or picrorhiza.

(Citrus and *Angelica sinensis* are already in the formula!)

Regarding diet, the spleen and stomach qi deficiency diet is recommended:

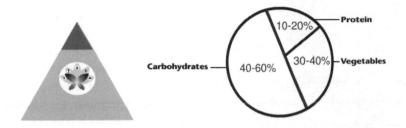

3. Act and Adapt

Try this approach for 30 to 60 days.

4. Reassess and Reevaluate

Retest and evaluate how you feel. Testing results may or may not change. How you feel is important.

5. Try and Try Again

Stick with the qi tonifying diet. Take a break from the formula or antiviral medication, as Epstein-Barr is a wily virus and it will adapt.

FOOD AS MEDICINE: **CLOVE**

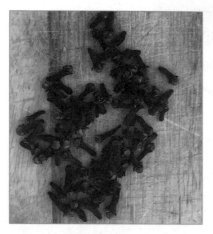

In Chinese medicine, clove is known as *ding xiang* or "spike fragrance," which is apt. It is considered acrid and warm, and it has an affinity for the kidney, spleen, and stomach.

Traditionally it is thought to warm the middle jiao, the area that encompasses the digestive system. Thus, it is used to treat a variety of digestive issues—for example, abdominal coldness and pain, vomiting, and hiccups.

It is also a yang tonic, and it tonifies kidney yang. Since hypothyroidism is considered, in some cases, yang deficiency, it can be helpful, especially in cold-type conditions.

Pharmacologically, clove is powerful.

- It increases bile and gastric acid secretions. It helps with vomiting, nausea, and belching. Drink one teaspoon of clove powder in warm water.

- It is a broad-spectrum antibiotic and has an inhibiting effect on a number of bacteria, including salmonella, *E. coli,* and staph infections. It also inhibits cholera and diphtheria. In addition, it has been shown to have antiviral properties, and it has been shown to be anti-EBV.

- It is a potent analgesic and is great applied topically for toothaches. Just chew it over the affected tooth.

Clove is not bad for cooking either—just saying. It's a versatile spice. I like it on winter squash, with duck, and on sweet potatoes. Hey, don't be afraid to use it. It tastes good, and what's more, it's good for you!

Chapter 18

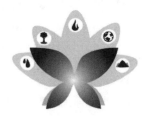

CANDIDIASIS

Candida or candidiasis is a common systemic infection that is sometimes an underlying problem with Hashimoto's patients. *Candida albicans* is the most common species. It is one of about 200 species of *Candida,* but it accounts for 75 percent of all Candida infections.[1]

It is a naturally occurring fungus in the body and one of those species that may actually have a symbiotic relationship with our guts when it's not out of control. Candida is thought to break down necrotic (dead) tissue in the digestive tract, and it may protect our digestive tract from other invaders.

We start to have problems when the balance with other microorganisms in the gut gets out of whack. The conventional Western medical approach to Candida is to not treat it unless it becomes manifest as a vaginal yeast infection or when immuno-compromised patients (like people suffering from HIV) develop it.

In the functional medical model, it is one of those underlying infections that is thought to lead to leaky gut, and it can be a player in the breakdown of the gut lining and gut mucosa, contributing to systemic problems such as autoimmunity and food sensitivities.

Some of the most common causes of Candida overgrowth is a history of antibiotic use, steroid use, oral contraception (birth control pills), recurrent vaginal yeast infections, and a diet high in sugar, alcohol, and/or refined carbohydrates.

Symptoms of Candida can be an awful lot like symptoms of Hashimoto's and hypothyroidism. These include:

- Brain fog or feeling spacey
- Fatigue
- Muscle soreness, heaviness or weakness, wandering pains
- Abdominal distention, bloating, or gas
- Chronic diarrhea or alternating constipation and diarrhea

- Depression, mood swings, anger, confusion, restlessness, disordered thought patterns
- Fluid retention
- Endometriosis
- Infertility
- Vaginal burning or itching
- Sinus congestion

TESTING

One way to check for Candida overgrowth is to test for it. It is commonly part of stool tests, and it can also be tested via urine or blood tests. I use a couple of different labs. Genova Diagnostics has a stool panel called GI Effects, and BioHealth Laboratory has a GI panel that also tests for it.

USE THE A.P.A.R.T. SYSTEM TO DIAGNOSE AND TREAT CANDIDA

1. Ask and Assess

Determine if you have the symptoms mentioned above. Get a stool test and see if you have Candida. If both are positive, do the following:

Try the damp heat diet and herbs to treat Candida, or do a course of pharmaceutical antifungal treatment such as nystatin or fluconazole. Personally, I'm not a big fan of conventional antifungal treatments because they are so hard on the liver. However, that's up to you and your practitioner.

2. Prioritize and Plan

If you choose to do the conventional treatment, do the damp heat diet during treatment, followed by the spleen qi and stomach qi deficient diet because antifungal medication is very cold and it will damage spleen and stomach qi.

If you choose to go the natural route, come with me, I'll show you what to do. First, the damp heat diet:

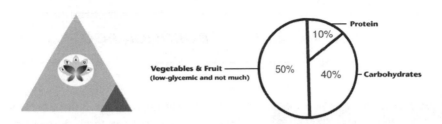

Regarding herbal formulas, there are two that I like. Yin Qiao San is a very popular formula that's easy to find, and research has found that it has broad-spectrum inhibitory effects on *Candida albicans*.[2]

The other, which I recommend for the vaginal-discharge type of Candida, may require that you consult an herbalist because it is harder to find. I know of one (that would be me). This is really effective for clearing damp heat in the lower jiao, which is another way of saying the urinary tract.

It's called Wan Dai Tang, and it has the following herbs: bai zhu, shan yao, ren shen, cang zhu, chen pi, che qian zi, bai shao, chai hu, jing jie, and gan cao. You might notice it has a lot of the herbs that are also in Bu Zhong Yi Qi Tang. Both formulas are effective in treating mucus and phlegm.

In addition, the following herbs kill Candida: melia, huang bai, psuedolaricis, huang qin, sophora, and subprostrata.[3]

3. Act and Adapt

Follow the instructions and see what happens.

4. Reassess and Reevaluate

Check on your symptoms and do another stool test. If you have improvement, return to the spleen and stomach qi deficient diet.

If it didn't work, consult a physician or someone who is experienced in treating Candida.

5. Try and Try Again

Make diet and lifestyle changes so that you don't encourage the return of damp heat and Candida (avoid refined sugar and carbohydrates). And follow the spleen and stomach qi diet.

FOOD AS MEDICINE: **BURDOCK ROOT**

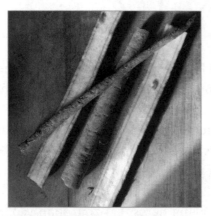

When I was a kid growing up in upstate New York and running like a madman through the fields, one plant that would often return home with me was burdock.

Its burs stick to your clothing like nothing else, and my mother was not happy with me when I came home covered in them.

This plant is one of those quiet heroes in the realm of remedies, as it doesn't do a lot that's dramatic, but it is remarkably effective. It covers a whole bunch of territory with equal success.

And it certainly excels in liver and gallbladder issues, which (if you've been paying attention) we have previously discussed.

Burdock root is kind of tough and is considered somewhat bitter and pungent, cool, dry, dissolving, stimulating, and restoring. In Japanese cuisine it is sometimes served as a side dish called gobo, and it's delicious.

Burdock root promotes detoxification, resolves damp, and dissolves deposits (yes, gallstones). It can also relieve eczema and irritation. So it helps detoxify internally and is fantastic for your skin.

It clears toxic heat and reduces infections and inflammation. It has a balancing effect on the immune system and can be helpful in reducing allergic reactions. It is rich in inulin and can also be beneficial for diabetes.

Burdock root is effective in treating urinary tract issues and was traditionally used to treat incontinence. It also promotes sweating and can be helpful in treating early onset colds and flus.

For those of us with poor gallbladder function, burdock root is effective for stimulating digestion, promoting bile flow, and relieving fullness.

Finally, it benefits the skin and hair and can promote tissue repair. It's effective for treating wounds and ulcers (like herpes).

This is truly an amazing herb! In Chinese medicine the seeds are also used, and they have a stronger ability to promote sweating and resolve upper respiratory infections than the root.

The root's polysaccharides are helpful in immune modulation, proving that you can effectively use more than one part of an herb to get even better results. Don't you just love it? (I do, geeking out right about now.)

Chapter 19

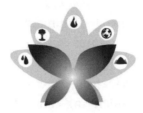

BLASTOCYSTIS HOMINIS

One digestive infection that is not as well known as some of the others is *Blastocystis hominis* or, as I like to affectionately call it, "Blasto." It is a parasite that's very common in our guts. It's considered the most common parasitic infection in the United States and infects an estimated 23 percent of the population.[1]

Blasto is interesting because it seems to overlap a number of other conditions. Leaky gut, hives, and Epstein-Barr virus all have links to it. It's not surprising, as all three are quite common among people with Hashimoto's.

There are a lot of studies linking autoimmune thyroid disease and hives.[2] I don't know if you've ever had them. I have and they are super itchy; they can cover your whole body and come and go randomly. No fun.

Hives are also often linked to histamine intolerance. And this is quite common with people with Hashimoto's. (I have devoted a chapter to this in Part III.) Research has shown that anywhere between 45 and 55 percent of people with chronic idiopathic urticaria (a chronic unknown form of hives) already have some kind of autoimmune condition.[3]

One theory about how this might happen involves people with Hashimoto's making antibodies to IgE anti-TPO antibodies. These bind to immune cells (mast cells and basophils) and trigger an autoallergic reaction. So the immune system attacking the thyroid actually triggers a secondary autoimmune allergic response!

We've also seen the link between autoimmunity and leaky gut. Hashimoto's is, of course, an autoimmune disease. And we have seen the possible links between Epstein-Barr and Hashimoto's. One theory about the link between Blasto and Epstein-Barr is that the virus feeds on arginine, and this amino acid can help suppress Blasto.

A 2015 article in *The Journal of Infection in Developing Countries* titled "Eradication of Blastocystis Hominis Prevents the Development of Symptomatic Hashimoto's Thyroiditis" reported on common root causes of Hashimoto's, hives, and irritable bowel syndrome (IBS).[4]

The researchers stated that evidence suggested the three commonly associated conditions may have the same underlying cause. Some recent case studies showed that infection with Blasto was linked to chronic hives, and one study found that it was present in 60.6 percent of patients affected by chronic hives. One clinical pilot study of a link between the parasite and IBS found that *Blastocystis hominis* was increased in all IBS patients.

The research revealed that killing the parasite often led to the remission of symptoms of chronic hives and IBS that commonly occur with Hashimoto's. It also showed that this treatment resulted in improvements in Hashimoto's. So, it may be possible to improve all three conditions at once.

Let's take a look at how we can treat Blasto.

USING THE A.P.A.R.T. SYSTEM TO DIAGNOSE AND TREAT BLASTO

1. Ask and Assess

First we want to test for Blasto. Stool tests are available although one problem in detecting it is that it can take on different forms in its life cycle. Stool tests look for the parasite and its eggs. Endoscopy is another, more invasive way of looking for it. Finally, blood tests for Blasto are now available, though they aren't commonly ordered.

Common symptoms include:

- Diarrhea

- Nausea

- Abdominal cramps

- Bloating

- Gas

- Hives

- Loss of appetite

- Fatigue

2. Prioritize and Plan

Again, as with other conditions we have seen, there's the conventional pharmaceutical route or a natural approach.

According to Dr. Izabella Wentz, pharmaceutical treatment includes:[5]

- Triple therapy used in Australia: diloxanide furoate, trimethoprim/sulfamethoxazole, and secnidazole* OR

- Alinia for three days on, then off for two weeks, repeated twice*

Dr. Wentz notes: "The key is to use these treatments long enough, or in a pulsed fashion to fully eradicate Blasto. Blasto can take on four different forms during its lifecycle, and some of the forms are resistant to treatment.

"*Keep in mind that antiprotozoal medications can lead to a yeast overgrowth, and a treatment with anti-yeast herbs or a medication like Nystatin may be necessary to rebalance the gut."

I think by now you know my feelings about conventional treatment. Let's look at an alternative approach.

According to the Blastocystis Research Foundation, "Some patients are able to manage symptoms with an extensive exclusion diet, which may include exclusion of refined sugar, wheat, dairy products, rice, corn, carbonated drinks, tea, coffee, alcohol, and fruit."[6]

This is, essentially, the autoimmune paleo approach we have already looked at in depth. Let's take a look at some natural treatment options.

Here are some Chinese herbs that are effective in treating Blasto: mume, anemone pulsatilla, crategus, agrimonia, artemesia apiacea, coptis, phellodendron, scutellaria, sophora root, melia, portuclaca, rhubarb, cinnamon bark, torreya, granatum, areca, and blechnum.[7]

In addition, oil of oregano may be effective.

H. pylori, a bacteria that can cause problems in the stomach and intestines, can be present at the same time as Blastocystis. Some of the herbal treatments I have recommended can treat both infections simultaneously.

3. Act and Adapt

Do whatever it is you decide to do. Go the conventional route, or join me and Li Dong-yuan in the traditional route.

Parasites are considered a Gu syndrome. So the diet for that is a damp heat diet.

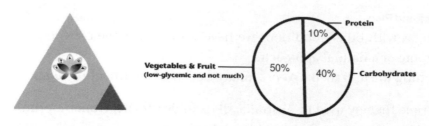

4. Reassess and Reevaluate

Try your approach and retest. And assess whether or not you have improvement with your symptoms.

If you do, celebrate and go back to the spleen and stomach qi deficient diet.

If you have no improvement, seek professional advice. I'm here for you.

5. Try and Try Again

Hopefully, by now, you know where we're going with this. A spleen and stomach supporting diet is our default return. It's the gift that keeps on giving. Don't abandon it.

FOOD AS MEDICINE: **COCONUT**

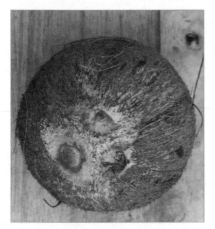

In Chinese medicine, the coconut is considered warm and sweet. It strengthens the body, reduces swelling, stops bleeding, kills worms, and activates heart function.

It was used traditionally to treat edema, weakness, nosebleeds, and intestinal and/or skin worms.

Traditional remedies include:

• For worms: Every morning on an empty stomach, drink the juice and eat the meat of half a coconut; wait three hours before eating anything else.

• For edema due to a weak heart: Drink lots of coconut juice.

Of course, coconut oil has many benefits as well.

It can be helpful with weight loss because it contains medium chain triglycerides that are metabolized differently from other oils. It can raise your good cholesterol (HDL). And it has broad-spectrum antiviral, antibacterial, and antifungal properties because it contains auric acid, capris acid, and caprylic acid.

Coconut oil is also helpful for magnesium and calcium absorption and for balancing blood sugar. Topically, it's great for both your hair and skin.

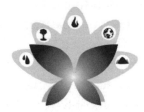

Chapter 20

HELICOBACTER PYLORI (H. PYLORI)

Helicobacter pylori (H. pylori) is a bacteria found in or attached to the gastric mucosa layer of the stomach. It causes more than 90 percent of duodenal ulcers, and up to 80 percent of gastric ulcers.[1]

It can damage the stomach lining by releasing an enzyme called urease, which produces ammonia. Ammonia is very basic, so it neutralizes stomach acid. *H. pylori* can contribute to low stomach acid, which, as we have seen, is also a common problem among those with hypothyroidism and Hashimoto's. If you have both conditions, it can compound the problem.

The problem with too little stomach acid is that food doesn't get broken down properly. And even though it's counterintuitive, this can actually lead to symptoms of acid reflux and heartburn, because the food can back up and cause acid to leak into the lower esophagus.

Too little stomach acid can also damage cells in the gut downstream from the stomach, leading to leaky gut. In addition, when food doesn't get broken down properly, the proteins (or amino acid fragments of proteins) can cause immune system activation. This is how food sensitivities develop.

H. pylori is a naturally occurring bacteria, and some researchers believe it plays a beneficial role when it is kept in balance. Testing is often required to find it, as people can have the bacteria and not have any symptoms.

If an ulcer or acid reflux that is caused by *H. pylori* is treated with a medication that suppresses stomach acid (like a proton pump inhibitor), symptoms may be temporarily relieved but will come back because the root cause has not been addressed.

H. pylori is transmitted from person to person or even from pets via saliva. If you test positive, it is a good idea to test your partner. Sometimes you have to treat the whole family or the infection may be passed back and forth again.

H. pylori can also be contracted by eating contaminated foods or fluids and from poor hygiene (yet another reason to wash your hands). Researchers believe that most people infected with *H. pylori* probably got infected through the mouth during childhood.[2]

H. PYLORI INFECTION AND THYROID ANTIBODIES

In the medical literature there is some conflicting information about the correlation between Hashimoto's and *H. pylori* infection.

On the one hand, there are a number of studies that suggest that *H. pylori* infections and Hashimoto's have a significant connection. In a meta-analysis published in 2017 that looked at more than 15,000 cases, patients with autoimmune thyroiditis were more susceptible to *H. pylori* infections, especially the C-agA positive strain of the bacteria (this strain is common in non-ulcer type infections).[3]

Another study showed that people with a high titer of Anti-TPO Ab were significantly affected by *H. pylori,* and treating and eradicating the bacteria caused a significant reduction in TPO and TgAb antibody levels.[4] So if you have high antibodies (700 or more), it is worth testing and treating the bacteria if you find it.

In contrast, a different study published in 2016 could not find a definite correlation between *H. pylori* and Hashimoto's. In this study they looked at 201 women; half had been diagnosed with Hashimoto's, and the other half, the control group, had not. The authors acknowledged that some of the women in the control group were hypothyroid and could have had Hashimoto's. In addition both the control group and the group with Hashimoto's had about a 45 percent rate of infection.[5]

In my opinion, in spite of this study there clearly is evidence of a connection to thyroid autoimmunity (the correlation may be stronger to Graves' disease) and *H. pylori*, so testing for it and treating it may not only help your stomach symptoms (if you have them), it may also help your Hashimoto's and reduce antibody levels.[6]

PARIETAL CELL ANTIBODIES (PCA) AND *H. PYLORI*

An additional place where there is a connection to both Hashimoto's and *H. pylori* is another autoimmune disease in which the immune system attacks cells in the stomach called parietal cells. Parietal cells are responsible for producing intrinsic factor, which is necessary for the absorption of vitamin B12.

This condition was previously reported to affect 10 to 40 percent of people with Hashimoto's. A 2014 study looked at the co-occurring rates of parietal cell antibodies in people with Hashimoto's; this study was conducted to examine this autoimmune disease because it can adversely affect absorption of thyroid hormone.[7]

It was found that about 34 percent of patients with autoimmune thyroid disease had PCA, and this can contribute to both poor absorption of thyroid hormone and anemia.

Another study found autoimmune gastritis (AIG) to be present in a third of people with autoimmune thyroid disease. AIG can cause low stomach acid. Anti-parietal cell antibodies were correlated with TPO antibodies, and parietal cell antigens in the stomach are very similar to the thyroid peroxidase enzyme.[8]

I think that's another important point regarding *H. pylori,* PCA, and hypothyroidism. All three can result in low stomach acid. So it's a fair question to ask whether or not the low stomach acid caused by hypothyroidism could have created an environment in the stomach that promotes the overgrowth of *H. pylori.*

It's a kind of like the "chicken or the egg" situation where one condition may lead to another. This emphasizes the importance of having proper levels of stomach acid. And this goes back to what we learned from Li Dong-yuan—that proper stomach qi is essential to protect the body from a myriad of diseases.

USING THE A.P.A.R.T. SYSTEM TO DIAGNOSE AND TREAT *H. PYLORI*

1. Ask and Assess

Hopefully by now you know my MO (modus operandi). Test first! In this case, obviously, you will test for *H. pylori.*

TESTING FOR *H. PYLORI*:

There are a several different tests for *H. Pylori,* including blood tests, breath tests, and stool tests. In my opinion, the best is a stool antigen test. For my clients I order a GI Pathogen Screen with *H. pylori* Antigen from BioHealth Labs.

The reason I prefer the stool antigen test is because it tests for *H. pylori* as well as other pathogens like parasites and Candida. In testing for *H. pylori,* you might discover other infections as well. This test must be ordered by a physician.

Next, ask if you have any symptoms of *H. pylori* infection.

COMMON SYMPTOMS OF *H. PYLORI* INFECTIONS:

- An ache or burning pain in your abdomen
- Bloating
- Loss of appetite
- Nausea
- Frequent burping
- Unintentional weight loss

2. Prioritize and Plan

Now depending on what the testing and symptoms tell you, create a plan to treat it. Yup, this is how we roll. First, diet. What's your guess?

Think about it. *H. pylori* attacks the stomach. What have we learned? The Earth phase is the spleen and stomach.

Based on these symptoms, the best diet is the spleen and stomach deficiency diet:

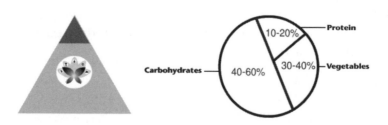

In addition, herbs that eradicate *H. pylori* include Sophora root, saussurea, corydalis, *Curcuma longa,* licorice, magnolia bark, lonicera, peony, forsythia.[9]

You know, sometimes in Chinese medicine (and in life) you can find elegant and simple solutions to problems—if you know where to look for them. There happens to be such a formula for treating *H. pylori* called Zuo Jin Wan.

It's just two herbs: huang lian and wu zhu yu. We've seen huang lian already in this narrative. It's rich in berberine, a natural antibiotic. Wu zhu yu addresses the liver. This is the Wood phase attacking the Earth phase. It's liver qi stagnation leading to stomach heat.

What does that tell us? There's an emotional component to *H. pylori.* Why? I do not know, but it is true. Research has demonstrated that Zuo Jin Wan was associated with successful treatment of *H. pylori* in 86 of 133 patients (that's 64.7 percent for those of you keeping score).[10]

Another natural supplement that is successful in treating *H. pylori* is mastic gum. I recommend 500 mg: take two capsules three times per day (breakfast, lunch, and dinner).

Also the probiotic *S. boulardii*: two to three times per day.

While it's ultimately up to you and your practitioner as to the right protocol to choose, I generally advise trying the natural approach first. Call me crazy, or call me practical.

Another thing I have found helpful is cabbage juice, as it's rich in glutamine that can help support gut healing and suppress the *H. pylori* bacteria, promoting healing.

3. Act and Adapt

Do what you want to do. But may I suggest you follow my recommendations?

4. Reassess and Reevaluate

Retest *H. pylori.* If it is resolved, go back to the spleen and stomach supporting diet. If it is not resolved, consult a physician or practitioner who has experience in treating *H. pylori.*

5. Try and Try Again

Get back to the spleen and stomach supporting diet. It's where we always return to.

FOOD AS MEDICINE: **MOLASSES**

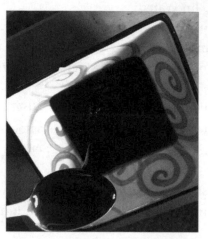

I've always loved molasses. My favorite cookies at Christmastime were always molasses cookies, and my mother made the most delicious recipe. With milk they were just heavenly. Now I make them with gluten-free flour and coconut milk.

Molasses is considered warm and sweet.

It tonifies qi, strengthens the spleen, lubricates the lungs, and stops cough. It is used to treat stomach and abdominal pain, qi deficiency, and cough.

For cough, dice carrots. Mix with molasses and leave overnight; take 2 teaspoons three times daily.

For stomach ulcers, take 2 teaspoons in warm water to stop the pain.

Chapter 21

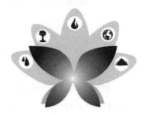

LYME DISEASE

While Lyme disease is not normally associated with digestive complaints, it is a Gu syndrome and can be a common underlying disease that can impact people with Hashimoto's.

Moreover, the long courses of treatment with antibiotics that are often prescribed to treat Lyme can really do a number on the digestive system. So let's take a look at Lyme disease and also look at what to do if you've had conventional Lyme treatment.

Lyme disease is a spirochetal inflammatory disorder caused by a bacteria of the *Borrelia* type transmitted by ticks. It begins with a distinctive rash called erythema migrans that may be followed by neurological, joint, and cardiovascular issues. It was first recognized in 1975 in Lyme, Connecticut, and has since been reported in 49 states with 90 percent of the cases occurring from Massachusetts to Maryland and in Wisconsin, Minnesota, California, and Oregon. It also occurs in Europe, Russia, China, and Japan.[1]

Western treatment for Lyme disease is antibiotic therapy. This can last anywhere from 21 to 30 days. Aspirin and NSAIDs are also often prescribed to relieve pain. This can result in damage to the spleen and stomach qi and can cause major digestive issues.

USE THE A.P.A.R.T. SYSTEM TO DIAGNOSE AND TREAT LYME DISEASE

1. Ask and Assess

There are five groups of symptoms for Lyme disease. These include:

1. The hallmark symptom is a red rash that appears between the 3rd and the 32nd day of being bitten by a tick. About 25 percent of people don't develop a rash. The red area usually expands; soon after about 50 percent of people develop additional, smaller red lesions.

2. The second group of symptoms are flu-like, including fatigue, chills, fever, malaise, headache, stiff neck, and muscle and joint pain. These symptoms usually come and go, and yet some can linger for weeks (especially the fatigue and malaise).

3. The third group of symptoms are neurological in nature. These can affect the brain and cause inflammation in the brain. About 15 percent of those infected experience this.

4. The fourth group of symptoms affect the heart. These can cause myocardial abnormalities such as conduction issues that can impact normal heart rhythms. These affect about 8 percent of patients.

5. The final group of symptoms cause arthritis and joint-related issues. About 60 percent of people with Lyme disease develop swelling and pain in the large joints, especially the knees. Joints can get painful and swollen, but not usually red.

Testing for Lyme disease is very controversial. Frequently, inconclusive Lyme disease test results will result in large doses of antibiotic therapy.

This type of treatment, I hope you have realized by now, results in major trauma to the microbiota. And in my way of looking at things, that can be an outcome that leaves people with more complications than it resolves.

So we need a clear head here. Lyme disease is a serious infection, but overzealous treatment is not good, either. Let's be smart and try a gentler approach. First, let's try the nonnuclear option. It's important not to let fear govern your decision-making process.

2. Prioritize and Plan

Okay, there are a ton of herbs that treat the bacteria that leads to Lyme disease (*Borrelia*) and these include stepahnia, forsythia, dandelion, clematis, acanthopanax, smilax, portulaca, lonicera, akebia, siler, *Gentiana macrophylla*, gardenia, phelloden- dron, scutellaria, istatis root, salvia, lycopodium, stemona, loranthus, andrographis, coptis, pyloria, coix, baphicanthes, anemone pulsatilla, artemesia apiacea, sophora root, *Chrysanthemum indicum*, sophora flower, tricsanthes root, lonicera stem, and picrorhiza.[2]

There are a couple of formulas that are quite effective for treating Lyme disease, but first we have to figure out whether the disease is acute or recent, or chronic and long term:

Acute: If it's a recent exposure, Bob Flaws and Philippe Sionneau recommend (in their book *The Treatment of Modern Western Medical Diseases with Chinese Medicine*) that you try Wu Wei Xiao Du Yin. This formula has the following herbs: dandelion, honeysuckle flower, zi hua di ding, poria fungus, che qian zi, chrysanthemum flower, Niu xi, Tian kui zi.[3]

Chronic: This is a more difficult decision because there may be different degrees of inflammation and deficiency. This may be one area where you need to consult with someone with experience in treating Lyme disease.

That being said, one formula called Tuo Li San Jia Jian has a balanced heat- clearing/pathogen-killing attack as well as some gentle support. This formula con- tains the following herbs: uncooked rehmannia root, astragalus, honeysuckle flower, ophiopogonis root, qiang huo, fang feng, dang gui, scutellaria, codonopsis, zhu ling, mu gua, achyranthis root, huang bai, zhi zi, citrus peel, licorice root, and huang lian.[4]

Notice that the herbs huang qin, huang bai, and huang lian are also part of this for- mula. These all contain berberine compounds, which are potent antibacterial agents.

3. Act and Adapt

For the diet, again you have two options. If you elect to do antibiotic therapy, then a spleen and stomach qi (and possibly yang) deficient diet must follow the rehabilita- tion process.

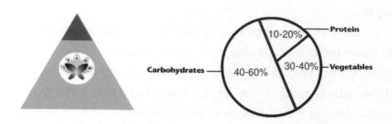

Probiotics and butyrate are also recommended supplements.

If you elect to go the natural route, a damp heat–clearing diet is recommended with the herbal treatment followed by the spleen and stomach qi deficient diet.

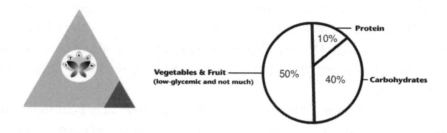

4. Reassess and Reevaluate

Try your approach and retest. Assess whether or not you have improvement with your symptoms.

If you do, celebrate and go back to the spleen and stomach qi deficient diet.

If you have no improvement, seek professional advice.

5. Try and Try Again

A spleen and stomach supporting diet is our default return. It's what we should always return to.

FOOD AS MEDICINE: **HAWTHORN BERRY**

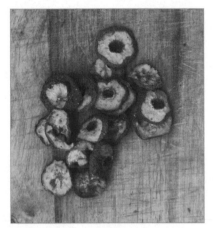

Hawthorn berry is a fruit that has a long tradition in both Chinese medicine and in Western herbalism. And it was used differently in both traditions. In TCM it is known for its digestive properties helping to alleviate indigestion and relieve food stagnation (especially from eating meat). In Western herbal medicine, it is a potent cardio tonic.

Austrian researchers have found that hawthorn actually decreases fat acids and lactic acid by stimulating digestive enzymes.

It's very beneficial for the heart. Both the berry and the flowers can be used. It tonifies heart qi, vitalizes heart blood, and strengthens the heart.

It is considered sweet, sour, and astringent. It's nourishing, restoring, calming, astringing, softening, and dissolving.

Hawthorn berries can also tonify heart yin and promote rest. They're a mild treatment for insomnia, palpitations, and anxiety.

It also promotes urination and drains water, making it a good remedy for cardiac edema.

It's nourishing for heart muscle and is slightly stimulating, which makes its overall impact on the whole cardiovascular system a positive one. It can also help reduce atherosclerosis. From a Western viewpoint, it is one of the leading remedies for essential hypertension and can be helpful in regulating heartbeat in arrhythmias and tachycardia.

It's pretty mild and nontoxic—even in high doses—so it can be taken regularly.

It's usually prepared with a decoction or tincture. You can simply soak hawthorn berries in vodka to make a tincture.

The best and most potent application is the fresh juice of hawthorn berries. The freeze-dried extract is also good. Functional heart disorders tend to respond more quickly than organic and degenerative heart disorders. Because it is mild, the treatment should be two months at minimum.

This is truly an herb that the fire element loves!

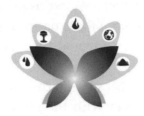

Chapter 22

YERSINIA ENTEROCOLITICA

Yersinia enterocolitica is a bacteria that causes yersiniosis. It is usually caused by eating raw or undercooked meat (usually pork), or by drinking contaminated water or unpasteurized milk or milk products. It is also possible to get the infection from another person if they don't thoroughly wash their hands before preparing food.

You can also get yersiniosis from a blood transfusion. And some animals are carriers, including cats, dogs, birds, deer, rodents, rabbits, sheep, cattle, and horses. Children can get infected if they put their hands in their mouth after playing with an infected puppy or kitten. About 117,000 people every year in the U.S. get the Yersinia infection.[1]

Yersinia is similar to food poisoning and generally affects the intestines.
Common symptoms include:

- Fever that usually lasts three to seven days

- Diarrhea (usually watery or bloody)

- Abdominal pain (Yersinia can also cause right-sided abdominal pain that may be confused for appendicitis.)

A skin rash called erythema nodosum (red or purple lesions) is sometimes present 2 to 20 days after infection mainly on the legs and torso in women, but it usually resolves on its own within a month.

Joint pain can also develop, which can last from one to six months. This is called reactive arthritis. *Yersinia enterocolitica* feeds on iron, so infection could be problematic if someone has iron deficiency anemia. It could make replenishing iron stores more difficult.

There are a number of studies that support the connection between *Yersinia enterocolitica* and Hashimoto's.[2] As we saw with the Epstein-Barr virus, one theory about why certain infections lead to autoimmunity is molecular mimicry.

This happens when your immune system targets the bacteria and mistakes it for your own body tissue such as the thyroid gland. As long as the infection is active in your body, your immune system will continue to attack the thyroid gland.

Yersinia has also been linked to Graves' disease, which, as you probably know, is another form of autoimmune thyroid disease.

USING THE A.P.A.R.T. SYSTEM TO DIAGNOSE AND TREAT YERSINIA

1. Ask and Assess

Check to see if you have any of the symptoms described above and test for the infection.

The most common test for Yersinia is a stool test. It is usually positive two weeks after the initial infection. Blood tests are also sometimes ordered with symptoms like colitis and reactive arthritis. IgG and IgA antibodies are commonly tested. These are also helpful for identifying chronic infections that didn't resolve on their own.

2. Prioritize and Plan

Yersinia is usually mild and self-limiting, meaning it resolves itself.

If Yersinia comes back positive in a stool analysis, it is most commonly treated conventionally with antibiotics.

Broad-spectrum antibiotic herbs like those we have seen that are rich in berberine (huang qin, huang bai, huang lian) can be quite effective in treating Yersinia. The formula that I mentioned previously, Huang lian jie du tang, is an excellent choice.

Oil of oregano and grapefruit seed extract can also be effective.

3. Act and Adapt

If you decide to take antibiotic or herbal antibiotics, do so for two to three weeks. Once you have completed treating the bacteria, employ the spleen and stomach qi (and possibly yang) tonifying diet.

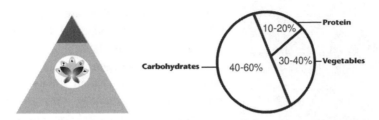

Probiotics and butyrate are also recommended supplements.

4. Reassess and Reevaluate

Try your approach and retest. Assess whether or not you have improvement with your symptoms. If stool or blood test was positive, retest to determine whether or not you still have the infection.

If you don't and symptoms have improved, celebrate and go back to the spleen and stomach qi deficient diet.

If you have no improvement, seek professional advice.

5. Try and Try Again

A spleen and stomach supporting diet is our default return. Once again, it's what we should always return to.

In this next section of the book, I have provided you with treatment options for a variety of common symptoms and conditions. Many of these can have multiple causes. So it's important for you to use the A.P.A.R.T. System to determine which scenario might be yours (and I have provided you with solutions for each possible scenario as well).

FOOD AS MEDICINE: **CHINESE DATE (RED OR BLACK JUJUBE)**

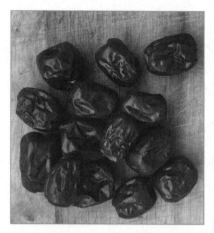

Chinese dates can be found in farmers markets and Asian markets when they are in season. They are delicious both fresh and dried, and they're not as sweet as conventional dates.

In Chinese medicine, they are considered neutral and sweet, and have an affinity for the spleen and stomach. Traditionally, they are thought to strengthen the spleen, tonify yin, nourish the body, lubricate the lungs, stop cough, and stop diarrhea. They are used to harmonize or make herbal formulas more palatable.

Chinese dates are used with yin deficient conditions, weak digestion, cough, night sweats, weakness, anemia, blood in the urine, bruises, and anxiety.

Pharmacologically they have been found to protect the liver, have anticancer properties, and are mildly sedating.

Combine with fresh ginger in a tea to treat a mild to moderate cold.

Make a tea from dried dates or eat fresh ones to help resolve diarrhea.

PART III

Using Diet to Treat
COMMON COMPLAINTS

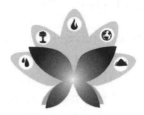

Chapter 23

GINGIVITIS/PERIODONTAL DISEASE

Gingivitis and periodontal disease are conditions involving inflammation or degeneration of the gums and the tissue that support the teeth. Usually it begins as gingivitis and then progresses into periodontitis.

It is actually an autoimmune disease triggered by infectious organisms and an abnormal response to collagen. In addition, there is evidence that it is more common among people with other autoimmune diseases.[1]

The inflammation and tissue destruction is caused by the immune system attacking bacterial plaque. Bleeding gums when brushing or flossing is one of the first signs of the disorder. The gums may also appear swollen and recede from the teeth.

If left untreated the disease can progress, and affected gums can separate from the teeth, causing periodontal pockets to form. Ultimately, if left unchecked large portions of the gums are destroyed, and the bones surrounding the roots can deteriorate and abscesses form.

Several bacteria and some viruses have been linked to periodontal disease. *P. gingivalis* and *A. actinolycetemcomitans* are both responsible for aggressive periodontal disease. *P. gingivalis* produces an enzyme that may disrupt immune function and lead to tissue destruction.

Beside bacteria, a number of herpes viruses have been implicated in periodontal autoimmune disease. These include herpes simplex, cytomegalovirus, and Epstein-Barr virus. Antibodies to collagen have been found to be more common in people with existing autoimmune diseases.

HASHIMOTO'S AND PERIODONTITIS

Researchers have looked into the links between Hashimoto's and periodontal disease. They did so because they noted that people with Hashimoto's did not respond to treatment in the same way that other people did.[2]

There are a couple of theories as to why. First, hypothyroidism can cause diminished circulation, particularly in very small blood vessels like capillaries. These capillaries in the gums are important for the defense of that tissue. This coupled with the low-grade inflammation that is a constant part of Hashimoto's can result in damage to the gums.

A number of other factors such as delayed wound healing, slower than normal salivary secretion, poor periodontal health in general, and osteoarthritis of the temporomandibular joint have all been found.

Those same researchers have also found that decreased levels of thyroid hormones may make periodontitis-related bone loss worse, as a function of an increased number of resorbing cells, whereas, the tooth-supporting alveolar bone seems to be less sensitive to alterations in hormone levels.

Stress is also a factor in periodontal disease and, as we all know, emotional stress and physiological stress are hallmarks of Hashimoto's.

WESTERN MEDICAL CAUSES

Western medical causes of gingivitis and periodontitis include:[3]

- Diabetes
- Smoking
- Stress
- Genetic vulnerability
- Poor oral hygiene and buildup of plaque on the teeth
- HIV infection
- Fungal, bacterial, or viral infections (i.e., Candida, herpes, and streptococcal)
- Malnutrition
- Osteoporosis
- Trauma
- Heavy metals
- Medications: dilantin, cyclosporine, calcium channel blockers, or any medication that reduces saliva secretion

CHINESE MEDICINE CAUSES

In Chinese medicine the mouth is under the sphere of influence of the Earth, Fire, and Water phases, specifically the spleen and stomach, heart and kidney.

The mouth itself is thought to be governed by the spleen, especially the lips and cheeks. As we have seen, microcirculation is important for gum health and the spleen governs the blood. The health of spleen blood can be seen in the color of the lips, and the state of fluid metabolism can be seen in the tongue and cheeks. The spleen channel spreads out over the top surface of the tongue.

The gums are thought to be governed by the stomach both via the stomach meridian and directly via the organ system. Heat and/or dryness in the stomach can damage the gums. Two common patterns related to gingivitis and periodontitis are yin deficiency and stomach heat.

The tongue is considered the sprout of the heart and mouth; ulcers on the tongue are attributed to heart fire or heart yin deficiency (which can turn into heat).

The teeth are thought to be under the sphere of influence of the kidneys, as the kidneys govern the bones. Kidney jing is responsible for healthy teeth and bones. Loose or easily chipped or broken teeth can be a sign of kidney weakness.

While not directly affecting the mouth, the liver channel encircles the inside of the lips. And, as we have seen, liver qi stagnation can lead to heat, which can affect the heart through the mother/son relationship and the stomach and spleen through the controlling cycle.

SYMPTOMS

The main symptoms of gingivitis are:

- Red, inflamed gum tissue at the base of the teeth
- Swelling and bleeding with flossing or brushing

As it progresses to periodontitis, the symptoms are:

- Deepening pockets between the gums and the teeth
- Enlarged calcium deposits
- Loss of attachment of the gums, teeth, and supporting bone

USING THE A.P.A.R.T. SYSTEM TO TREAT GINGIVITIS AND PERIODONTITIS:

1. ASK AND ASSESS

From a Chinese medicine perspective, there are a couple of different scenarios that can lead to this condition. The first involves heat or fire in the stomach, and the second involves qi and blood deficiency.[4]

So once again, ask the question, "Is it excess or deficiency?"

Let's start with the excess pattern.

Stomach heat is most often associated with diet. Eating too many spicy, hot foods and drinks or overconsumption of hot herbs can lead to this. Liver fire caused by stagnation in the liver is another possible cause. This tends to be a chronic condition.

Symptoms of stomach heat/fire include:

- Redness, swelling, and pain in the gums
- Bad breath, dry mouth, thirst, bad taste in the mouth
- Frontal headaches

- Ravenous, gnawing hunger
- Red face, red lips
- Tendency to be constipated
- Concentrated or dark urine
- Epigastric pain or discomfort

In contrast, the deficient pattern is more often associated with poor nutrition or malabsorption. Symptoms of qi and blood deficiency gum issues are:

- Atrophy of the gums revealing the roots of the teeth
- Pale gums and loose teeth that bleed easily with brushing, flossing, or even chewing
- Easy bruising

- Heavy menstruation
- Pale complexion, pale lips
- Loss of appetite
- Abdominal distention
- Fatigue, weakness, shortness of breath
- Insomnia, restless sleep
- Palpitations

2. PRIORITIZE AND PLAN

Decide which scenario best fits you. If you aren't sure, consult a practitioner to help you figure it out.

Obviously, the heat pattern requires a cooling diet and cooling herbs. The deficient pattern requires a spleen and stomach deficiency diet and herbs that nourish qi and blood. These are two very different approaches.

3. ACT AND ADAPT

Determine which dietary approach you are going to try. Review the symptoms above to make your decision. If you aren't sure, consult a practitioner.

HEAT AND/OR FIRE DIET

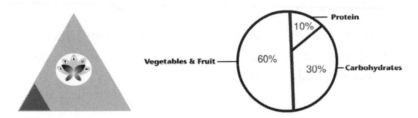

A good formula for stomach heat/fire is Qing wei san. It contains huang lian, sheng ma, mu dan pi, dang gui, and sheng ma. If the heat is very severe, you could use Huang lian jie du tang, the formula we have already discussed. If you are unsure, consult a practitioner.

Sometimes yin deficiency of the stomach and/or kidneys can also be at the root of this heat. In this case, you might have additional symptoms:

- Dryness of the mucous membranes
- Dizziness, blurred vision, or poor memory

- Night sweats
- Hot sensation in the face, palms, and soles
- Lower backache

In this case a formula called Yu nu jian is recommended. This formula contains shi gao, rehmannia, zhi mu, mai men dong, chuan niu xi, and nu zhen zi. Or try the Chinese formula called Lui wei di huang wan, which is helpful for oral tolerance (see Appendix 3).

As you can see, this can get complicated so be sure to consult with a practitioner if you are unsure and need help. But the basic cooling diet will help if you have a stomach heat/fire condition.

For the qi and blood deficiency scenario, the spleen and stomach qi deficiency diet is appropriate.

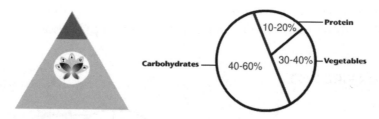

A good herbal formula for this condition is a Ba Zhen tang, which contains herbs that tonify both qi and blood. This formula contains rehmannia, codonopsis, dang gui, peony root, bai zhu, fu ling, chuan xiong, and gan cao.

4. REASSESS AND REEVALUATE

After trying one of the treatment options above for 15 to 30 days, review the symptoms and see if you have had improvement. If you have, celebrate and move back to or stay with the spleen and stomach deficiency diet.

If not, consult a practitioner.

5. TRY AND TRY AGAIN

Never give up and never lose hope. The solution is there, sometimes it just takes a little more digging.

FOOD AS MEDICINE: **AMERICAN GINSENG**

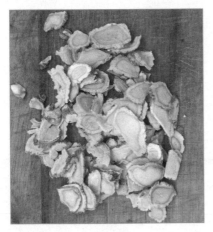

Make America Ginseng Again. That's the #MAGA I'm talking about.

This herb does so many good things.

In Chinese medicine ginseng tonifies qi and nourishes yin. So for deficient conditions, it covers most of the bases. It also clears fire and generates body fluids, making it the perfect antidote for yin fire. In addition, ginseng sedates heat in the intestines and stops bleeding.

Pharmacologically, American ginseng has been found to be a sedative to the central nervous system, making it helpful for resetting your circadian rhythms. And it was found to relieve fatigue, calm urgency to urinate, and increase resistance to hypoxia, which means it helps get more oxygen to your tissues.

And wait there's more . . . ginseng has been found to be effective in helping reduce side effects from both chemo and radiation therapy. It's always good to have that ace in your pocket. I mean, what are the odds that you get exposed to chemicals or radiation?

A good herbal combination for yin fire is American ginseng, fresh rehmannia, dendrobia, and schisandra. That will get your yin right.

Ginseng is also a great herb to make into flour and add to other flours that you bake with. It's sweet and much better for you than sugar.

Chapter 24

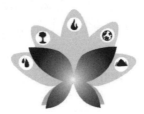

ABDOMINAL DISTENTION

Abdominal distention refers to a sense of discomfort, fullness, blockage, or obstruction felt anywhere in the abdomen (upper, lower, or across the whole abdomen).

When people speak about distention, they often use words like *bloating, fullness,* or *discomfort*. It's usually a subjective feeling of being uncomfortably full. It may also be accompanied by actual visible swelling of the abdomen; however, this is not always the case.

It can be localized to a specific part of the abdomen, and it can move around to different places. Distention is generally not felt with pain. It can also be acute or chronic.

Acute distention is usually caused by dietary choices or by food-borne pathogens like viruses or bacteria. Chronic distention can be caused by a number of things and is relatively common with Hashimoto's and hypothyroidism.

WESTERN MEDICAL CAUSES

Possible biomedical causes of abdominal distention include:[1]

- Anxiety and/or depression
- Chronic gastritis
- Chronic peptic ulcer
- Hiatal hernia
- Eating disorders
- PMS
- Chronic pancreatitis
- Chronic colitis
- Gallstones

- Hormone replacement therapy, oral contraception
- Hepatitis or cirrhosis
- Irritable bowel syndrome (IBS)
- Motility disorders: gastroparesis, intestinal pseudo obstruction, neuropathies, and myopathies

- Opiate medication
- Vagus nerve disorders
- Mesenteric artery insufficiency
- Cancer: gastric, pancreatic, colonic

CHINESE MEDICINE CAUSES

From a Chinese medicine perspective, there are three main mechanisms:

- Spleen and stomach qi deficiency
- Damp and/or phlegm accumulation/fluid retention
- Liver qi stagnation

In Chinese medicine there is also a term called "food stagnation" that is a common cause of abdominal distention. It's caused by diet or behaviors around eating. For example, eating too much or binging, eating irregularly, and eating at odd hours (especially at night) can all lead to this.

And as we have seen, if the spleen and stomach qi is compromised, then large, heavy meals are often very difficult to digest. This leads to obstruction in the gut and can also lead to constipation.

Too much cold or raw food can also weaken the spleen and stomach qi and lead to food stagnation. As can eating too much or eating too many rich foods or too many spicy, warming foods. This can lead to stagnation and to damp and/or damp heat conditions.

Food stagnation can also lead to other more chronic problems, especially in people just becoming accustomed to feelings of being bloated, belching, bad breath, and gas. Sometimes these symptoms are just so commonplace that we accept them as normal.

This is also a perfect example of one mechanism giving rise to others. If these symptoms are repeatedly ignored and the spleen and stomach are habitually overloaded, it can lead to inflammation in the gut and food lingering longer in the intestines where it rots and ferments.

This in turn can lead to more heat (more inflammation) as well as dampness and/or phlegm. As we have seen in the five-phase model, this can then spread to other systems. It can attack the cardiovascular system and become plaque or chest pain. It can affect the lungs and the skin and lead to cysts, swelling, sores, and even thyroid nodules.

It can affect the nervous system and lead to anxiety, insomnia, vertigo, tremors, and more. Heat or damp heat can also injure the intestines and intestinal lining and lead to leaky gut and stagnation of blood, which can cause polyps, tumors, and nodules.

EMOTION ALSO A BIG FACTOR (AGAIN)

This is another example of emotions playing a large role, especially in chronic distention. This is liver qi stagnation, and it can impact the abdomen in a number of different ways. From the five-phase model, we know that the Wood phase can invade the Earth phase and disrupt natural flow and activity.

When this happens the spleen's ability to process fluids can be compromised and fluids accumulate in the abdomen (in the form of excess mucus, for example). Or it can create dampness or phlegm as we have already seen. When these fluids stagnate they can easily transform into heat, and this can cause injury of yin or blood.

Liver qi stagnation is often caused by frustration, anger, resentment, and the repressing or not expressing of these emotions. And as we saw in the chapter on the brain and the gut, this has an impact on the HPA axis, as well as the smooth muscles of the gut.

People who have this kind of chronic qi stagnation in their gut often know that they store emotion in their gut in the form of stomach cramps, a "knot" in the stomach, loss of appetite over conflict, and bowel disturbances that are made worse by emotional upset.

This type of stagnation tends to come and go and is very much related to stress levels. In addition to those emotions mentioned above, feelings like worry, obsessive thinking, and prolonged studying or concentration in combination with a sedentary lifestyle and poor dietary choices can damage the spleen qi and this can set up an invasion of liver qi.

As we have so often noted, everything is connected and what the five-phase system teaches us is that everything also leads to everything else. Nothing is happening in a vacuum. Vicious cycles are real, and they cause and create other vicious cycles.

Another example of this is problems with the Metal phase. Emotions that affect the lung element like feelings of isolation, feelings of abandonment, or feelings of being an outsider can cause lung qi to stagnate and accumulate.

If you are like me or many of the people I have worked with, there may have been times when having Hashimoto's has left you feeling like an outsider.

Because many of us can't eat certain common foods like gluten and dairy, etc., it can make going out to dinner or going to family gatherings really difficult. And then there is the added anxiety of having to worry about being accidentally exposed to something and the fallout from that.

In addition, overwhelming fatigue can make the idea of doing something or going out feel like it's not worth all the effort. You might be concerned that you'll be wiped out for days afterward.

And then there is guilt added on top of that that you are lazy. Or that people think you're lazy. Even though you know you do a lot under the circumstances.

Sometimes you outwardly look okay, while you inwardly feel like crap. And you start to worry that people might think you are a hypochondriac or that you're making it up just to get attention.

Have you ever had any of those feelings?

I definitely have and as someone who is already kind of an introvert, it can all add up to making us feel isolated and alone. And these feelings sometimes harken back to deep-seated childhood memories and behavior.

If these feelings weaken the lung qi and they are exacerbated by lack of exercise, then this can affect the large intestine and cause stagnation and constipation. Lung disorders can cause people to hunch forward, slouch, and roll their shoulders internally in an effort to reflexively protect the lungs.

USE THE A.P.A.R.T. SYSTEM TO TREAT ABDOMINAL DISTENTION:

PROPER TREATMENT REQUIRES PROPER DIAGNOSIS

As you can see, abdominal distention can be the result of excess or deficiency or a combination of both as it has progressed through the five-phase system.

As always, we must first determine which is most predominate for you.

1. Ask and Assess

By now, you should know the drill. Is this caused by excess or deficiency?

Abdominal distention that's caused by deficiency means the whole digestive process is not working properly. This can include symptoms such as:

- Abdominal distention, fullness, and discomfort that decreases with warmth and pressure

- Distention worsening after eating raw or uncooked food

- Poor appetite

- Fatigue, muscle weakness

- Loose stools or a tendency for sluggish bowel movements

- Puffiness around the eyes or in the fingers

- Pale complexion and lips

- Shortness of breath, weak, low voice

If there is also yang deficiency, symptoms may include:

- Cold intolerance and cold extremities

- Diarrhea with undigested food in the stools

- Edema

In contrast, excess patterns include the following symptoms:

For liver qi stagnation type of distention:

- Abdominal distention, fullness, and discomfort that is worse with stress and emotional upset

- Acid reflux, heartburn

- Belching, lots of sighing, gas

- Discomfort in the hypochondriac region (just under the ribs, especially on the right)

- Loss of appetite, indigestion

- Alternating constipation and diarrhea

Damp heat abdominal distention includes:

- Distention in the upper abdomen
- Generally worse after eating
- Nausea
- Dry mouth
- Thirst, but no desire to drink
- Fullness and stuffiness in the chest
- Restlessness, irritability
- Red complexion
- Possibly strong body odor
- Heavy sensation in the body
- Loose stools or sluggish stools or constipation

2. Prioritize and Plan

Decide which pattern fits you. In the beginning of this chapter we identified three main mechanisms:

- Spleen and stomach qi deficiency
- Damp and/or phlegm accumulation/fluid retention
- Liver qi stagnation

3. Act and Adapt

Choose the appropriate diet for your scenario. See these below and the herbal formulas that are recommended with them.

For deficiency, this would be the spleen and stomach qi (and/or yang) deficiency diet (see pages 151 and 156).

For damp and phlegm, choose the damp heat diet (see page 166).

For liver qi stagnation, choose the liver qi stagnation diet (see page 163).

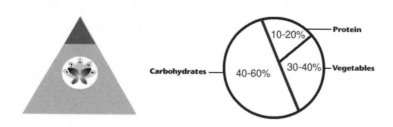

A good herbal formula for this type of distention is one we've already been introduced to: Li Dong-yuan's Bu Zhong Yi Qi Tang. This, if you recall, treats all three aspects of the Tummy Triangle in a balanced way.

If there is a lot of dampness or phlegm with the digestive weakness, another good formula is Xiang sha liu jun zi tang.[2] This formula more strongly tonifies qi and relieves stagnation. It includes codonopsis, bai zhu, fu ling, ban xia, citrus peel, sha ren, mu xiang, licorice root, cang zhu, and hou po.

In contrast the excess diet would be a liver qi stagnation or a damp heat resolving diet:

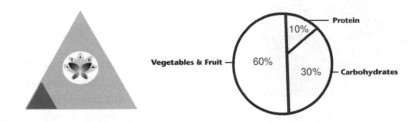

A good formula for this (especially with the emotional component of being uptight and irritable with muscle tension in the neck and upper back, cold fingers and toes, and tension headaches and achiness in the hypochondriac region) is called Chai hu shu gan san.[3]

This contains chai hu, bai shao, xiang fu, zhi zi, chuan xiong, and licorice root.

For damp heat distention, choose the damp heat diet:

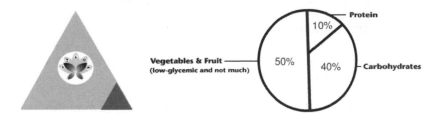

A good herbal formula for this is Lian po yin.[4] It's gentle yet effective. It contains huang lian, hou po, zhi zi, dan dou chi, shi chuang pu, ban xiia, and lu gen.

FOOD AS MEDICINE: *PAPAYA*

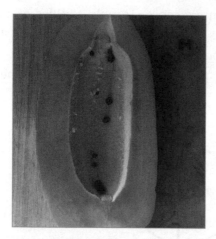

Papaya is one of my favorite fruits. Some of my fondest memories are of eating it right off the tree in the Caribbean. There's nothing better than eating fresh papaya in the shade on a hot day. It's the fruit of the angels!

Papaya contains an enzyme called papain, which is a powerful digestive aid. It is very effective in breaking down proteins. This is a very good thing. The more we break down proteins, the less we react to them.

Papain is effective in breaking down meat fibers and has been traditionally used to tenderize meat in South America. Papain will completely break down cells. It is used by some people to pass urine tests for cannabinoids. It sometimes works because it breaks down the proteins and makes them undetectable.

In Chinese medicine, papaya is neutral, sweet, and sour. It strengthens the stomach and spleen, aids digestion, clears summer heat, lubricates the lungs, stops cough, aids irritability, kills worms, and increases milk production.

It was used to treat coughs, indigestion, stomachache, eczema, skin lesions, and intestinal worms.

Some remedies are:

- Stomachache and Indigestion: Cook papaya and eat it with or after meals.

- Cough: Peel and steam papaya, then add honey. Eat and relax.

- Skin Lesions: Apply fresh papaya.

- Intestinal Worms: Sun dry green papaya, grind it into a powder, and take 2 teaspoons on an empty stomach every morning.

There's a Thai restaurant in my neighborhood that makes the most delicious green papaya salad. Ask for it at your local restaurant—it's another great way to enjoy it.

Chapter 25

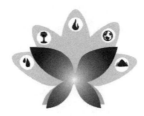

ACID REFLUX

Acid reflux, and its cousin GERD (gastroesophageal reflux disease), share the same symptoms. GERD usually has more severe symptoms. Both are conditions in which gastric acids ascend up the esophagus and cause a burning sensation in the lower esophagus or higher up.

This can be experienced with other symptoms including stomach pain, abdominal distention and discomfort, nausea, and gnawing hunger. It can also be the only symptom. Acid reflux can also progress to GERD.

Acid reflux is a very common complaint for people with Hashimoto's and hypothyroidism. Hypothyroidism can cause less gastrin (the hormone that causes stomach acid to be released) to be produced, and this can result in too little stomach acid.

Even though it's a bit counterintuitive, too little stomach acid leads to acid reflux because the stomach fails to properly break down foods and transform them, which results in a kind of traffic jam that sends gastric acid back up the esophagus in the wrong direction.

WESTERN MEDICAL CAUSES

Some other common causes of acid reflux include:

- Peptic ulcer

- Cardiac sphincter scarring

- Gastritis (both chronic and acute)

- Dyspepsia

- Chronic alcohol and tobacco abuse

- Hiatal hernia

- Pregnancy

- Obesity

- Anticholinergic drugs

- Calcium channel blockers

CHINESE MEDICINE CAUSES

In Chinese medicine, reflux is generally associated with rebellious stomach qi. Stomach qi should travel down the digestive tract, carrying the chyme and partially broken down food through the intestines. It will rise if something interferes with proper digestion (as in the case with hypothyroidism).

Stomach qi will also rise if it is forced by heat or if it is too weak to descend (also possibly caused by hypothyroidism). It can be blocked by weakness in the Earth phase, by qi stagnation, or by dampness or phlegm.

Chronic acid reflux and heartburn can cause other issues over time. If gastric contents end up in the lungs, which sometimes happens during sleep, it can cause asthma or bronchitis. If they reach the throat, it can lead to hoarse voice or sore throat. If the esophagus becomes damaged or scarred, it can result in dysphagia or an uncomfortable sensation when swallowing.

DIET IS KEY

Diet plays a major role in the production of acid reflux and heartburn. Eating large amounts of food that are warming in nature can create heat in the liver and stomach. Acidic foods like coffee, tomatoes, citrus fruits, uncooked peppers, radishes, onions, and garlic and spicy foods like chilies and other hot spices, can all lead to this. Alcohol can also exacerbate acid reflux.

In addition, eating at odd hours or very late at night or while feeling rushed or stressed can disrupt the function of the stomach and weaken the stomach and spleen.

Overeating can also cause stagnation and obstruction in the stomach. When this is combined with hypothyroidism, it can result in the generation of dampness, phlegm, and/or constipation. Ironically, excessive amounts of cold and raw foods that weaken the qi of the stomach and spleen can lead to dysfunction in the stomach.

Very cold herbs and medications (such as antibiotics) also weaken the spleen and can lead to dampness. In addition, extreme restriction in food intake (as a result of severe dieting or in eating disorders like bulimia or anorexia or in times of famine) can all result in serious damage to the spleen and stomach qi.

EMOTION IS ALSO A BIG FACTOR

Once again emotion can play a big role in acid reflux and heartburn. Liver qi stagnation impacts the abdomen in a number of ways.

From the five-phase model, we know that the liver qi can invade the spleen and stomach and disrupt proper digestion. It can impair the spleen's ability to transform and transport nutrients, vitamins, and minerals properly.

And this can result in the accumulation of mucus and dampness. This dampness can, in turn, prevent the proper flow of fluids in the digestive tract leading to constipation and a backing up of the whole process.

Liver qi stagnation can be caused by repressed anger, frustration and resentment, and buried emotions. These unexpressed emotions can affect the function of smooth muscles of the gut and lead to spasms or tension.[1]

Other emotions can also impact the spleen and stomach. Worry, obsessive thinking, and many of the habits of modern living like sedentary living or excessive sitting will weaken the spleen. The weakened spleen creates circumstances for the liver to invade, and this further disrupts the stomach qi.

COMMON MEDICATION CAN ALSO CAUSE PROBLEMS

Acid reflux is frequently treated with antacid medication. These over-the-counter drugs usually have some metal ion in them (aluminum, calcium, magnesium, or sodium), which provides temporary relief. However, they don't address the underlying problem.

OTCs can also cause problems with thyroid hormone medication absorption because thyroid hormone tends to bond quite easily to these ions.

Other drugs like proton pump inhibitors are also frequently prescribed by doctors even though studies have shown that these treatments aren't effective. In fact, in a 2009 article published in the journal *Gastroenterology,* the authors remarked: "Treating gastroesophageal reflux disease with profound acid inhibition [which is exactly what proton pump inhibitors do] will never be ideal because acid secretion is not the primary underlying defect."[2]

For decades the medical establishment has been focusing on how to reduce stomach acid secretion in people suffering from heartburn and GERD, even though it's common knowledge that these conditions are not caused by too much stomach acid.

As I mentioned, the real problem is too little stomach acid. So these drugs are ensuring that the people who use them must continue to use them indefinitely.

USE THE A.P.A.R.T. SYSTEM TO DIAGNOSE AND TREAT ACID REFLUX

1. Ask and Assess

In determining whether or not acid reflux is caused by a deficiency or excess condition (or a combination of both), it is helpful to determine the cause.

If the acid reflux is made worse by the items listed below, it may indicate the following sources (that is, if acid reflux is made worse by stress, it's usually caused by qi stagnation:

- Stress: liver qi stagnation
- Warming foods (coffee, alcohol, chocolate): stomach and liver heat
- Eating: Food stagnation, damp heat, or phlegm damp
- Bending or lying down: spleen deficiency
- Palpitations: blood stagnation, damp heat

If it is improved . . . it is usually caused by . . .

- Belching and releasing gas: food stagnation or qi stagnation

Next, determine if it is caused by excess or deficiency:

This comes down to liver qi stagnation and heat-related scenarios, damp heat/ phlegm, and spleen and stomach qi deficiency patterns.

Once again, this is another way of saying that there is an emotional component to the issue.

Symptoms include:[3]

- Acid reflux and heartburn that is worse with stress or emotional upset
- Hypochondriac pain, tenderness, fullness, or discomfort
- Irritability, moodiness, depression, anxiety, excessive worrying
- Tension headaches

- Bloating
- Alternating between constipation and loose stools
- Frequent sighing and belching
- Irregular menstruation
- PMS, including breast tenderness prior to period
- Neck and shoulder tension
- Cold hands and feet

With stomach fire, add:

- Symptoms that are worse with chocolate, coffee, or alcohol
- Sour or bitter belching

- Gnawing hunger
- Foul-smelling stools
- Irritable, easily angered, hot temper

Phlegm damp excess pattern is caused by stomach qi "rebelling" upward and can result in tasting stomach acid or bile in the mouth.

Symptoms include:

- Acid reflux, heartburn
- Poor concentration, foggy headedness
- May be overweight
- May have chronic mucous issues in lungs and sinuses

- Sensitive to smells
- Greasy skin, musty body odor
- Loss of appetite
- Tends toward loose stools or diarrhea

Deficient symptoms include:

- Chronic acid reflux that's worse with hard to digest or raw foods

- Worse with bending or abdominal pressure

- Bloating after eating

- Hypersalivation, drooling

- Fatigue, weakness, poor muscle tone

- Loose stools or diarrhea

- Cold extremities, sensitive to cold

2. Prioritize and Plan

Determine which pattern is yours. If you can't decide, consult a practitioner. Use the appropriate diet for your scenario.

Liver qi stagnation requires, of course, the liver qi stagnation diet:

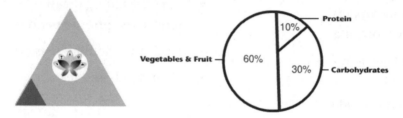

A good formula for this is Si ni san.[4] This regulates qi and harmonizes the liver and stomach, and it redirects stomach qi downward.

It contains chai hu, zhi shi, bai shao, licorice root, hai piao xiao, huang lian, and wu zhu yu.

For phlegm damp acid reflux, choose the damp heat diet:

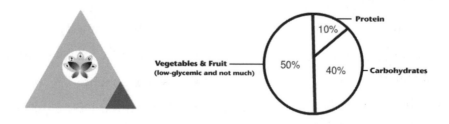

A good herbal formula for this is Ping wei san.[5] This is a great formula that works like a charm. It dries dampness and transforms phlegm, invigorates the spleen function, and harmonizes the stomach.

It contains cang zhu, hou po, chen pi, gingerroot, Chinese date, licorice root, and wu zhu yu.

For deficient acid reflux, use the spleen and stomach deficiency diet.

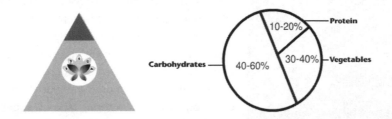

A great formula for deficient type acid reflux is one we have already seen: Xiang sha liu jun zi tang.[6] This formula warms and strengthens the spleen and harmonizes the stomach. It redirects qi downward and alleviates the reflux.

It contains codonopsis, bai zhu, fu ling, ban xia, citrus peel, mu xiang, sha ren, and licorice root.

3. Act and Adapt

Try your plan for 15 to 30 days.

4. Reassess and Reevaluate

Review your symptoms. If you have improved, return to a spleen and stomach supporting diet.

If symptoms do not improve, try to figure out why and tweak your plan or consult a practitioner for help.

5. Try and Try Again

Keep working on healing your stomach and spleen.

FOOD AS MEDICINE: **CILANTRO**

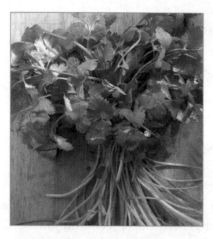

As we know, Chinese medicine has long had a tradition of using herbs, foods, and other natural substances as medicine. Let's take a closer look at the cilantro leaf and see what benefits it offers.

Cilantro leaves are slightly cool and pungent. They promote sweating, strengthen digestion, and encourage the flow of chi, or energy.

Cilantro has been used traditionally to treat the common cold, indigestion, lack of appetite, and chest and stomach fullness.

For the common cold in the early stages (what is known as wind cold), drink a tea made from ginger and cilantro (and sweat it out). To make the tea, cut a couple of slices of fresh organic ginger and loosely chop a handful of fresh organic cilantro. Boil 3 cups of filtered water and simmer ginger for 3 to 5 minutes. Remove from the stove and add cilantro. Let steep for 2 minutes. Enjoy!

For more advanced cold symptoms with sore throat and possibly fever (known as wind heat), drink a tea made of cilantro and mint. To make the tea, chop a handful of organic cilantro and mint. Bring 3 cups of filtered water to a boil, remove from the stove, add mint and cilantro. Let steep for 3 to 5 minutes. Enjoy!

For indigestion, make a tea of cilantro and orange peel. To make the tea, chop a handful of organic cilantro and one organic orange peel. Bring 3 cups of water to a boil and simmer orange peel for 3 to 5 minutes. Remove from flame and add cilantro. Let it steep for another 3 to 5 minutes. Yummy!

Chapter 26

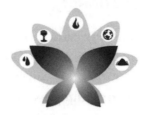

HISTAMINE INTOLERANCE

One common problem that I have seen repeatedly with patients who have Hashimoto's and food sensitivities is histamine intolerance. This is caused by high histamine levels in the body (often in the gut).

Histamine is a neurotransmitter that is used by the immune system, digestive system, and central nervous system. It is synthesized by various types of cells, including mast cells, basophils, platelets, neurons, and more. Histamine acts as a trigger for many different types of biological responses in the gut, brain, spinal cord, and uterus.

HOW DO YOU KNOW IF YOU HAVE HISTAMINE INTOLERANCE?

Depending on where it is found, histamine reactions can cause a whole bunch of different symptoms. The most common sign of histamine intolerance is a (usually unpleasant) reaction after eating fermented foods like sauerkraut.

In the gut this can lead to diarrhea, stomachache, or cramps. High histamine does not only produce gastrointestinal symptoms, however. It can also lead to skin problems like hives, itching, flushing, rashes, eczema, and psoriasis and even acne in some people.

Histamine intolerance has also been linked to headaches, menstrual issues, sinus congestion, asthma, vertigo, nausea and vomiting, and circadian rhythm disruption. When it impacts the cardiovascular system, it can cause hypertension, arrhythmias, and allergic reactions.

WHAT CAUSES HISTAMINE REACTIONS?

Technically, a histamine reaction is caused by a deficiency of an enzyme that breaks down histamine called diamine oxidase (DAO). And if a deficiency of this enzyme is what's causing it in you, then all you need to do is take the enzyme or something that stimulates it and your symptoms may improve.

Stinging nettle, quercetin, and ginger will all do that. You can also purchase formulations of the DAO enzyme. What I have found, however, is that like everything Hashimoto's related, this sometimes works but sometimes doesn't.

I think one possible reason that it doesn't always work is that the problem is not simply just a lack of this enzyme. For some people, an overzealous Th2 response that kicks in after meals may also be the culprit.

In addition, stress and an overactivated HPA axis can lead to histamine intolerance. It is very important to take the impact of stress seriously when treating histamine reactions. Here again, we see the clear manifestation of the role of emotions in disease that Li Dong-yuan so keenly observed and wrote about.

From a Chinese medicine perspective, histamine intolerance is a classic yin fire presentation. As Li noted, damage to the spleen and stomach and emotional stressors of anger, fear, and worry cause harm to the qi of the spleen and stomach (this is the equilibrium of the gut), and this results in heart fire becoming excessive on its own.

This fire in the heart is yin fire. Li wrote that "the heart does not reign [personally. Rather,] ministerial fire is its deputy. [It] is the fire of the pericardium developing from the lower burner. It is a foe to the original qi."[1] The original qi is the metabolic energy of the gut.

And what is histamine intolerance but this fire raging out of control. All of the symptoms we described above are forms of this immune fire (inflammatory response) raging out of control. Because equilibrium has been lost, there is nothing to contain it.

Li continues: "There is no yang to sustain the constructive and defensive or ying and wei." The *wei qi* is the Chinese term for the immune response. In that same passage he describes symptoms that are exactly the same as the symptoms I mentioned above.

And Li asks how we treat this: "The only choice is to apply acrid, sweet, warm ingredients to supplement the center and upraise yang with sweet, cold [ingredients] to drain fire."[2] As it turns out, these acrid (aromatic) herbs define molecules with a ring of organic atoms that provides for increased interaction of electrons with surrounding molecules.

Histadine, the aromatic amino acid that makes histamine, is just one of four aromatic amino acids (along with phenylaniline, tyrosine, and tryptophan), and some of the herbs that Li recommends contain potent aromatic hydrocarbons that are the main active ingredients.

In addition, other herbs in a formula he created (Bu Zhong Yi Qi Tang), which has been shown pharmaceutically to reduce IgE antibodies and reduce histamine in type I allergic responses as well as lower Th2 responses, have broad-spectrum antiviral and antibacterial properties and stimulate Th1 immune responses.

In other words, he perfectly describes how to treat histamine intolerance by treating it as a yin fire phenomenon. Mind blown again!

Other things to consider are a host of potential chemicals that are naturally occurring in foods that may also contribute to food reactions. These include gluten, lectins, amines, tannins, FODMAPS, salicylates, suplhites, and more.

The AIP diet is helpful in this regard because it removes all of the harmful lectins and, thus, eliminates that variable as we try to heal this problem.

However, some of the important foods in the AIP diet are also high in histamine—for example, bone broth and fermented foods. So we have a number of potential land mines to work around, and this is yet another example of why one diet doesn't work for everybody.

When trying to figure out what to do about histamine intolerance, we must first know which foods are high in histamine.

These include the following:[3]

HIGH HISTAMINE FOODS

- Fermented alcoholic beverages like wine, champagne, and beer
- Fermented foods like sauerkraut, vinegar, soy sauce, kefir, kombucha, yogurt, etc.
- Foods with vinegar like pickles, mayonnaise, olives, etc.
- Dried fruit like dates, apricots, prunes, raisins, etc.

- Smoked fish and certain species of fish like mackerel, tuna, anchovies, and sardines

- Cured meats like bacon, salami, pepperoni, hot dogs, etc.

- Aged cheeses, including goat cheese

- Nuts like cashews, peanuts, and walnuts

- Sour foods like sour cream, sour milk, sourdough bread, buttermilk, etc.

- Most citrus fruits

- Some vegetables like avocado, eggplant, spinach, and tomatoes

These foods also block the DAO enzyme and thus create the circumstances for histamine intolerance:

- Alcohol
- Black tea
- Maté
- Green tea
- Energy drinks

And these foods release histamine:

- Alcohol
- Chocolate
- Cow's milk
- Papaya
- Nuts
- Bananas
- Pineapple
- Shellfish
- Strawberries
- Tomatoes
- Wheat germ
- A number of food additives, artificial dyes, and preservatives

So what *is* left to eat? Quite a lot, actually. As a reminder, check out the charts in Chapter 13 on pages 180–183.

One thing that's important to understand with histamine intolerance is that histamine levels in cooked meat immediately start to rise. So it's best to get fresh meat and cook it and eat it as soon as possible. It's also important to freeze leftovers right away. In this way you can still batch cook and prepare larger meals.

Remember to apply the principles of a qi deficient diet to these histamine foods:

All food should be cooked and eaten warm. Slow cooking soups, stews, and broths is particularly effective. Chew food thoroughly. Try simple combinations of a few ingredients, eat frequent smaller meals, and set regular mealtimes.

Be sure to have a high proportion of complex carbohydrates and vegetables and use less meat (nutrient-dense meat like organ meat is recommended).

Avoid excessive fluids during meals, overeating, skipping meals, and multitasking during meals.

BENEFICIAL FOODS FOR QI DEFICIENCY:

Neutral or sweet, warm flavors: artichoke, mustard greens, pumpkin, sweet potato, celery root, squash, carrot, parsnip, yams, peas, string beans, beets, winter squash, okra, turnip, Jerusalem artichoke, coconut milk, papaya, apricots, figs, grapes, currants, coconut, stewed fruit, chicken, beef, lamb, liver, kidney, mackerel, tuna, and anchovy

Pungent flavors in small amounts help assist the natural function of dispersing and descending: onion, leek, garlic, turnip, pepper, fresh ginger, cinnamon, and non-seed kitchen spices (sage, savory, thyme, tarragon, etc.)

Complex sweet flavors (use with caution in damp and damp heat conditions): molasses, dates, coconut sugar

Helpful herbs: astragalus, codonopsis, red and black dates

Optional (only to be eaten once you have eliminated and reintroduced them successfully): light grains, especially rice and rice porridge, oats, chickpeas, black beans, walnuts

Optional spices (Same as above. Eliminate first, then reintroduce. Eat in moderation if tolerated): nutmeg, fennel

Avoid cold-natured, uncooked, and raw foods: salads, raw fruits (whole and juiced, especially citrus), wheat, raw vegetables, tomatoes, spinach, Swiss chard, tofu, millet, seaweed, salt, too many sweet foods and concentrated sweeteners, vitamin C (over 1 to 2 grams per day), beer, ice cream and dairy products (except a little grass-fed butter), sugar, chocolate, nuts and seeds (except walnuts), nut butters

ADDITIONAL KEYS TO SUCCESSFULLY TREATING HISTAMINE INTOLERANCE:

- Avoid foods high in histamine and those that cause histamine release (see above).

- Eat freshly prepared meat and freeze leftovers immediately to keep histamine levels low.

- Take herbs or supplements that boost DAO enzyme levels (stinging nettle, quercetin, and ginger).

- Avoid Th2-stimulating compounds:

  Caffeine

  Curcumin (found in turmeric)

  Genistin (found in soybeans)

  Green Tea Extract

  Lycopene (found in tomatoes and other red fruits excluding strawberries and cherries)

  Pine Bark Extract

  Pycnogenol (found in the extract of the French maritime pine bark and apples)

  Resveratrol (found in grape skin, sprouted peanuts, and cocoa)

  White Willow Bark

- Work on reducing stress and practicing stress-relieving hobbies, such as meditation, qi gong, and yoga.

- Consider trying Li Dong-yuan's formula Bu Zhong Yi Qi Tang. Research has shown that this formula suppresses IgE antibody production and lowers histamine in mice.[4]

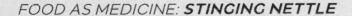

FOOD AS MEDICINE: *STINGING NETTLE*

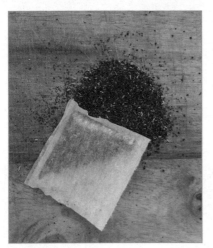

Nettle has been used since ancient times in the Western herbal tradition, and yet it is also considered a bothersome weed that some people just want to get rid of.

But they shouldn't because it has remarkable healing and restorative powers, especially for building blood.

From a Chinese medical viewpoint, it is considered sweet and salty and slightly cooling. It has an affinity for the liver, spleen, lung, and bladder meridians.

Stinging nettle has been used quite effectively to nourish liver blood, relieve fatigue, regulate metabolism, and strengthen connective tissue. It can also be helpful in restoring the adrenals and thyroid, and it promotes hair growth.

Stinging nettle nourishes and strengthens the lungs, resolves phlegm, and relieves coughing and wheezing. In addition, it promotes detoxification, resolves eczema, dissolves deposits and stones, and reduces tumors and nodules.

It can also promote urination and help to reduce edema anywhere in the body, including around the eyes. Stinging nettle has an immune-modulating effect, and as we have seen, it's one of the primary herbs to help boost DAO enzyme levels in histamine intolerance.

In short, this is a fantastic herb for many hypothyroid and digestive issues. I have stinging nettle on my short list of "must have" herbs in my herbal tea collection. And to think that for many it's just an annoying weed. Talk about magic hiding in plain sight!

Make a simple tea by adding 1 to 2 tablespoons of dried leaves per cup of hot water, and then letting them soak for 5 to 10 minutes. You can make a big batch and refrigerate it; it makes a wonderful iced tea too!

Chapter 27

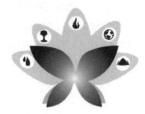

GALLSTONES/GALLBLADDER INFLAMMATION

Gallbladder-related issues are very common with Hashimoto's and hypothyroidism. Thyroid status clearly impacts the flow of bile from the gallbladder as well as its composition. The decrease in bile flow is due mostly to a decrease in bile salts.

Hypothyroidism also slows cholesterol metabolism and excretion of bilirubin though the bile is diminished. One theory is that increased cholesterol levels found in patients with myxedema is caused by too much cholesterol in the bile, and this can result in a higher incidence of gallstones.[1]

Gallstones obstructing the bile duct is the most common cause of gallbladder inflammation, which results in abdominal pain.

Common symptoms include:

- Pain that is usually severe, acute, and colicky; typically felt in the upper right quadrant of the abdomen and can radiate to the lower right scapula.

- Pain is sometimes accompanied by nausea and/or vomiting

Common risk factors include the classic "3 Fs" known to most medical students: fat (obese), female, and over 40. Obviously, these are common symptoms in women with Hashimoto's and hypothyroidism as well. About 75 percent of people with this condition have had the same symptoms at least once before.

The Western medical approach is to give antibiotics for the inflammation and pain and often to remove the gallbladder if symptoms persist (or even sometimes just as a precaution to prevent future flare-ups). In addition, antacids and anticholinergic drugs are also prescribed.

CHINESE MEDICINE VIEW

Gallbladder inflammation and gallstones are thought to be caused by several different factors in Chinese medicine. Overeating fried, oily foods can damage the spleen and cause dampness. As we have seen, this dampness can transform into heat, which then obstructs the flow of qi.

This qi and resulting blood stagnation leads to pain in the right ribs and abdomen. This is also a condition where Gu, or worms, has traditionally been thought to be a causative factor that leads to qi and blood stagnation. If dampness and heat develop, this can cause jaundice.

In addition, there is also thought to be an emotional component to gallbladder issues. Unfulfilled desires and anger or rage can damage the liver and lead to qi stagnation. If the liver attacks the stomach, stomach qi can be damaged resulting in nausea or vomiting.

If the liver attacks the spleen, this can weaken the spleen and dampness can accumulate as a result. This can combine with heat, and then you have damp heat making everything worse. There is a logic to it all, isn't there?

USING THE A.P.A.R.T. SYSTEM TO TREAT GALLBLADDER INFLAMMATION AND/OR STONES:

Like many of the other conditions, there are both excess and deficiency patterns for gallstones. These include liver/gallbladder qi stagnation, damp heat, and heat/fire conditions, as well as qi and blood deficiency.[2]

1. Ask and Assess

Liver/gallbladder qi stagnation symptoms include:

- Rib pain on the right side, possibly radiating to the upper back and right shoulder

- Chest pressure

- Nausea

- Aversion to oily, fried foods

- Reduced appetite

- Belching

- Bitter taste in mouth, dry mouth

- Emotional tension, short temper

- Irregular bowel movements

- Slight fever

These symptoms could occur during an acute episode or during a period of remission after passing stones.

Damp heat symptoms are similar and are usually experienced during a more severe acute attack or when gallbladder inflammation is complicated by infection. If you experience these symptoms, consult your doctor as soon as possible.

Symptoms include:

- Severe rib pain on the right side

- Abdominal distention and fullness, palpable pain in the area of the gallbladder

- Nausea, vomiting

- Dry mouth with a bitter taste

- Thirst with no desire to drink

- Feeling cold, hot, or heat and chills mixed

- Jaundice

- Dry stools

- Yellow urine

Deficiency symptoms include:

- Yellowing of the eyes and skin that comes and goes in severity

- Dizziness or vertigo

- Fatigue, lack of strength

- Rib-side distention

- Not wanting to speak

- Pain that comes and goes

- Reduced appetite and consumption of food

- Engorged sublingual veins

2. Prioritize and Plan

If you have severe symptoms, see your doctor right away, especially if you have a fever or are in intense pain. Otherwise, adopt the appropriate diet.

If you aren't sure which pattern fits you, consult a practitioner.

For liver/gallbladder stagnation, employ a liver stagnation/heat clearing diet (see page 163):

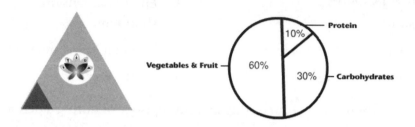

A good formula for treating gallstones is Xiao chai hu tang.[3] It clears heat, moves qi, and helps expel stones. Ingredients include chai hu, huang qin, ban xia, ginger-root, ginseng, licorice root, and Chinese date.

One study found that this formula combined with another Xiao cheng qi tang had an 85 percent success rate in passing stones.[4]

For damp heat, employ the damp heat diet.

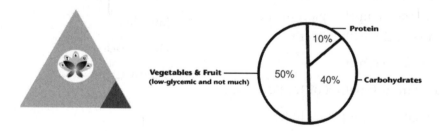

A formula that comes in patent form (patent meaning mass produced and you can purchase online or in any Chinese herb store) called Long dan xie gan tang could be used in this case.[5] Again, if this is severe, you should consult a doctor or physician.

For deficiency patterns, employ the deficiency diet.

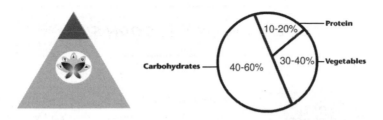

For this type of gallstone or gallbladder inflammation pattern, combining Si jun zi tang, which tonifies qi, with another formula for reducing gallbladder inflammation (like Wen dan tang or the other formula we have already seen), Huang lian jie du tang could be helpful.

3. Act and Adapt

This is a condition that can be tricky and can result in infection and rather severe pain. It is recommended to see a practitioner if you are unsure or if diet doesn't help. Gallstones can be quite painful to pass if they are too large.

In China a combination of Western medication and Chinese medical approaches are used to expel the stones if they are small enough. Very large stones are unnecessary to expel. In this case, preventative measures are used.

In mild to moderate cases, diet can sometimes be quite effective. Generally it's best to avoid sweet and sugary foods and oily, fried foods.

Where there is an emotional component, be sure to employ exercise and relaxation techniques. Qi gong can be very effective for treating the emotional part of this disorder.

4. Reassess and Reevaluate

After trying the recommended intervention, reevaluate your symptoms. Keep eating a damp heat and spleen and stomach qi supporting diet.

5. Try and Try Again

Keep going! Keep nourishing and healing your spleen and stomach.

FOOD AS MEDICINE: **CORN SILK**

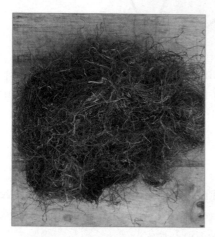

You know that stringy hair-like stuff that you pick off an ear of corn when you shuck it? Well, that's corn silk and as it turns out, you're throwing away an excellent herb for promoting urination and treating gallstones.

In Chinese medicine, corn silk is considered sweet, bland, and neutral and has an affinity for the urinary bladder, kidney, and liver.

Corn silk was used traditionally to treat edema and swelling (it's a natural diuretic). In addition, it is very effective in stimulating the production and excretion of bile acid, and it decreases its viscosity (thickness of bile). Gallstones can often develop in people with Hashimoto's and hypothyroidism because of sluggish bile flow.

Pharmacologically, corn silk has been found to be both a diuretic and a hypertensive (a good, natural alternative to some blood pressure medications if used under the supervision of a doctor). Obviously, be cautious with using it if you are already taking a diuretic such as Lasix.

Corn silk also contains vitamin K, so be cautious if you are taking Warfarin or other blood thinners.

An excellent remedy for gallstones is to make a tea with corn silk and the Chinese herb jin qian cao. Drink it daily.

Chapter 28

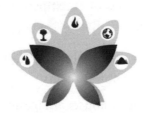

CONSTIPATION

Another very common symptom for people with Hashimoto's and hypothyroidism is constipation. Motility in the entire gut and thyroid hormone levels are closely linked. When you are hypothyroid or functionally hypothyroid (you have enough thyroid hormone in your system, but it isn't getting into the cells), one common result can be constipation.[1]

Constipation can be difficulty passing stools, prolonged periods between bowel movements, or a desire to defecate without being able to do so completely. Stools may be normal or hard, dry, and pebble-like. In addition, normal bowel frequency can vary.

For some people, a bowel movement once a week may be normal, while others might consider themselves constipated if they only go once a day. So it's important to consider what is normal for you and what has been normal historically for your body.

Once again, the key question with constipation, as in all issues, is to determine if it's caused by a deficient or an excess imbalance. Deficient patterns are often characterized by dryness from insufficient fluids lubricating the bowels, such as blood or yin, or lack of motility and movement through the bowel caused by a deficiency of qi and/or yang.

Excess conditions are normally caused by too much heat or phlegm. Or by a pathological buildup of qi that has blocked the proper movement of the bowels. Heat can be of internal or external origins.

There are many potential causes of constipation from a biomedical standpoint, and these include the following:[2]

- Lifestyle causes: low-fiber diet, sedentary lifestyle, lack of exercise, travel (especially air travel), poor bowel habits

- Medication: chronic laxative abuse, analgesics, aluminum-containing antacids, diuretics, iron supplements, opiates, tricyclic antidepressants, anticholinergic agents, antidiarrheal agents

- Endocrine: hypothyroidism, hyperkalemia (high blood levels of potassium caused by Addison's disease)

- Anal lesions (usually caused by trying to avoid pain): hemorrhoids, fissure, stenosis, diverticulosis, abscess

- Mental emotional: irritable bowel syndrome, depression, anorexia nervosa, anxiety, embarrassment around going to the bathroom

- Cancer or polyps in the colon: sigmoid colon or rectum or tumors outside the colon putting pressure on the colon

CHINESE MEDICINE CAUSES

YIN, BLOOD, AND FLUID DEFICIENCY

Yin, blood, and fluid deficiencies are quite common causes of constipation; it's simply that there are insufficient amounts of fluid in the intestine to lubricate and move stools through the bowels. These types of conditions are frequently found among elderly people and postpartum women, both of whom may have depleted yin.

Yin deficiency constipation can also follow some kind of external illness like a cold or flu. These can damage the yin of the lung, and this can in turn damage yin fluids in the intestines. Sometimes depletion of fluids can also result from overzealous treatments of cold, bitter, and drying herbs (or antibiotics, also considered cold in Chinese medicine) used to treat pathogens in the gut.

Blood deficiency can occur after prolonged breastfeeding, excessive sweating, hemorrhaging, or too little protein in the diet (leading to anemia). These can complicate spleen qi deficiency.

QI AND YANG DEFICIENCY

Qi and yang deficiency constipation is caused by a lack of qi movement through the intestines. Since yang is, in my opinion, another way of talking about endocrine activity, this could certainly be related to hypothyroidism and/or issues involving the adrenals and the HPA axis.

Cold in the intestines can also complicate yang deficiency and slow or constrict movement in the intestines as well. Stools are usually loose and moist with qi and yang deficiency. This is more of a problem of lack of peristalsis, or a desire to go to the bathroom.

Lack of exercise or excessive amounts of exercise as well as excessive worry or excessive mental activity can lead to deficiency of lung and spleen qi. And eating too much raw, cold, or damp-producing foods can also contribute.

Lung qi is also impacted by emotions (like unexpressed or unresolved grief) and by poor posture and shallow breathing. It's interesting to note that smoking cigarettes can sometimes help with constipation in the short term because it disperses lung qi and nicotine can stimulate peristalsis. But, obviously, this has many adverse health effects that include damaging both the lungs and large intestines, in addition to causing cancer.

Yang deficiency is especially common in older people because yang naturally declines as we age. As we have seen, spleen yang can be damaged by eating too many raw, cold foods or by taking drugs that are cold (such as antibiotics). Yang can also be damaged by serious illness or surgery to the gastrointestinal tract.

Caution: Be aware that sudden or recent onset of constipation that doesn't resolve itself among middle-aged or elderly people can be an indication of bowel cancer. Make sure to consult a doctor to rule this out if dietary and herbal interventions do not help. Thin or ribbon-like stools can be an indication of a physical obstruction of the bowel.

USE THE A.P.A.R.T. SYSTEM TO TREAT CONSTIPATION:

1. Ask and Assess

Like the other conditions we have seen, constipation can have a number of possible causes. Again, the question we must ask ourselves is, Is it deficient or excess in nature?

Excess patterns include heat-related patterns and liver qi stagnation (which, as we have seen, can also develop into heat).

Heat can cause constipation by drying out the intestines and the stool. Without sufficient water, you can't "float de boat," if you know what I'm saying. This can lead to obstruction in the intestines and hinder the stomach's ability to descend qi. The key symptom here is hard, dry, pellet-like stools.

There is also heat caused by pathogens, and these would be caused by a bacterial or viral infection in the intestines. This is a stomach bug or food poisoning type of problem causing constipation. This is rarer and can also lead to diarrhea (which we will cover in the next chapter).

Chronic heat constipation symptoms include:

- Chronic constipation with dry, hard stools
- Possible red complexion, bad breath, dry mouth, thirst, and concentrated urine
- With liver-related heat, there may be irritability, short temper, temporal headaches, red, sore eyes, hypochondriac pain, and/or dizziness

If there is dampness or phlegm combined with the heat, the following symptoms may occur:

- Chronic constipation with stools that may contain mucus
- Abdominal distention and discomfort
- Foggy headedness, poor concentration, poor memory
- Sleepiness, lethargy, heaviness in the body
- May be accompanied by chronic mucous production in the sinuses and lungs
- Greasy skin, musty body odor
- Tendency toward being overweight

In contrast, deficiency type constipation may be spleen and stomach qi and/or yang related or yin deficient.

Qi deficient constipation symptoms include:

- Constipation with stools that are difficult to pass, but not dry or hard

- Stools tend to be soft and thick

- Feeling of fatigue after bowel movement

- Pale complexion

- Fatigue

- Spontaneous sweating

- Soft voice, reluctance to speak

If there is yang deficiency, it will have the symptoms above and the following:

- Disordered fluid metabolism resulting in edema and/or frequent urination

- Cold extremities, sensitivity to cold

- Abdominal pain that is improved with warmth

- Low back and/or knee pain (which may be cold to the touch)

2. Prioritize and Plan

Determine whether or not your constipation is of an excess or deficient nature. If you are unsure, consult a practitioner with knowledge of these matters.

For heat type constipation, a heat/fire clearing diet is recommended:

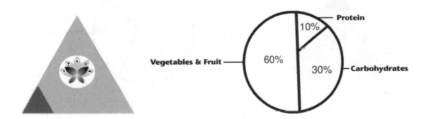

A popular formula for mild to moderate heat type constipation is called Ma zi ren wan.[3] It is named for one of its primary ingredients: huo ma ren (cannabis seed), which is helpful in promoting bowel movements.

It contains huo ma ren, da huang, zhi shi, hou po, bai shao, and xing ren.

As with any type of laxative, it is not recommended to take this formula for a long period of time because one may develop a dependency on it. One of the ingredients, da huang, is itself a powerful laxative herb.

When phlegm is a factor, a damp heat diet is appropriate:

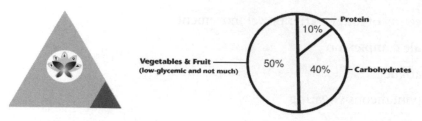

There are a couple of good formulas that are helpful for damp heat– and phlegm-related constipation. These include Er chen tang and a formula we have already seen, Ping wei san.

Er chen tang is a simple, elegant formula containing ban xia, ju hong, fu ling, and licorice root.[4]

An interesting sidenote: I found one study where Er chen tang was used to treat enlargement of the thyroid, and it reduced the size of the goiter in five out of seven patients. All of the patients received the classic formula without any modifications or any other treatment. It's not a very large sample size, but the results are interesting nonetheless.[5]

For qi and yang deficiency patterns, employ the deficiency diet.

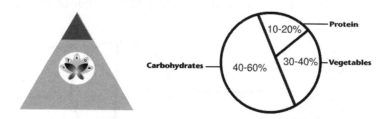

A good formula for deficiency type constipation is one we have already seen in a couple of other contexts: Li Dong-yuan's Bu Zhong Yi Qi Tang. This formula is effective in so many different situations because it is so well designed and balanced.

For yin deficiency type constipation, add yin deficiency diet variations (see page 159). It has the same basic food group proportions.

The formula that is effective for yin deficiency constipation is the one I mentioned in my discussion of oral tolerance (see Appendix 3): Liu wei di huang wan. And if you think about it, What is the yin of the stomach and intestines? It's the intestinal lining!

So it makes sense that something that would help rebuild the intestinal lining and improve oral tolerance would also treat yin deficiency of the digestive tract. It's also great for treating liver and kidney yin deficiency.

3. Act and Adapt

Decide which plan of action you are going to choose, and do it for 30 days. If you can't figure out which presentation is yours, consult a practitioner.

4. Reassess and Reevaluate

Once you have implemented your plan for 30 days, review your initial symptoms and see if they have improved. If they have, great! Celebrate with a terrific bowel movement and go back to a spleen and stomach supporting diet.

If they haven't improved, try to figure out why and tweak or make changes by reassessing your symptoms. If you can't figure it out, consult a practitioner.

5. Try and Try Again

Keep it going! Keep nourishing and healing the spleen and stomach.

FOOD AS MEDICINE: **MULBERRY**

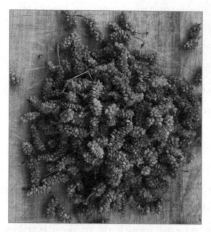

When I was a kid, we had a mulberry tree in the front yard. It was about 10 feet tall, and it formed a thick umbrella. You could stand inside it and hide—which I did when its berries were ripe. I would eat them up like a little bear. They're not as sexy as raspberries, but they're still delicious, and, oh, what wonderful things they can do.

In Chinese medicine, mulberries are considered slightly cold and sweet. They have an affinity for the heart, liver, and kidney. Mulberry is cool and gentle, and works well as a long-term tonic.

Traditionally, it was used to quench thirst, detoxify, nourish blood, tonify the kidneys, lubricate the lungs, relieve constipation, calm the spirit, and promote diuresis (make you pee).

And mulberry was used to treat dry mouth, excessive thirst and diabetes, anemia, constipation, back pain due to kidney weakness, alcohol intoxication, lymph node enlargement, and blurred vision.

Some natural remedies include:

- For insomnia: Boil mulberry tea and drink ½ cup before bed.

- For constipation: Drink mulberry juice (they're like little prunes).

- For cough: Take 2 teaspoons of mulberry syrup two times per day. To make mulberry syrup: cook mulberries on a low flame until they dissolve. Then add honey and cook down to desired thickness.

Chapter 29

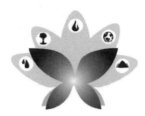

DIARRHEA/LOOSE STOOLS

Diarrhea is another condition that can impact Hashimoto's and hypothyroid patients. It is the increase in frequency of usually soft or fluid bowel movements. Emotionally, it can be draining and embarrassing and can cause anxiety and isolating behavior.

In Chinese medicine terms, diarrhea is frequently associated to dampness and the spleen. Dampness can come from external pathogens in the form of damp heat (these would be viral or bacterial infections) or internal ones, caused by spleen qi and/or yang deficiency.

As we have seen in every condition we've looked at thus far, emotion can also play a role in diarrhea. And as mentioned in Chapter 5 on the brain/gut connection, we can see that stress can impact the intestines and cause spasticity and too much movement through the gut.

WESTERN MEDICAL CAUSES

There are a number of causes of diarrhea, both acute and chronic.[1]

ACUTE

MEDICATION:

- Antibiotics
- Laxatives, purgatives
- Alcohol
- Vitamin C

- Levothyroxine
- Digitalis
- Antiviral medications, protease inhibitors

- Post-gastrointestinal surgery (can sometimes become chronic)

INFECTIONS:

- Viral
- Bacterial

- Protozoa
- Gastroenteritis

CHRONIC

- IBS (irritable bowel syndrome)
- Chronic parasitic infection (amoeba, giardia, cryptosporidium)
- Diverticular disease
- Celiac disease
- Lactose intolerance

- Ulcerative colitis
- Crohn's disease
- Graves' disease
- Diabetes
- Addison's disease
- Carcinoma of the bowel

CHINESE MEDICAL CAUSES

Diarrhea has a number of causes in Chinese medicine as well. And these include both external pathogens and internal causes.

The one thing that both internal and external causes have is dampness. The spleen is particularly vulnerable to dampness, and it can clog up the works and cause various problems. And a spleen weakened by dampness will often produce more dampness and, thus, a vicious cycle is born.

External sources of damp heat are infectious diseases caused by viruses, parasites, and bacteria. Chinese medicine also has a term called *summer heat,* which is a kind of external pathological heat. This often occurs in humid or wet weather and can also be similar to heatstroke or dehydration caused by severe heat.

DIET

Diet can be a major factor in developing diarrhea. Food poisoning caused by eating spoiled or contaminated food can cause explosive type diarrhea. And changes in normal dietary habits like traveling or emotional upset can also cause diarrhea in some people.

As we have already seen, too much cold or raw food can damage the qi and yang of the spleen. Drugs like antibiotics, laxatives, and herbs with antiviral and antibacterial properties (heat-clearing herbs) can also damage the qi of the stomach and spleen.

In addition, yo-yo dieting, fads like the HCG diet (a diet of 500 calories per day combined with injections of human chorionic gonadotropin), and a history of eating disorders (like bulimia, anorexia, binge eating, etc.) can all cause damage to the spleen and stomach. As we saw in Chapter 24 on abdominal distention, eating at irregular times, skipping meals, and eating late at night or at odd hours can all also potentially weaken the spleen and stomach qi.

EMOTION

Emotion can also play a big role in various digestive complaints, and diarrhea is no exception. Stress has a huge impact on the gastrointestinal system. And sensitivity in this area can be passed down through generations. Researchers have found that certain gastrointestinal diseases have a genetic component (such as polyps, colon cancer, hemochromatosis, autoimmune liver disease, Wilson's disease, and more).[2]

In addition, digestive weakness can also be passed down, perhaps in part because our behavior around the table is so deeply ingrained and habituated.

You may recall from five phase interactions that qi stagnation is a major factor in spleen and stomach weakness. Repressed emotions cause the liver to stagnate, and via the controlling cycle it invades the spleen and stomach.

As we learned from Li Dong-yuan, this liver qi stagnation can develop into heat and systemic inflammation. Long-term qi stagnation can develop into blood stagnation, which can lead to masses, nodules, and tumors. The damage to the spleen and stomach can also easily lead to dampness, and thus, we have a common triad of liver qi stagnation, spleen and stomach weakness or deficiency, and dampness.

This triad plays out again and again as a causative factor in many different digestive complaints. And we must treat all three aspects of this triad in order to resolve it.

Otherwise, one problem will continue to lead to the others over and over again. But this same tendency can be turned on its head, and we can develop healing momentum by reversing that vicious cycle and getting all the parts of the triad working together to heal.

SPLEEN AND STOMACH QI DEFICIENCY

Other behavior and emotions that can affect the spleen and stomach include working too much, obsessive thinking, worrying, not exercising, and eating junk food. These can all weaken the spleen and stomach.

Prolonged inactivity and sitting, especially while doing tasks that require sustained mental focus and concentration, can also damage the spleen and stomach. That describes pretty much every modern worker in the 21st century. And, of course, this applies to almost every student.

Students are particularly vulnerable to spleen and stomach qi deficiency because of a combination of the factors that I just described, especially if they combine poor diet habits with a sedentary life of studying.

Another factor to be cautious about is treatment of infections, digestive or respiratory, with antibiotics or herbs and supplements that have antibiotic and antiviral properties. These treatments are very cold and can damage the spleen and stomach long term.

This is why it is so important to be cautious about taking antibiotics and also to make sure you utilize the approaches that you are learning here to rebuild the metabolic health (qi) of the spleen and stomach after those kinds of therapy.

SPLEEN AND KIDNEY YANG DEFICIENCY

This type of diarrhea is often chronic and linked to endocrine dysfunction like hypothyroidism and/or adrenal or pancreatic weakness and dysfunction. Kidney yang deficiency can also be caused by age, chronic illness (like autoimmunity), and too much exercise (excessive lifting or standing).

In women, many pregnancies, or not being able to fully recover from pregnancy, can result in kidney yang deficiency. As you probably know, onset of Hashimoto's frequently happens in the postpartum period.

One thing that spleen and kidney yang deficiency can lead to is fluid accumulation (edema) or myxedema, when mixed with hypothyroidism. And this imbalance of fluids can cause diarrhea as well.

USE THE A.P.A.R.T. SYSTEM TO TREAT DIARRHEA:

1. Ask and Assess

You know the drill. Is the condition of excess or deficient origins? With diarrhea, excess conditions are mostly damp or damp heat related.

These include a seasonal type of diarrhea called summer heat or summer damp. It's thought to be weather induced and usually happens in humid or wet weather, often in late summer or autumn, though it could happen any time of year.

The main difference between these summer heat patterns and regular damp heat or cold damp patterns is that there are some cold or flu-like symptoms with summer heat.

Summer heat diarrhea symptoms include:[3]

- Acute diarrhea with rumbling in the tummy, possible abdominal cramping and pain

- In severe cases, diarrhea may be watery and urgent

- Chills, possible fever

- Generalized muscle ache

- Possible dull occipital or general headache

- Nausea and vomiting

- Malaise, heaviness in the head and body

- Foggy head

- Fullness in the chest and abdomen

Damp heat diarrhea symptoms include:

- Acute or recurrent, frequent, urgent foul-smelling diarrhea, possibly with burning anus
- Possible tenesmus or constant feeling like you have to go
- Fever or afternoon fever unrelieved by sweating
- Sweating that tends to come in the afternoon or worse in the afternoon
- Restlessness and irritability
- Cramping, abdominal pain
- Concentrated, scanty urine
- Thirst

Liver qi stagnation can also lead to diarrhea. As we have learned, the most important part of this type of condition is the emotional component.
Symptoms include:

- Recurrent diarrhea that may be urgent and preceded by cramping abdominal pain
- May alternate with constipation
- Irritability, moodiness, depression
- Cold hands and feet
- Abdominal distention
- Hypochondriac pain
- Heartburn, indigestion
- Gas and/or burping
- Shoulder and neck tension and/or pain
- PMS and breast tenderness prior to period

In contrast, deficient conditions include:

Cold damp diarrhea is something that can occur with hypothyroidism. This can also be caused by antibiotic therapy or other cold medications. In addition, eating too many raw foods, juices, or teas can also result in cold damage.

Symptoms include:

- Acute or chronic recurrent diarrhea: could be loose stools to watery and urgent

- Cramping or colicky abdominal pain

- Better with warmth and warm foods or fluids

- Fullness and distention in the abdomen

- Nausea

- Increased desire to sleep

- Heavy sensation in the body

- Clear urine

Spleen and stomach qi deficient diarrhea is common in children and in people who have really rigid or inappropriate diets. Like cold damp above, it can be caused by antibiotic treatment, high doses of vitamin C, or other cold-natured drugs.

Symptoms are the same as above plus:

- Poor appetite

- Weak, tired limbs

- Pale complexion

- Puffiness around the eyes and/or fingers

- Weight loss

- Fatigue

- Abdominal distention or dull ache, relieved by warmth

2. Prioritize and Plan

Decide if your diarrhea has a deficient or excess origin. If you can't decide, consult a practitioner. Choose the appropriate diet and herbal formula.

For summer heat and damp heat conditions, use the damp heat diet:

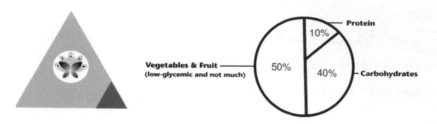

A great formula for summer heat, damp heat, and any type of food poisoning or stomach flu (or even hangovers!) is called Huo xiang chen qi wan.[4]

Over the years I have literally used this formula hundreds of times in dozens of different situations, and it's worked every time. It works for kids too. This should be in your herbal medicine cabinet.

This brilliant formula contains huo xiang, fu ling, hou po, zi su ye, ban xia, da fu pi, bai zhu, citrus peel, bai zhi, jie geng, licorice root, and gingerroot.

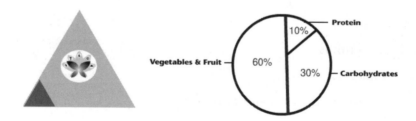

A good formula for liver qi stagnation is a simple one called Tong xie yao fang.[5] It harmonizes the liver and spleen, regulates liver qi, and supports and strengthens the spleen.

It contains four herbs: bai shao, bai zhu, chen pi, and fang feng. Another choice that could work is xiao yao san, a formula we have already seen, or a variation of it called jia wei xiao yao san, which is better for liver qi stagnation and heat.

For cold damp qi and yang deficiency patterns, employ the deficiency diet.

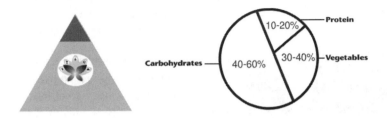

For cold damp diarrhea and qi and yang deficiency diarrhea, there are a couple of formulas. Ping wei san, which we have seen in a couple of different contexts already, is a good choice. As is Shen ling bai zhu san.[6]

This formula tonifies the spleen qi and dries damp and diarrhea. It contains dang shen, bai zhu, yi yi ren, fu ling, bian dou, shan yao, lian zi, jie geng, sha ren, and licorice root.

3. Act and Adapt

Decide which plan of action you are going to choose, and do it for 30 days. If you can't figure out which presentation is yours, consult a practitioner.

4. Reassess and Reevaluate

Once you have implemented your plan for 30 days, review your initial symptoms and see if they have improved. If they have, great! Celebrate and go back to a spleen and stomach supporting diet. If they haven't, try to figure out why and tweak or make changes by reassessing your symptoms. If you can't figure it out, consult a practitioner.

5. Try and Try Again

Keep it going! Keep nourishing and healing the spleen and stomach.

FOOD AS MEDICINE: *ASTRAGALUS ROOT*

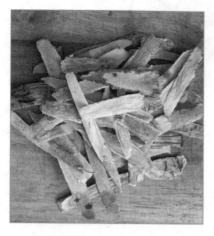

Here's another great herb that is a classic qi tonic. Its common name is Mongolian milkvetch.

Astragalus has a nice, sweet flavor and can be added to soups and porridges (it is too fibrous to eat, but you can cook with it and then remove it before serving).

Astragalus tonifies digestive qi, promotes absorption, and relieves fatigue. It's also a mild diuretic and helps to detoxify and relieve edema.

It is also astringing and is used traditionally to treat excessive sweating and bleeding. Finally, it promotes tissue repair and stimulates immunity. The immune-stimulating properties mean that it should be used with caution with autoimmunity.

Astragalus is considered a Th1 stimulant. So if you have an overzealous Th1 system, you need to be careful.

Traditionally, this herb has been used since the earliest times to treat weak or deficiency conditions involving metabolic or digestive functions, such as diarrhea caused by deficiency of spleen qi.

Modern research has revealed that it enhances cellular metabolism, making energy more available. It has adaptogenic functions and has been found to be restorative to the adrenals. It's also restorative to the liver, aiding assimilation, storage, and detoxification.

Astragalus is also rich in saponins, which help rejuvenate red blood cells and aid in better digestive absorption. This includes enhanced calcium and silicon utilization, which means it's also helpful for preventing bone loss.

You can purchase the root and make your own tea (which is what I do), or buy it in tincture or capsule form.

For cooking, I like to throw two or three slices into a pot of soup or gluten-free porridge. May the qi be with you!

Chapter 30

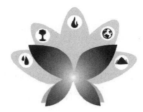

HEMORRHOIDS

Hemorrhoids are another condition I have seen in several Hashimoto's and hypothyroid patients. This is basically a blood clot in the veins around the anus. They are thought to be due to increased pressure in the veins that drain the rectum and anus; sometimes there is also weakness or loss of tone in the walls of the veins.

Because constipation and vascular weakness are common symptoms of Hashimoto's and hypothyroidism, this condition can sometimes develop.[1] Hemorrhoids can have no symptoms or can become painful and swollen, and can cause bleeding. Pain usually develops when they have ulcerations or get very large.

There are two kinds: internal and external, which are based on their geography. Internal hemorrhoids are found in the upper two-thirds of the anal canal (above what is known as the dentate line). These are covered by the mucosa of the rectum. External hemorrhoids are below that line and can sometimes extrude outside the anus.

There are three stages or degrees of hemorrhoids, and these describe their size and how much they have prolapsed. The first two stages tend to respond best to natural treatment. Third-degree hemorrhoids sometimes require surgery.

Stage 1 are small; they don't protrude and sometimes bleed.

Stage 2 are larger; they protrude with defecation, but retract or get smaller spontaneously. These may also bleed.

Stage 3 are large; they protrude with any kind of abdominal pressure, including sneezing or coughing as well as with walking, standing, or defecating. These may also bleed and require surgery to remove them.

CHINESE MEDICINE VIEW

According to Chinese medicine, emotions can contribute to the formation of hemorrhoids because of stagnation to liver qi. Again, we see the familiar sequence of liver qi stagnation leading to damage of the spleen and the buildup of dampness.

Over time, stagnation can result in heat, which leads to damp heat. This stagnates blood, which backs pressure on the portal system and increases pressure on the rectal veins. In addition, excessive worry or prolonged concentration can deplete spleen qi. Add poor dietary habits and too much sitting, and you have a recipe for more stagnation of blood flow.

Diet, of course, also plays a large role. Poor dietary habits, such as a diet high in refined sugars and fats, can lead to dampness and damp heat in the intestines. The spleen then has difficulty holding in the blood in the vessels and maintaining muscle tone, which can lead to constipation or diarrhea.

Overconsumption of warming, damp-causing foods and drinks like alcohol, and rich and hot-natured foods can lead to accumulation and stagnation of food and result in damp heat in the intestines.

And lastly, a sedentary lifestyle with lots of sitting can impact the flow of blood and qi in the anal region. Prolonged standing and jarring exercise like long-distance running or heavy lifting may exhaust the qi and muscles and weaken the spleen.

This in turn can weaken muscle tone and cause prolapsed hemorrhoidal veins. Hemorrhoids may also occur during pregnancy due to pressure of the growing fetus on blood flow in the pelvic region. In addition, the tremendous amount of pressure on the anus during labor can cause extreme strain on the blood vessels in that area resulting in hemorrhoids.

USING THE A.P.A.R.T. SYSTEM TO DIAGNOSE AND TREAT HEMORRHOIDS

1. Ask and Assess

Once again, we must ask, Is this condition due to excess or deficiency? Hemorrhoids can have both scenarios.

Excess conditions include damp heat and blood stagnation.

Symptoms of damp heat hemorrhoids include:[2]

- Hemorrhoids with bleeding of fresh red or plum-colored blood

- Hemorrhoids may be swollen or painful (could be stage 2 or 3)

- Itch, discomfort, distention, burning, irritation, or pain in the anus

- Tenesmus (feeling like you have to go number two)

- Abdominal distention

- Thirst

- Concentrated urine

Blood stagnation is a more severe condition. It tends to be chronic and may require surgery. If you suspect you have this type of hemorrhoid, it may be appropriate to see a doctor.

Symptoms include:

- Hemorrhoids with relatively severe or continuous anal pain

- Hemorrhoids may be large and appear dark purple

- There may be bleeding; fresh red or purple

- Hypochondriac pain, tension, or discomfort under the ribs

- Dry mouth

- Dry, scaly skin

- Dark rings around the eyes

- Dark or purplish lips

In contrast, spleen qi deficiency hemorrhoids are usually less severe and correspond to stage 2 or 3. These are common with people with poor muscle tone. The main characteristic is a prolapsing nature of the hemorrhoids because weakness in the spleen results in prolapse.

Symptoms include:

- Hemorrhoids that easily protrude with defecation, coughing, sneezing, or prolonged standing or walking

- Intermittent, dull abdominal pain that is alleviated with warmth and pressure

- Abdominal distention

- Tendency to loose stools or diarrhea

- Loss of appetite

- Pale complexion

- Fatigue, weakness

- Shortness of breath

- Spontaneous sweating

2. Prioritize and Plan

Determine which type of hemorrhoids you have. If you are not sure or have difficulty, consult a practitioner. If they are very painful and do not resolve (stage 3), they may require surgery.

For damp heat type hemorrhoids, a damp heat diet is appropriate:

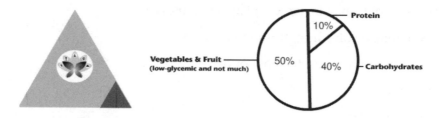

A very effective formula for damp heat type hemorrhoids is Huai hua san.[3] This clears damp heat from the intestines and cools blood and stops bleeding.

It contains huai hau, ce bai ye, jing jie, zhi ke, and huang bai; huang qin and hu lian are sometimes added if there is severe bleeding. You will recall these are the primary herbs of Huang lian jie du tang.

For blood stagnation type hemorrhoids, first determine whether or not this requires surgery. If not, a liver qi stagnation diet is appropriate.

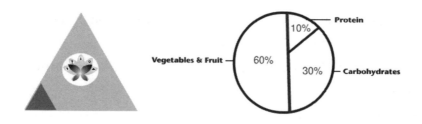

A good formula for blood stagnation type hemorrhoids is Xue fu zhu yu tang.[4] This is an effective formula for both relieving pain and stopping bleeding.

It contains dang gui, sheng di huang, chi shao, chuan xiong, tao ren, hong hua, chai hu, licorice root, zhi ke, jie geng di yu, and haui hua.

If surgery is required, a formula called Yunnan bai yao is quite helpful for recovery.

For spleen qi deficient hemorrhoids, a spleen and stomach qi diet is recommended:

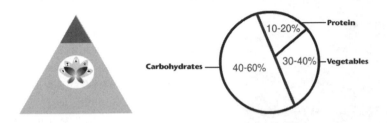

And once again, Li Dong-yuan's brilliant formula, Bu Zhong Yi Qi Tang, is quite effective because it is so balanced.

3. Act and Adapt

Choose which scenario is best for your case. If you don't know or are uncertain, consult a practitioner. If you suspect that your hemorrhoids may be stage 3, consult a doctor.

If they are mild to moderate, try the approach suggested above for 15 to 30 days.

4. Reassess and Reevaluate

Check your symptoms after following the recommendations. If you were successful in resolving the hemorrhoids, celebrate. And then return to a spleen and stomach supporting diet.

If you were not successful, try to determine why. If you are unable to, consult a doctor or practitioner.

5. Try and Try Again

Keep going! Keep continuing to support and heal the stomach and spleen.

FOOD AS MEDICINE: *PARSNIP*

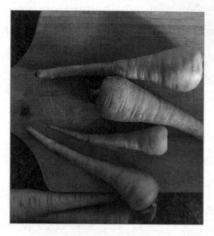

Parsnip is a delicious root vegetable that is an excellent carbohydrate source. I love to add it to soups and roast it with other root vegetables like carrots and turnips.

In Chinese medicine, parsnip is considered warm and pungent. It promotes sweating, dispels wind and dampness, and relieves pain. When it's cooked until it is charred (actually burned), it was traditionally used to stop bleeding.

Parsnip can be used to treat the common cold if it is mild and there is no fever. It can also be used to treat headache, muscle ache, dizziness, and arthritis.

- A simple recipe for treating the common cold is a tea made of ginger and parsnip.

- For cold-type arthritis (one that doesn't have a lot of redness and swelling, but it's worse with cold), combine parsnip, cinnamon, black pepper, and dried ginger into a tea and drink it. (That will warm you up!)

- For nosebleeds and abdominal bleeding (consult a doctor if abdominal bleeding persists), make a tea from charred parsnips and drink it.

HASHIMOMENT: Embracing Change

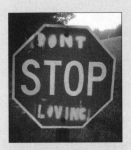

The only thing that is certain is change. Hard times will pass, and good times will pass. You may go through phases of flare-ups and have good days and bad ones. Nothing will ever stay the same forever.

Nowhere is this truer than in dealing with diet and Hashimoto's.

You may find something that works for you, but over time if it's too restrictive, it may lead to unintended consequences, like more food sensitivities.

And you may also be unwilling to make some of the changes that you need to make. Eventually, these can develop into other problems and you run the risk of encouraging the progression of Hashimoto's or causing other health problems.

So, we must wrap our minds around the inevitability of change and get in touch with our bodies so that when they signal or warn us, we can make the necessary changes.

You have the tools—all you need is the resolve.

I know change can be scary and it can be difficult, but when you embrace it and accept it, it's often much easier than you think.

Keep a journal, meditate, and exercise. Learn to listen to what your body tells you. You might be pleasantly surprised by how rewarding this type of living can be. And if you aren't, this too will change.

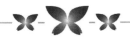

Conclusion

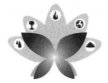

We did it! We made it through a maze of possibilities and challenges and arrived here at the end. An end that is really just the beginning of what I hope will be a life-long exploration into what is possible with using food to heal.

Hopefully, by now, you have gotten a good sense of how to apply the principles in this book to your specific situation, and you have gotten a glimpse of just how many options there are to use diet effectively. In addition, I hope that we can put to rest once and for all the ignorant notion that diet doesn't matter when it comes to treating Hashimoto's and autoimmunity.

One thing that writing and researching this book has done for me is to make me firmly convinced that diet is not just the foundation of health and well-being—it's the vehicle to get us there. And it really should be the first thing we examine when we are faced with a health challenge, not the last.

Another insight I think is incredibly important is that diet choices need to have some degree of flexibility, and we must be open to making changes as the situation dictates. Temporary conditions like colds and flus, infections, and stressful life events are opportunities to make adjustments. And those adjustments can help us overcome the challenges more quickly.

In addition, it's important to continue to stay in touch with your body so that you can sense when you need to alter your routine to get through a challenging period or phase. And as I have recommended on a number of occasions, keeping a journal is a great way to do this.

If you are feeling overwhelmed or still aren't sure what you need to do, here are some things to keep in mind. First, remember that the easiest way to simplify this process is to determine if your current situation is a problem of excess or one of deficiency.

Excess problems include the buildup of any pathological process like phlegm or dampness that can result in nodules or stones, as well as excessive heat (inflammation) or cold (due to poor circulation and/or yang deficiency) within the body. They may also include some type of systemic infection. These conditions may include an emotional component leading to anxiety or depression as well.

Deficient conditions, in contrast, are those primarily characterized by weakness and metabolic fatigue or exhaustion. Hypothyroidism, adrenal fatigue, iron deficiency, and other nutrient or mineral deficiencies are all examples.

And if there is an element of both, which sometimes happens, you will need to make a decision about which is the priority. This may mean cycling between a diet that supports deficiency and one that helps resolve the underlying challenge.

Bear in mind that treatment for deficient conditions tends to be longer in duration than treatment for excess conditions. In fact, it is not recommended to do any sort of excess treatment approach for a prolonged period.

Furthermore, since the underlying condition is ultimately one of metabolic weakness or deficiency, the spleen qi deficient diet is the default that should be returned to after any other type of intervention. It is where you want to have your "home base."

Finally, I think it's important to remember that this is a long-term project. There is plenty of room for experimentation and even letting things go for a period of time, as long as you return with renewed vigor and dedication.

And don't forget to look for opportunities everywhere in life where you might be able to do less, because by emptying your cup, you will allow the universe to fill it up again with the things that rejuvenate you like family, friends, experiencing nature, creative hobbies, exercise and more.

You can do this, by gently making this process a permanent part of your life and trusting the inherent wisdom that your body has been blessed with. I wish you the best on your journey. Be good, be kind, and remember to have compassion for everyone, including yourself.

Yours in health,

Marc

Appendix 1

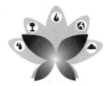

HASHIMOTO'S HEALING DIET:
Keys to Success

Here are a few important questions to ask yourself as well as some guidelines and reminders to ensure your success on this journey!

1. WHERE CAN YOU DO LESS?

From the beginning of writing this book, I have come to believe that this is a powerful theme. And please don't confuse doing less with being deprived or shrinking your life to fit Hashimoto's. On the contrary, by simplifying we create more space to transform, grow, and enlarge the possibilities.

Many health-related issues involve doing too much/consuming too much: too much sugar, too much coffee, too many carbs, too much stress, too much work, too much anger, too much clutter, too much stuff, too much meat, too much television, too much (you fill in the blank).

It's important to do everything in moderation (including moderation). It's just common sense; you can't maintain something in excess, as it's not sustainable. "Too much" will burn you out, and in some cases, it may even kill you.

There are a few exceptions to this rule, but I think it's a valuable guiding principle. By doing less we allow more space for things that matter, including family, friends, sleep, relaxation, meditation, exercise, qi gong, yoga, etc. And these are the bricks in the road to remission and the building blocks of a long, happy, and fulfilling life.

2. ARE YOUR HEALTH ISSUES CAUSED BY EXCESS OR DEFICIENCY?

This is a really important question. Are your issues problems of excess like "too much" of the things mentioned above or perhaps excess bacterial overgrowth or excess fungal overgrowth or excess inflammation or excess cortisol or excess thyroid hormone or excess iron or excess alcohol or excessive drug use or . . . ?

Or if we think about it in Chinese medical terms, excess dampness, excess heat, excess stagnation, excessive emotions, excess fire . . .

For problems of excess, we must do less and/or minimize and treat those excessive problems in order to reduce them. It's very logical. If it's a problem of too much, reduce whatever that too much is.

On the other hand, are your health issues problems of deficiency like too little thyroid hormone, too little cortisol, too little iron, too little magnesium, too little sleep, too little time, too little exercise, too little social interaction, too little absorption of nutrients, too little circulation, etc.?

Or in Chinese medical terms, are your issues caused by too little qi, too little blood, too little yin, too little of the proper nourishment, too little blood flow, too little peace, etc.?

For problems of deficiency, we must build up and/or tonify or target nutrition toward those areas where there is too little. Again, it's very logical and simple.

The difficulty is when we have some of both, like adrenal fatigue and dampness or excess stagnation in the liver and blood deficiency or iron deficiency and excess inflammation. In these cases, we have to address both areas.

3. DO YOU KNOW WHEN TO CHANGE YOUR APPROACH?

This is another vital question. This is why you have to pay attention, because circumstances will change. Your body will change, you might get a cold or need surgery, something that's been developing may suddenly become manifest, or you may have to stop a certain approach and make adjustments.

Autoimmune disease is also progressive. Where are you in the progression? What if you take steps and reverse that progression? Or what if, God forbid, you progress to the next level? You need to be able to make adjustments accordingly.

This can be difficult, especially when we find something that works. We may be afraid to change. I see this in a lot of people who have success with the autoimmune paleo diet. And it makes sense; it can really help and improve your quality of life, and you don't want to mess with that.

The problem is that never deviating from something can, itself, be a form of excess and lead to problems. This can happen with the autoimmune paleo diet. I have seen it time and time again, and the result can be an increase in food sensitivities.

Never changing what you eat and eating the same foods every day can result in an overgrowth of certain bacterial species; deficiencies in certain nutrients, vitamins, and minerals; or excessive amounts of certain enzymes like beta-glucuronidase.

BETA-GLUCURONIDASE: THE TROUBLEMAKING ENZYME

Beta-glucuronidase is an enzyme that aids in the breakdown of complex carbohydrates (like rice or pasta). It is found in many different tissues in the body. It is important for helping the body to get rid of environmental toxins.

But it also helps break down sugar molecules so that they can be used by the body to create energy in the cells. It's also necessary for converting thyroid hormone from T4 into T3, which is the form the body uses.

Beta-glucuronidase plays a major role in vitamin D and estrogen recirculation. But this enzyme can also cause problems by reversing converted toxins and hormones and sending them back into circulation in the bloodstream.

DYSBIOSIS IN THE GUT CAUSES MORE BETA-GLUCURONIDASE TO BE MADE

When you have dysbiosis (an imbalance of gut bacteria), this can cause increases in beta-glucuronidase and can increase its activity.

And by dysbiosis, I mean a couple of things: too little diversity and overgrowth of species that aren't helpful.

Diversity in the gut is significant because it leads to more balanced growth. When you eat too many of the same foods all the time, you can develop a lack of some populations.

This is why it's vital to explore variety in your diet.

Now that you've asked yourself the important questions, here are some simple guidelines to follow to help you make the most of your experience.

RESPECT MEALTIME

Digestion is a process that demands energy. If that energy is diverted from the Earth phase to some other place when it should be concentrated in the gut, then there is just less available to transport and transform our food.

Even activities that seem innocent, like watching TV while eating, can take away from proper digestion. And much more so with working breakfasts, eating on the run, and working through lunch. These can have a major negative impact on digestive function.

I think this is a very important point. In our society today, for a variety of reasons, the ritual of having a meal has sometimes been lost. Traditionally, sharing a meal has been a powerful part of many different cultures. In a sense, it's a tradition that's as old as human society.

Nowadays, people watch television while they eat or text or surf the web on their smartphones, they eat in their cars, they have fast food and don't even sit down, they skip meals, and they eat on the run.

If we are to believe that the Earth phase is the center and it has that much importance on our health, we have to consider that meals, themselves, the times that we get our food for digestion, are also pretty important.

For our health and well-being, for proper digestion, and for the harmony of the Earth phase, we need to give meals the reverence they deserve.

BE PRESENT FOR YOUR MEALS

Stop multitasking during mealtime. You can take 15 to 30 minutes off from television or your smartphone, tablet, iPad, or your computer a few times a day. Treat meals like a meditation, and focus on what you are doing.

It's also a great chance to spend time with family, friends, and loved ones. Take advantage of that opportunity.

CHEW YOUR FOOD THOROUGHLY

Digestion begins in your mouth, so be sure to chew your food thoroughly and completely. Don't race to finish. Take your time and enjoy it.

DON'T DRINK EXCESSIVE AMOUNTS OF LIQUIDS WHEN EATING

Having a moderate amount of water or a little tea to aid digestion is a great idea. Drinking 16 to 32 ounces of sugar-laced soda, however, is destroying the nutritional value of your food.

Even drinking a lot of water may also be a problem because it can lower stomach acid levels. Remember that we need sufficient amounts of stomach acid to break down our food and to release bile and pancreatic enzymes.

A little water with apple cider vinegar, ginger tea, or lemon in water can all help boost stomach acid. Too much liquid is going to compromise that. This is another opportunity to do less.

AVOID DRAMA DURING MEALTIME

For me, one of the biggest takeaways from studying Li Dong-yuan was realizing just how profound the impact of emotion is on disease and the health of the Earth phase.

For example, having lots of drama during meals can really compromise your digestion. Try to avoid controversial topics, such as politics or religion. Keep the conversation light and positive. If you are dining alone, stay off social media and avoid reading or watching upsetting news stories.

BE PATIENT

For many of us, food plays an important social role in our lives. It can be something we use to bond over, something we use in celebrations or in rituals, and something we use for comfort emotionally.

Major changes in diet can cause a big psychological shock and can upend our lives. So we need to remember that this is a long-term project, and like the process of healing our Hashimoto's, it's a journey.

The modifications, additions, and subtractions you will inevitably have to make should be made in such a way so that they provide you with the space for both physical and emotional adaptation. Go easy on yourself and be gentle.

Also keep in mind that changes may be accompanied by digestive symptoms as your body adjusts. Make sure you keep a journal to chronicle these changes and so that you can learn from the experience.

Appendix 2

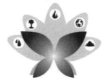

HASHIMOTO'S HEALING DIET:
for Vegetarians and Vegans

One area where there seems to be some controversy and very little guidance is on a vegetarian and/or vegan version of the autoimmune paleo diet. The basic challenges remain the same: How do we reduce systemic inflammation and heal the gut?

And the diagnostic criteria are also the same: Is the health challenge excess or deficient in nature? There are, however, some unique challenges for vegetarians and vegans.

Namely, these are as follows: What are safe sources of protein (ones that won't further damage the gut)? And how does one get sufficient amounts of B12? The concern with proteins is that the common sources of protein in a vegan and vegetarian diet are grains, legumes, dairy, soy products, and nuts and seeds.

All of these are potentially problematic because they can damage the gut and cause an inflammatory or immune response. And soy products can be goitrogenic and impair thyroid function.

So, in my opinion, the problem comes down to this:

- Is a vegetarian or vegan diet without those major sources of vegetable-based protein sufficient to provide enough nutrition to heal Hashimoto's?

- Can you work with some of those foods that are eliminated and avoid immune flare-ups and triggers?

First, there is no question in my mind that a vegetarian diet can provide sufficient nutrients for health and well-being. And some vegetarians also eat fish, eggs, dairy, and sometimes fowl. So for them, I don't think it's an issue.

This is a perfectly sustainable diet and is actually very close to what I have proposed in terms of proportions of food, etc.

For those following a strict vegan diet, the question becomes more difficult. Traditionally, in China there aren't a lot of records of strict vegan sects, though some Taoists were primarily vegan. I think what they had going for them is extensive knowledge and use of herbs to supplement their diets. And even some of them raised chickens and caught fish for those in their community who were sick.[1]

What that tells us is that there were times when judiciously using animal protein to heal was recommended. And some in the autoimmune paleo community (like Mickey Trescott) were vegans for many years and then made the transition to eating meat. For Mickey and others, it helped her to heal when other interventions did not.

So I think it's important to be open to the possibility that you may get to a point where you may need to incorporate high-quality animal protein in order to heal. And I think this may be a question of asking how far your autoimmunity has progressed and how weak and deficient you are.

As I noted in my first book, there are three stages of autoimmunity. If you have progressed to the third stage, which is quite severe and involves the breakdown of multiple systems, then you should consider doing everything you can to recover.

On the other hand, if you are in an earlier stage, simply incorporating more herbs and using the same principles I have taught you may be perfectly fine. And I have had people share with me that a vegan diet really helped them.

There's no question that a well-balanced vegan diet (one that isn't a junk-food, sugar-based vegan diet) can be very healing and anti-inflammatory.

So what does that diet actually look like, and what herbs can you incorporate to make up for what you may lose from the foods that are problematic?

I think the basics of the diet that I have laid out in Chapter 13 and Chapter 14 still apply. I would first do an elimination diet, followed by the reintroduction/restoring oral tolerance diet. And I would look to see how deficient you are.

I would also recommend the spleen and stomach qi supporting diet as a base diet. Be cautious about eating too many salads and raw foods, however. I think that could really compromise your health if you are already depleted.

Let's review that diet:

1. QI DEFICIENCY DIET

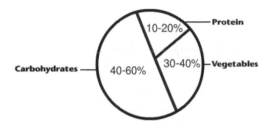

A diet that focuses on strengthening the spleen qi consists of well-cooked, simple meals. The basis of the diet is complex carbohydrates with some high-quality protein and lightly cooked vegetables. Fresh, locally grown seasonal food is preferable, as it will have the most vibrant qi.

Food should be lightly cooked, with vegetables steaming or blanching just enough to preserve a light crunch is recommended. Green leafy and delicate vegetables like broccoli and beans are best cooked this way. Heavier root vegetables and grains should be cooked longer and slowly so that they retain their qi, shape, and texture.

Easily digested carbohydrates, such as sweet potatoes and starchy root vegetables, should make up a larger proportion of the diet (40 to 60 percent). The remainder should be cooked greens and red and yellow vegetables (30 to 40 percent). Since animal protein will be avoided, here are some options for protein.

During the elimination phase (30–60 days): Chlorella, spirulina, and wild blue-green algae are good sources of both protein and vitamin B12. Nutritional yeast can also be helpful for both (be cautious if you have Candida or damp heat conditions). Miso and tempeh in moderation might also be helpful.

During the reintroduction phase (30–60 days): You can start reintroducing grains (with the exception of wheat and gluten-containing grains, of course) and beans. Follow the reintroduction/boost oral tolerance guidelines. I would continue to be very cautious about soy; fermented soy products (like tempeh and miso) are fine on occasion, in my opinion, and tofu may be as well. But I would not recommend highly processed soy-based meat substitutes at all. Nor would I recommend gluten-based meat substitutes.

As the spleen becomes stronger, you can shift and add other elements. Salads may be added (but not several per day) as the spleen gets stronger or if you are in a hot climate. Be aware that this larger proportion of carbohydrates can lead to dampness, and adjustments may have to be made accordingly (see the diet for dampness in Chapter 12).

Soups and stews are particularly beneficial for qi deficient conditions. You can also batch cook on weekends to last the entire week. Taking time to cook your own food can be healing and therapeutic on its own.

From the Earth phase system, we learned about the important relationship between the Earth and Metal phases. Targeting nutrition for the spleen will also benefit the lungs and visa versa. Qi gong exercises are also excellent and vital for helping to build qi. (See my first book *How to Heal Hashimoto's: An Integrative Road Map to Remission* for some powerful, restorative qi gong exercises.)

Here are a few specific qi deficiency dietary recommendations:

GENERAL RECOMMENDATIONS:

All food cooked and warm, slow cooking of soups, stews, and broths are particularly effective. Chew your food thoroughly. Simple combinations of a few ingredients; more frequent, smaller meals, and regular mealtimes.

High proportion of complex carbohydrates and vegetables; less meat (nutrient-dense meat like organ meat is recommended).

Avoid excessive fluids during meals, overeating, missing meals, and multitasking during meals.

BENEFICIAL FOODS FOR QI DEFICIENCY:

Neutral or sweet, warm flavors. Artichoke, mustard greens, pumpkin, sweet potato, celery root, squash, carrot, parsnip, yams, peas, string beans, beets, winter squash, okra, turnip, Jerusalem artichoke, coconut milk, papaya, apricots, figs, grapes, currants, coconut, stewed fruit.

Pungent flavors in small amounts help assist the natural function of dispersing and descending: onion, leek, garlic, turnip, pepper, fresh ginger, cinnamon, and non-seed kitchen spices (sage, savory, thyme, tarragon, etc.).

Complex sweet flavors (use with caution in damp and damp heat conditions): molasses, dates, coconut sugar.

Helpful herbs: astragalus, codonopsis, red and black dates.

Optional (only to be eaten once you have eliminated and reintroduced them successfully): light grains, especially rice and rice porridge, oats, chickpeas, black beans, walnuts.

Optional spices (same as above; eliminate first, then reintroduce; eat in moderation if tolerated): nutmeg, fennel.

Avoid: cold-natured, uncooked, and raw foods; salads, raw fruits (whole and juiced, especially citrus), wheat, raw vegetables, tomato, spinach, Swiss chard, tofu, millet, seaweed, salt, too many sweet foods and concentrated sweeteners, vitamin C (over 1 to 2 grams per day), beer, ice cream and dairy products (except a little grass-fed butter), sugar, chocolate, nuts and seeds (except walnuts), nut butters.

2. YANG DEFICIENCY DIET

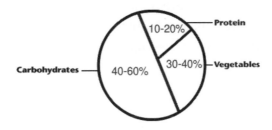

GENERAL RECOMMENDATIONS:

Spleen yang deficiency foods are the same as spleen qi deficiency foods plus more warming ingredients like parsnip, sweet potato, onion, leek, stocks and broths (miso), stewed fruit, and chestnut.

In addition, more warming spices like ginger, clove, cinnamon, rosemary, and turmeric are recommended.

For kidney yang deficiency, add clove, fenugreek, black pepper, cinnamon bark, dry ginger (more warming than fresh ginger), rosemary, chestnut, lamb, salmon, onion, leek, chives.

In addition, more warming spices like ginger, clove, cinnamon, rosemary, and turmeric are recommended.

For kidney yang deficiency, add clove, fenugreek, black pepper, cinnamon bark, dry ginger (more warming than fresh ginger), rosemary, chestnut, lamb, salmon, onion, leek, chives.

Avoid for both: raw fruits and vegetables, sprouts and salads, tomato, spinach, tofu, soybean, millet, kelp, excessive salt and sweet foods, dairy products, nuts and seeds, soymilk, refrigerated or iced drinks.

And just as anyone else, you must keep track and make adjustments as necessary. If you develop too much heat or dampness, incorporate heat-clearing, dampness-reducing elements.

Some herbs to consider for overcoming weakness include:

Herbs that tonify qi: ginseng, atractylodes, Chinese dates (black), shan yao, Siberian ginseng, codonopsis, licorice root, American ginseng, polygonatum root, pseudosteallaria root.

Herbs that tonify blood: rehmannia, dang gui, angelica root, longan fruit, lycii berries (though these are nightshades), Chinese dates (red), white peony root.

Other beneficial herbs: cordyceps, stinging nettle, he shou wu, drynaria root.

REGARDING B12:

The danger with strict veganism is that you could wind up becoming B12 deficient over time. It's very important to test vitamin B12 levels periodically.

Some things that deplete B12 include:

- Antibiotics and birth control pills

- Recreational drugs and intoxicants (alcohol, cigarettes, coffee, cocaine, methamphetamine, etc.)

- Stress from any source (emotional or physiological—i.e., injury, surgery, or trauma)

- Liver disease or chronic illness (like Hashimoto's)

As we have seen, proper levels of stomach acid and intrinsic factor are critical for B12 absorption. Autoimmunity to parietal cells can cause major B12 deficiencies.

PLANT SOURCES OF B12

- Fermented foods: miso, tempeh, pickles, amasake, and nut and seed yogurts. These will have at least trace amounts of B12.

- Algae, micro-algae, and seaweed: caution must be used with these as they contain iodine and may cause flare-ups of Hashimoto's.

- Nutritional yeast (brewer's yeast): It doesn't contain large amounts of B12; be cautious in damp conditions like Candida.

- Supplement with sublingual B12 and/or B12 injections.

BOTTOM LINE:

In my opinion, a vegan and/or vegetarian approach can be used with success. However, if you choose to go this route, you must be extra vigilant about B12 levels and keep close track of your symptoms and results in a journal.

Follow the same basic principles of excess or deficiency, making changes as necessary. And finally, if testing and symptoms reveal that it is not working for you, consider incorporating some quality animal protein for a period of time as an experiment to see how much better it makes you feel.

Appendix 3

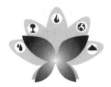

How to Improve Oral Tolerance

Before we look at what to do to improve oral tolerance, let's examine some of the mechanisms for developing and maintaining it.

MECHANISMS OF ORAL TOLERANCE

IL-10 AND ORAL TOLERANCE: IL-10 is an **anti-inflammatory** cytokine because it decreases various immune cells such as Th1 *and* Th2 cells. It also inhibits NF kappa beta, which is important in destructive inflammation. It inhibits COX 2 and mast cells and decreases insulin and leptin resistance.

IL-10 is something we want to increase.[1]

IL-12 AND ORAL TOLERANCE: IL-12, which is part of the Th1 family of cytokines, can block oral tolerance in Th1 conditions. It is responsible for helping cytotoxic lymphocytes (natural killer cells) mature, and it also supplies growth factor to help certain cells grow into the killers that they are.

IL-12 is involved in turning on genes that result in attacks on specific organs, which has been implicated as an important player in Hashimoto's. IL-12 is something we want to reduce.

TREGS AND ORAL TOLERANCE: Tregs comprise about 5 to 10 percent of T-helper cells.[2] There are two types of Tregs: "induced" (iTregs) and "natural" (nTregs). Both types are anti-inflammatory. *Induced* means that they are created outside the thymus. There are two kinds of induced Tregs: Th3 and Tr1. *Natural* means that they are part of the cells naturally produced in our thymus gland.

Tregs calm and suppress Th1, Th2, and Th17 cells and their cytokines, as well as many other immune cells and proteins, such as basophils, eosinophils, mast cells, and IgE. They also influence migration of inflammatory cells to tissues.

Tregs are directly anti-inflammatory. However, they need to be "activated" in order to have their suppressor functions. Exposure to a dietary protein or an antigen is one of the ways that they get activated. Obviously, increasing Tregs in a balanced way is a good idea with autoimmunity.

But, as with all things, if you do this too aggressively, there is the risk of becoming less able to defend against some infections. And unfortunately, one of those infections is a viral infection like herpes and Epstein-Barr.

MUCUS IN THE INTESTINES AND ORAL TOLERANCE: Researchers have found that mucus plays an important role in maintaining the barrier of the gut and in modulating homeostasis (or balance) in the gut. Having a healthy amount of mucus in the gut is also a good idea.[3]

DENDRITIC CELLS AND ORAL TOLERANCE: Dendritic cells (DCs) main function is to process antigen material and present it on the cell surface to the T cells of the immune system. They act as messengers between the innate and the adaptive immune systems.[4]

Dendritic cells are necessary for immune tolerance because they can adapt to proteins or enhance the attack on them. At low levels these proteins help dendritic cells to adapt, but if proteins become excessive and aren't cleared, this can result in dendritic cells attacking and consuming the protein (and in some cases our own tissue). **With dendritic cells, we want to encourage as much variety (especially lots of different vegetables) as we can and make sure that the bowels are moving and that we aren't eating too much animal protein.**

cAMP is a signaling molecule that relays messages to T cells to not respond and proliferate to a protein. This, essentially, trains the immune cells to not respond. **Increasing cAMP may be beneficial.**[5]

Oral tolerance is dependent on good bacteria in the gut. The more we learn about intestinal bacteria and the microbiome, the more valuable they become and the more irresponsible excessive antibiotic treatment becomes. **Gut bacteria should be treated like an endangered species and be tended to and watched over carefully.**

HIGH–PROTEIN DIETS AND ORAL TOLERANCE: This was a very interesting finding in recent research: Diets that are lower in protein reduced both Th1 and Th2 and were effective in helping promote oral tolerance. **Thus, reducing dietary protein (especially animal protein) may help reduce sensitivity; here's where we see direct evidence of the importance of shifting proportions in the diet.**

THINGS THAT CAUSE DECLINES IN ORAL TOLERANCE: A number of things may lead to declines in oral tolerance. Obviously, these are things we want to avoid:

ALCOHOL: Sorry, booze fans. Alcohol has been shown to reduce intestinal mucosa and to disrupt immune regulation in the gut, resulting in a decline in oral tolerance.

CITRUS PECTIN: Pectin occurs naturally in the cell walls of most plants and especially concentrated in the peel and pulp of citrus fruits (lemons, limes, oranges, and grapefruits), plums, and apples. Recently, scientists have been able to modify and break down pectin's long, branched chains of polysaccharides into shorter, unbranched lengths of soluble fiber molecules that dissolve easily in water.[6]

The result, modified citrus pectin (MCP), is a substance that is rich in galactose residues, which are easily processed by the digestive system and absorbed into the bloodstream. It has shown promise in some cancer treatments. It has also been found to inhibit oral tolerance to certain types of proteins.

H. PYLORI: *Helicobacter pylori,* as we have learned, is a bacteria that can cause declines in stomach acid and can lead to ulcers and GERD. It has also been linked to lower oral tolerance.[7]

PALMITATE: Palmitate is derived from palm oil and is used in soaps and cosmetics. It can bind to dietary proteins and inhibit tolerance.[8]

BOTTOM LINE:

In summary, you can see that many factors contribute to the development and maintenance of oral tolerance, and that they are critical for dampening immune reactions.

The loss or decline of tolerance may be an important factor in autoimmunity and in sensitivity reactions to dietary proteins.

But, as with everything, carefully balancing oral tolerance is vital when dealing with autoimmune disease and reactions to dietary proteins.

WHAT IMPROVES ORAL TOLERANCE?

This is a question that's not so easy to answer. Creating tolerance is different depending on what it is you want to create tolerance for.

Creating tolerance for a Th2 system issue like almonds or peanuts, for example, in IgE type allergies is very different than creating tolerance for someone with a Th1 condition (which some people with Hashimoto's have).

TREGS ARE IMPORTANT FOR INTESTINAL TOLERANCE

Intestinal tolerance requires the T regulatory cells and T cells found in the intestinal lining. These T regulatory cells are created in response to proteins that pass through the intestines.

One important vitamin that encourages these T regulatory cells to travel to the gut is **vitamin A.**

T regulatory cells that are created in the gut suppress the local immune response.

Basically, what happens is this: Immune cells in the gut take proteins to lymph nodes (which are numerous in this part of our body) with the help of other molecules (vitamin A, TGF beta, etc.). These cells program T cells to be T regulatory cells.

These T regulatory cells then spread throughout the gut and suppress the local immune response. This means that they turn off the immune reaction to these proteins.

Because the lymphatic system travels throughout the body, the theory is that this information gets shared with the entire immune system, and it stops the attack on this protein.

Two immune proteins that are critical for this process are TGF beta and IL-10. In researching this topic, I discovered there are a number of Chinese herbs that have been identified as increasing IL-10 (more on that in a moment).

SUPPLEMENTS THAT CAN HELP CREATE TOLERANCE

BUTYRATE: A short-chain fatty acid that is an important food for cells lining the colon. It is very important for the maintenance of oral tolerance. There's a product called Enterovite that I carry in my online store (hashimotoshealing.com /hashimotoshealthstore) that contains butyrate, vitamin E, and calcium, which help feed the good bacteria in the colon.[9]

COD LIVER OIL: Contains vitamin A and D3 and DHA; these vitamins are critical for oral tolerance and immune balance.[10]

PROBIOTICS: Research has identified these species: *B. infantis, Lactobacillus casei,* and *Lactococcus lactis.*[11] These species of intestinal bacteria play an important role in inducing and maintaining oral tolerance. Research has shown that deficiencies in these bacteria can lead to more allergies.

URSOLIC ACID: Commonly found in fruit peels, rosemary, and thyme, it's helpful in maintaining oral tolerance and can be used in the treatment of obesity. Clears out T cells that attack the body; an interesting finding, given that modified citrus pectin, which also comes from fruit peels, has the opposite effect.[12]

THE CHINESE HERBAL FORMULA LIU WEI DI HUANG WAN: This is a base formula with over a dozen variations. One of the main ingredients, rehmannia, has been shown to benefit the thyroid and to modulate immune cells in a number of positive ways. For example, it has been shown to boost cAMP and IL-10.[13]

Some additions to this formula can enhance its ability to modulate the immune and endocrine systems. Cinnamon cortex (rou gui) and immature orange peel (zhi shi) have both been shown to modulate mechanisms that lead to enhanced oral tolerance. Zhi shi has been shown to boost Tregs.[14]

This was a very interesting discovery for me because this formula is not normally thought of in the context of digestive or autoimmune issues in Chinese medicine.

However, the pharmacology of the formula reveals that it is effective in modulating the immune response, in clearing out circulating immune complexes, and in helping to reestablish oral tolerance.

Other herbs that have been found to be helpful are curcumin, quercitin, cinnamon, and slippery elm (this is helpful with the intestinal mucosa, which is responsible for oral tolerance).

EXERCISE: Exercise has been shown to accomplish exactly what is needed to improve oral tolerance. It is an effective means of inducing reduction in CRP, IL-1, IL-6, and INF-gamma levels, as well as increase IL-10.[15]

For the gut, moderate exercises that stimulate and strengthen the core and abdomen are quite helpful. Fire breathing (a form of rapid, vigorous breathing used in yoga) and qi gong are both excellent examples. In addition, the amount and intensity of exercise you do matters.

Doing too much, for too long is counterproductive and weakens immune function. But doing it regularly is clearly beneficial.[16]

One large review and consensus statement on exercise sums it up like this: Of note, IL-6 infusion totally mimics the acute anti-inflammatory effects of a bout of exercise both with regard to induction of IL-1ra and IL-10 and with regard to suppression of endotoxin-stimulated increases in TNF-α levels.[17]

During acute exercise there is also a marked increase in adrenaline (epinephrine), cortisol, growth hormone, prolactin, and other factors that have immunomodulatory effects. **Taken together, it appears that each bout of exercise induces an anti-inflammatory environment.**

Endnotes

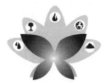

Introduction

1. Scorecard: The Pollution Information Site. (n.d.). Pollution locator: Toxic chemical releases. Retrieved from www.scorecard.goodguide.com/env-releases/us-map.tcl

2. Food and Agriculture Organization of the United Nations, Intergovernmental Technical Panel on Soils. (2015). *Status of the world's soil resources* (Main Report). Retrieved from http://www.fao.org/3/a-i5199e.pdf

3. Lao Tzu. (1990). *Tao teh ching.* (John C. H. Wu, Trans.) (p. 71). Boston, MA: Shambhala Publications.

4. Kochanek, K. D. et al. (2016). Deaths: Final data for 2014. *National Vital Statistics Reports* 65(4).

5. Collin, P. et al. (1994). Autoimmune thyroid disorders and coeliac disease. *European Journal of Endocrinology*, *130*, 137–140.

6. Stojanovich, L., & Marisavljevich, D. (2008). Stress as a trigger of autoimmune disease. *Autoimmunity Reviews 7*(3), 209–13.

Chapter 1

1. Kendall, D. E. (2002). *Dao of Chinese medicine: Understanding an ancient healing art.* (p. 89). Oxford: Oxford University Press.

2. Ibid, p. 94.

3. *Li Dong-yuan's treatise on the spleen & stomach: A translation of the* Pi Wei Lun. (2004). (Bob Flaws, Trans.). Boulder, CO: Blue Poppy Press.

4. Naschitz, J. E. et al. (2000). Heart diseases affecting the liver and liver diseases affecting the heart. *American Heart Journal*, *140*(1), 111–120.

5. Laugero, K. D. (2001). A new perspective on glucocorticoid feedback: relation to stress, carbohydrate feeding, and feeling better. *Journal of Neuroendocrinology*, *13*(9), 827–835.

6. Reinehr, T., & Andler, W. (2004). Cortisol and its relation to insulin resistance before and after weight loss in obese children. *Hormone Research*, *62*(3), 107–112.

7. Sherman, S. (n.d.). Li Dong-yuan and the earth school in Chinese medicine [blog post]. Retrieved from https://www.philadelphia-acupuncture.com/li-dong-yuan/

8. Flaws, B., & Sionneau, P. (2001).*The treatment of modern western medical diseases with Chinese medicine: A textbook and clinical manual* (p. 15). Boulder, CO: Blue Poppy Press.

9. Ibid, p. 16.

10. Breines, J. G. et al. (2014). Self-compassion as a predictor of interleukin-6 response to acute psychosocial stress. *Brain, Behavior, and Immunity, 37*, 109–114.

Chapter 2

1. Patil, B. S., Patil, S., & Gururaj, T. R. (2011). Probable autoimmune causal relationship between periodontitis and Hashimoto's thyroiditis: A systemic review. *Nigerian Journal of Clinical Practice, 14*(3), 253.

2. Scadding, G. K. (1990). Immunology of the tonsil: A review. *Journal of the Royal Society of Medicine,* 83.

3. Ji, J. et al. (2016). Tonsillectomy associated with an increased risk of autoimmune diseases: A national cohort study. *Journal of Autoimmunity, 72,* 1–7.

4. Draborg, A. H., Duus, K., & Houen, G. (2013). Epstein-Barr virus in systemic autoimmune diseases. *Clinical and Developmental Immunology,* 2013.

5. Dittfeld, A. et al. (2016). A possible link between the Epstein-Barr virus infection and autoimmune thyroid disorders. *Central-European Journal of Immunology, 41*(3), 297–301.

6. Rafsanjani, F. N. et al. (2003). Effects of thyroid hormones on basal and stimulated gastric acid secretion due to histamine, carbachol and pentagastrin in rats. *Saudi Medical Journal, 24*(4), 341–346.

7. Gebhard, R. L. et al. (1992). Thyroid hormone differentially augments biliary sterol secretion in the rat. I: The isolated-perfused liver model. *The Journal of Lipid Research, 33,* 1459–1466.

8. Gropper, S. S., Smith, J. L., & Groff, J. L. (2005). The digestive and absorptive processes. *In Advanced nutrition and human metabolism* (5th ed.) (p. 51). Belmont, CA: Wadsworth, Cengage Learning.

9. Ibid, p. 53.

10. Magge, S., & Lembo, A. (2012). Low-FODMAP diet for treatment of irritable bowel syndrome. *Gastroenterology & Hepatology, 8*(11), 739–745.

11. Spahn, T. W. et al. (2001). Induction of oral tolerance to cellular immune responses in the absence of Peyer's patches. *European Journal of Immunology, 31*(4), 1278–87.

Chapter 3

1. Stulberg, E. et al. (2016). An assessment of US microbiome research. *Nature Microbiology 1,* Article ID: 15015. doi: 10.1038/nmicrobiol.2015.15

2. Roesslein, M. (2017). How I Came to Love MegaSporeBiotic, the World's Best Probiotic. Rebel Health Tribe. Retrieved from https://rebelhealthtribe.com/probiotic/

3. Ichinohe, T. et al. (2011). Microbiota regulates immune defense against respiratory tract influenza A virus infection. *PNAS, 108*(13), 5354–5359. doi: 10.1073/pnas.1019378108

4. Blaser, M. J., & Falkow, S. (2009). What are the consequences of the disappearing microbiome? *Nature Reviews Microbiology, 7*(12), 887–94. doi: 10.1038/nrmicro2245

5. Siezen, R. J., & Kleerebezem, M. (2011). The human gut microbiome: Are we our enterotypes? *Microbial Biotechnology, 4*(5), 550–553. doi: 10.1111/j.1751-7915.2011.00290.x

6. Arumugam, M. et al. (2011). Enterotypes of the human gut microbiome. *Nature, 473,* 174–180. doi: 10.1038/nature09944

7. Cabrera-Rubio, R. et al. The human milk microbiome changes over lactation and is shaped by maternal weight and mode of delivery. *American Journal of Clinical Nutrition,* 2012; *96*(3): 544.

8. Ho, J. T. et al. (2015). Systemic effects of gut microbiota and its relationship with disease and modulation. *BMC Immunology 16*(21). doi: 10.1186/s12865-015-0083-2

9. Mathis, D., & Benoist, C. (2011). Microbiota and autoimmune disease: The hosted self. *Cell Host & Microbe, 10*(4), 297–301. doi: 10.1016/j.chom.2011.09.007

10. Chervonsky, A. V. (2013). Microbiota and autoimmunity. *Cold Spring Harbor Perspectives in Biology, 5*(3). doi: 10.1101/cshperspect.a007294

11. Grand View Research. (2016, September). Probiotics market analysis by application and segment forecast to 2024. Retrieved from http://www.grandviewresearch.com/industry-analysis/probiotics-market

Chapter 4

1. Maoshing Ni. (1995). *The Yellow Emperor's Classic of Medicine.* (p. 1). Boston, MA: Shambhala Publications.

2. *Li Dong-yuan's treatise on the spleen & stomach: A translation of the* Pi Wei Lun. (2004). (Bob Flaws, Trans.). (p. 3). Boulder, CO: Blue Poppy Press.

3. Ibid, p. 9

4. Ibid, p. 13

5. Ibid, p. 20.

6. Swirski, F. K. et al. (2009). Identification of splenic reservoir monocytes and their deployment to inflammatory sites. *Science, 325*(5940), 612–616. doi: 10.1126/science.1175202

7. Watanabe, K. et al. (1995). Long-term effects of thyroid hormone on lymphocyte subsets in spleens and thymuses of mice. *Endocrine Journal, 42*(5), 661–668.

8. Keown, D. (2014). *The spark in the machine: How the science of acupuncture explains the mysteries of western medicine* (pp. 202–203). Philadelphia, PA: Singing Dragon.

9. Robinson, R. (2009). Serotonin's role in the pancreas revealed at last. *PLOS Biology, 7*(10): e1000227. doi: 10.1371/journal.pbio.1000227

10. Isaac, R. et al. (2013). Selective serotonin reuptake inhibitors (SSRIs) inhibit insulin secretion and action in pancreatic β cells. *The Journal of Biological Chemistry, 288*(8), 5682–5693. doi: 10.1074/jbc.M112.408641

Chapter 5

1. Allen, A.P. et al. (2017). A psychology of the human brain-gut-microbiome axis. *Social and Personality Psychology Compass, 11*(4):e12309. doi: 10.1111/spc3.12309

2. Kelly, J. R. et al. (2015). Breaking down the barriers: The gut microbiome, intestinal permeability and stress-related psychiatric disorders. *Frontiers in Cellular Neuroscience, 9*(392). doi: 10.3389/fncel.2015.00392

3. Abdallah, I. N. et al. (2001). Frequency of Firmicutes and Bacteroidetes in gut microbiota in obese and normal weight Egyptian children and adults. *Archives of Medical Science: AMS, 7*(3), 501–507. doi: 10.5114/aoms.2011.23418

4. Braniste, V. et al. (2014). The gut microbiota influences blood-brain barrier permeability in mice. *Science Translational Medicine, 6*(263):263ra158. doi: 10.1126/scitranslmed.3009759

5. Guarner, F. et al. (2006). Mechanisms of disease: The hygiene hypothesis revisited. *Nature Clinical Practice Gastroenterology & Hepatology, 3*, 275–284. doi: 10.1038/ncpgasthep0471

6. Claesson, M. J. et al. (2012). Gut microbiota composition correlates with diet and health in the elderly. *Nature, 488*(7410), 178–184. doi: 10.1038/nature11319

7. Söderholm, J. D. et al. (2002). Neonatal maternal separation predisposes adult rats to colonic barrier dysfunction in response to mild stress. *American Journal of Physiology-Gastrointestinal Liver Physiology, 283*(6), G1257–G1263. doi: 10.1152/ajpgi.00314.2002

8.   Ait-Belgnaoui, A. et al. (2014). Probiotic gut effect prevents the chronic psychological stress-induced brain activity abnormality in mice. *Neurogastroenterology & Motility, 26*(4), 510–520. doi: 10.1111/nmo.12295

9.   Hueston, C. M., & Deak, T. (2014). The inflamed axis: The interaction between stress, hormones, and the expression of inflammatory-related genes within key structures comprising the hypothalamic-pituitary-adrenal axis. *Physiology & Behavior, 124,* 77–91. doi: 10.1016/j.physbeh.2013.10.035

10. Carroll, I. M. et al. (2011). Molecular analysis of the luminal- and mucosal-associated intestinal microbiota in diarrhea-predominant irritable bowel syndrome. *American Journal of Physiology-Gastrointestinal Liver Physiology, 301*(5), G799–G807. doi: 10.1152/ajpgi.00154.2011

11. Pinto-Sanchez, M. I. et al. (2015). Anxiety and depression increase in a stepwise manner in parallel with multiple FGIDs and symptom severity and frequency. *The American Journal of Gastroenterology, 110*(7), 1038–1048. doi: 10.1038/ajg.2015.128

12. Berger, M., Gray, J. A., & Roth, B. L. (2009). The expanded biology of serotonin. *Annual Review of Medicine, 60,* 355–366. doi: 10.1146/annurev.med.60.042307.110802

13. Keszthelyi, D. et al. (2014). Serotonergic reinforcement of intestinal barrier function is impaired in irritable bowel syndrome. *Alimentary Pharmacology & Therapeutics, 40*(4), 392–402. doi: 10.1111/apt.12842

14. Yano, J. M. et al. (2015). Indigenous bacteria from the gut microbiota regulate host serotonin biosynthesis. *Cell, 161*(2), 264–276. doi: 10.1016/j.cell.2015.02.047

15. Plöger, S. et al. (2012). Microbial butyrate and its role for barrier function in the gastrointestinal tract. *Annals of the New York Academy of Sciences, 1258,* 52–59. doi: 10.1111/j.1749-6632.2012.06553.x

16. Sánchez-Villegas, A. et al. (2012). Fast-food and commercial baked goods consumption and the risk of depression. *Public Health Nutrition,15*(3), 424–432. doi: 10.1017/S1368980011001856

17. Kim, K. A. et al. (2012). High fat diet-induced gut microbiota exacerbates inflammation and obesity in mice via the TLR4 signaling pathway. *PLOS One, 7*(10):e47713. doi: 10.1371/journal.pone.0047713

18. Dinan, T. G., Stanton, C., & Cryan, J. F. (2013). Psychobiotics: a novel class of psychotropic. *Biological Psychiatry, 74*(10), 720–726. doi: 10.1016/j.biopsych.2013.05.001

Chapter 7

1.   Fasano, A. (2012). Leaky gut and autoimmune diseases. *Clinical Reviews in Allergy & Immunology, 42*(1), 71–78. doi: 10.1007/s12016-011-8291-x.

Chapter 8

1.   Ahmed, S. H. et al. (2013). Sugar addiction: Pushing the drug-sugar analogy to the limit. *Current Opinion in Clinical Nutrition & Metabolic Care, 16*(4), 434–439. doi: 10.1097/MCO.0b013e328361c8b8

2.   Ryan, M. (2015). Celiac disease and Hashimoto's. Retrieved from https://hashimotoshealing.com/celiac-disease-and-hashimotos/

3.   Zhang, J. et al. (2014). A classification of Hashimoto's thyroiditis based on immunohistochemistry for IgG4 and IgG. *Thyroid, 24*(2), 364–370. doi: 10.1089/thy.2013.0211

4.   Asik, M. et al. (2014). Decrease in TSH levels after lactose restriction in Hashimoto's thyroiditis patients with lactose intolerance. *Endocrine, 46*(2), 279–284. doi: 10.1007/s12020-013-0065-1

5.   Cellini, M. et al. (2014). Systematic appraisal of lactose intolerance as cause of increased need for oral thyroxine. *The Journal of Clinical Endocrinology & Metabolism, 99*(8), E1454–8. doi: 10.1210/jc.2014-1217

6. Ruchała, M. et al. (2012). The influence of lactose intolerance and other gastro-intestinal tract disorders on L-thyroxine absorption. *Endokrynologia Polska, 63*(4), 318–23.

Chapter 9

1. Mclean, W. & Littleton, J. (2002) *Clinical Handbook of Internal Medicine, Volume 2 Spleen and Stomach* (page 862). Australia: University of Western Sydney Press.

Chapter 10

1. Pitchford, P. (1993) *Healing with Whole Foods, Asian Traditions and Modern Nutrition* (p. 274). Berkeley, CA: North Atlantic Books.

2. Ibid, p. 276.

3. Ibid, p. 276.

4. Ibid, p. 273.

5. Ibid, p. 272.

6. Mclean, W. & Littleton, J. (2002) *Clinical Handbook of Internal Medicine, Volume 2 Spleen and Stomach* (page 866). Australia: University of Western Sydney Press.

7. Avena, N.M., Rada, P., & Hoebel, B.G. (2008). Evidence for sugar addiction: Behavioral and neurochemical effects of intermittent, excessive sugar intake. *Neuroscience & Biobehavioral Reviews, 32*(1), 20–39. doi: 10.1016/j.neubiorev.2007.04.019

Chapter 11

1. Maclean, W., & Lyttleton, J. (2002). *Clinical handbook of internal medicine: The treatment of disease with traditional Chinese medicine. Volume 2: Spleen and stomach* (pp. 870–872). Penrith, Australia: University of Western Sydney.

2. Ibid, p. 873.

3. Ibid, p. 874.

4. Saunders, C. W. (1926). The nutritional value of chlorophyll as related to hemoglobin formation. *Experimental Biology and Medicine, 23*(8), 788–789. doi: 10.3181/00379727-23-3172

5. Maclean, W., & Lyttleton, J. (2002). *Clinical handbook of internal medicine: The treatment of disease with traditional Chinese medicine. Volume 2: Spleen and stomach* (pp. 874). Penrith, Australia: University of Western Sydney.

6. Ibid, pp. 876–877.

Chapter 12

1. Ibid, pp. 879

2. Paul Pitchford, Healing with Whole Foods, Berkeley, California, North Atlantic Books, 1993, p.286.

3. Maclean, W., & Lyttleton, J. (2002). *Clinical handbook of internal medicine: The treatment of disease with traditional Chinese medicine. Volume 2: Spleen and stomach* (pp. 880-881). Penrith, Australia: University of Western Sydney.

4. Ibid, pp. 882–883.

Chapter 13

1. Ballantyne, S. (2013). *The Paleo Approach: Reverse autoimmune disease and heal your body.* Las Vegas, NV: Victory Belt Publishing.

2. Groven, S. et al. (2017). Rapid improvement in symptoms and quality of life among patients with inflammatory bowel disease following an autoimmune protocol diet. *Gastroenterology, 152*(5), S410.

3. Konijeti, G. G. et al. (2017). Efficacy and tolerability of the autoimmune protocol diet for inflammatory bowel disease. *Gastroenterology,152*(5), S401–S402.

4. Esposito, T. et al. (2016). Effects of low-carbohydrate diet therapy in overweight subjects with autoimmune thyroiditis; possible synergism with ChREBP. *Drug Design, Development and Therapy*, 10, 2939–2946.

5. Trescott, Mickey. (2016). *The autoimmune paleo cookbook.* (p. 18). McMinnville, OR: Trescott, LLC.

6. Ibid, p. 19.

7. Beinfield, H., & Korngold, E. (1991). *Between heaven and earth: A guide to Chinese medicine.* (p. 335). New York: Ballantine Books.

8. Ibid, p. 335.

Chapter 14

1. Wang, X. et al. (2013). Mechanism of oral tolerance induction to therapeutic proteins. *Advanced Drug Delivery Reviews, 65*(6), 759–773. doi: 10.1016/j.addr.2012.10.013

2. David, T. J. (1984). Anaphylactic shock during elimination diets for severe atopic eczema. *Archives of Disease in Childhood, 59*(10), 983–986.

3. Friedman, A., & Weiner, H.L. (1994). Induction of anergy or active suppression following oral tolerance is determined by antigen dosage. *Proceedings of the National Academy of Sciences of the United States of America, 91*(14), 6688–6692.

4. Scheppach W. (1994). Effects of short chained fatty acids on gut morphology and function, *Gut, 35*(1), S35–S38.

5. Kresser, C. (2014, August 14). How resistant starch will help to make you healthier and thinner. Retrieved from https://chriskresser.com/how-resistant-starch-will-help-to-make-you-healthier-and-thinner/

6. Laird, E. (2014). *Reintroducing foods on the paleo autoimmune protocol: A step-by-step guide with recipes.* e-book: Eileen Laird.

7. Ibid, p. 8.

8. Bode, C. (1997). Alcohol's Role in Gastrointestinal Tract Disorders, *Alcohol, Health and Research World, 21*(1). Retrieved from https://pubs.niaaa.nih.gov/publications/arh21-1/76.pdf

9. LoConte, Noelle K. et al. (2018). Alcohol and Cancer: A Statement of the American Society of Clinical Oncology, *Journal of Clinical Oncology, 36*(1), 83–93.

10. Netting, M. et al. (2013). Heated allergens and induction of tolerance in food allergic children. *Nutrients, 5*(6), 2028–2046. doi: 10.3390/nu5062028

11. Chen, John and Chen, Tina, Chinese Medical Herbology and Pharmacology, 2004, City of Industry, CA, Art of Medicine Press, page 768.

Chapter 15

1. Fruehauf, H. (1998). Driving out demons and snakes: Gu syndrome, a forgotten clinical approach to chronic parasitism. *Journal of Chinese Medicine, 57.*

2. Quinn, B., with Moreland, E. (2008). Gu syndrome: An in-depth interview with Heiner Fruehauf. Retrieved from https://classicalchinesemedicine.org/gpa/gu-syndrome-in-depth-interview-with-heiner-fruehauf/

3. Fruehauf, H. (1998). Driving out demons and snakes: Gu syndrome, a forgotten clinical approach to chronic parasitism. *Journal of Chinese Medicine, 57.*

Chapter 16

1. Ryan, M. (2017). *How to Heal Hashimoto's: An integrative road map to remission* (p. 301). Carlsbad, CA: Hay House.

2. Grace, E. et al. (2013). Review article: Small intestinal bacterial overgrowth—prevalence, clinical features, current and developing diagnostic tests, and treatment. *Alimentary Pharmacology & Therapeutics, 38*(7), 674–688. doi: 10.1111/apt.12456

3. Cooper, J. G. et al. (2005). Ciprofloxacin interacts with thyroid replacement therapy. *The BMJ, 330*(7498), 1002. doi: 10.1136/bmj.330.7498.1002

4. Ibid, pp. 321–322.

5. Lauritano, E. C. et al. (2008) Small intestinal bacterial overgrowth recurrence after antibiotic therapy. *American Journal of Gastroenterology, 103*(8), 2031–2035.

6. Maoshing N. & McNease, C. (1987). *The Tao of Nutrition* (p. 48). Santa Monica, CA: Seven Star Communications Group.

Chapter 17

1. Fujinami, R. S. et al. (2006). Molecular mimicry, bystander activation, or viral persistence: Infections and autoimmune disease. *Clinical Microbiology Reviews, 19*(1), 80–94. doi: 10.1128/CMR.19.1.80-94.2006

2. Cusick, M. F., Libbey, J. E., & Fujinami, R. S. (2012). Molecular mimicry as a mechanism of autoimmune disease. *Clinical Reviews in Allergy & Immunology, 42*(1),102–111. doi: 10.1007/s12016-011-8294-7

3. Pender, M. P. (2012). CD8+ T-cell deficiency, Epstein-Barr virus infection, vitamin D deficiency, and steps to autoimmunity: A unifying hypothesis. *Autoimmune Diseases,* Article ID 189096. doi: 10.1155/2012/189096

4. Blanc, M. et al. (2011). Host defense against viral infection involves interferon mediated down-regulation of sterol biosynthesis. *PLOS Biology, 9*(3): e1000598. doi: 10.1371/journal.pbio.1000598

5. Van Benschoten, M. M. *Chinese herbal therapy* , Lecture, Emperor's College of Oriental Medicine, 2004.

6. Lab Tests Online, AACC (2018). Retrieved from https://labtestsonline.org/understanding/analytes/ebv/tab/test/

Chapter 18

1. Jenkinson, H. F., & Douglas, L. J. (2002). Interactions between Candida species and bacteria in mixed infections. In K. A. Brogden & J. M. Guthmiller [Eds.], *Polymicrobial diseases* (p. 357). Washington, DC: ASM Press.

2. Chen, J. K. & Chen, T. T. (2009). *Chinese Herbal Formulas and Applications* (p. 93) City of Industry, CA: Art of Medicine Press.

3. Van Benschoten, M. M. *Pharmacology of Chinese herbs with Biomedical Applications,* Lecture, Emperor's College of Oriental Medicine, June 21, 2003.

Chapter 19

1. Markell, E. K., & Udkow, M. P. (1986). Blastocystis hominis: Pathogen or fellow traveler? *The American Journal of Tropical Medicine and Hygiene, 35*(5), 1023–1026.

2. Verneuil, L. et al. (2004). Association between chronic urticaria and thyroid autoimmunity: A prospective study involving 99 patients. *Dermatology, 208*(2), 98–103. doi: 10.1159/000076480

3. Kolkhir, P. et al. (2017). Comorbidity of chronic spontaneous urticaria and autoimmune thyroid diseases: A systematic review, *Allergy, 72*(10),1440–1460. doi: 10.1111/all.13182

4. Rajiⵉ, B. et al. (2015). Eradication of Blastocystis hominis prevents the development of symptomatic Hashimoto's thyroiditis: A case report. *The Journal of Infection in Developing Countries 9*(7), 788–791. doi: 10.3855/jidc.4851

5. Wentz, I. (2015, September 29). The common root cause of Hashimoto's, Hives, and IBS. Retrieved from https://thyroidpharmacist.com/articles/the-common-root-cause-of-hashimotos-hives-and-ibs/

6. Blastocystitis Research Foundation. (n.d.) Diagnosis. Retrieved from http://bhomcenter.org/wp/diagnosis

7. Van Benschoten, M. M. (2004). *Pharmacological properties of Chinese herbs* [Lecture notes].

Chapter 20

1. NIH Consensus Conference. (1994). Helicobacter pylori in peptic ulcer disease. NIH Consensus Development Panel on Helicobacter pylori in Peptic Ulcer Disease. *The Journal of the American Medical Association, 272,* 65–69.

2. Hunt, R. H. (1996). Helicobacter pylori: from theory to practice. Proceedings of a symposium. *The American Journal of Medicine*; 100 (5A) supplement.

3. Hou, Y. et al. (2017) Meta-analysis of the correlation between Helicobacter pylori infection and autoimmune thyroid diseases. *Oncotarget, 8*(70), 115691–115700. doi:10.18632/oncotarget.22929

4. de Luis, D. A. et al. (1998). Heliobacter pylori infection is markedly increased in patients with autoimmune atrophic thyroiditis. *The Journal of Clinical Gastroenterology, 26*(4), 259–263.

5. Shmuely, H., Shimon, I., & Gitter, L. A. (2016). Helicobacter pylori infection in women with Hashimoto thyroiditis: A case-control study. *Medicine*, 95(29), e4074. doi :10.1097/MD.0000000000004074

6. Bassi, V., Santinelli, C., Iengo, A., & Romano, C. (2010) Identification of a correlation between Helicobacter pylori infection and Graves' disease. *Helicobacter, 15*(6), 558–62. doi: 10.1111/j.1523-5378.2010.00802.x

7. Gerenova, J.B., Manolova, I. M., & Tzoneva, V. I. (2013). Clinical significance of autoantibodies to parietal cells in patients with autoimmune thyroid diseases. *Folia Medica (Plovdiv), 55*(2), 26–32.

8. Centanni, M. et al. (1999). Atrophic body gastritis in patients with autoimmune thyroid disease: An underdiagnosed association. *Archives of Internal Medicine, 159*(15), 1726–1730.

9. Van Benschoten, M. M. (2004). *Pharmacological properties of Chinese herbs* [Lecture notes].

10. Zhe Jiang Zhong Yi Zha Zhi. (1998). *Zhejiang Journal of Traditional Chinese Medicine, 3*(40).

Chapter 21

1. Flaws, B., & Sionneau, P. (2001).*The treatment of modern western medical diseases with Chinese medicine: A textbook and clinical manual* (p. 329). Boulder, CO: Blue Poppy Press.

2. Van Benschoten, M. M. (2004). *Pharmacological properties of Chinese herbs* [Lecture notes].

3. Flaws, B., & Sionneau, P. (2001).*The treatment of modern western medical diseases with Chinese medicine: A textbook and clinical manual* (p. 330). Boulder, CO: Blue Poppy Press.

4. Ibid, p. 330.

Chapter 22

1. Chakraborty, A. et al. (2015). The descriptive epidemiology of yersiniosis: A multistate study, 2005–2011. *Public Health Reports, 130*(3), 269–277. doi: 10.1177/003335491513000314

2. Shenkman, L., & Bottone, E. J. (1976). Antibodies to Yersinia enterocolitica in thyroid disease. *Annals of Internal Medicine, 85*(6), 735–739.

Chapter 23

1. Hirsch, H. Z. et al. (2006). Autoimmunity to collagen in adult periodontal disease. *Journal of Oral Pathology & Medicine, 28*, 456–459.

2. Patil, B. S., Patil, S., & Gururaj, T. R. (2011). Probable autoimmune causal relationship between peri-odontitis and Hashimoto's thyroiditis: A systemic review. *Nigerian Journal of Clinical Practice, 14*(3), 253–61.

3. Maclean, W., & Lyttleton, J. (2002). *Clinical handbook of internal medicine: The treatment of disease with traditional Chinese medicine. Volume 2: Spleen and stomach* (p. 384). Penrith, Australia: University of Western Sydney.

4. Flaws, B., & Sionneau, P. (2001).*The treatment of modern western medical diseases with Chinese medicine: A textbook and clinical manual* (pp. 409–410). Boulder, CO: Blue Poppy Press.

Chapter 24

1. Maclean, W., & Lyttleton, J. (2002). *Clinical handbook of internal medicine: The treatment of disease with traditional Chinese medicine. Volume 2: Spleen and stomach* (p. 2). Penrith, Australia: University of Western Sydney.

2. Chen, J., & Chen, T. (2008). *Chinese herbal formulas and applications: Pharmacological effects & clinical research* (p. 533). City of Industry, CA: Art of Medicine Press.

3. Ibid, p. 238.

4. Ibid, p. 1099.

Chapter 25

1. Mayer, E. A. (2011). Gut feelings: The emerging biology of gut-brain communication. *Nature Reviews Neuroscience, 12*(8), 453–466. doi: 10.1038/nrn3071

2. Reimer, C. et al. (2009). Proton-pump inhibitor therapy induces acid-related symptoms in healthy volunteers after withdrawal of therapy. *Gastroenterology, 137*(1), 80–87.e1. doi: 10.1053/j.gastro.2009.03.058

3. Maclean, W., & Lyttleton, J. (2002). *Clinical handbook of internal medicine: The treatment of disease with traditional Chinese medicine. Volume 2: Spleen and stomach* (p. 104). Penrith, Australia: University of Western Sydney.

4. Chen, J., & Chen, T. (2008). *Chinese herbal formulas and applications: Pharmacological effects & clinical research* (p. 233). City of Industry, CA: Art of Medicine Press.

5.   Ibid, p. 1068.

6.   Ibid, p. 531.

Chapter 26

1.   *Li Dong-yuan's treatise on the spleen & stomach: A translation of the* Pi Wei Lun. (2004). (Bob Flaws, Trans.). (p. 83). Boulder, CO: Blue Poppy Press.

2.   Ibid, p. 85.

3.   Maintz, L., & Novak, N. (2007). Histamine and histamine intolerance. *The American Journal of Clinical Nutrition, 85*(5), 1185–1196.

4.   Suzuki, T. et al. (1999). Suppressive effects of Hochu-ekki-to [the Japanese name for Bu Qi Zhong Yi Qi Tang] on IgE production and histamine release in mice immunized with ovalbumin. *Biological and Pharmaceutical Bulletin, 22*(11), 1180–1184. doi: 10.1248/bpb.22.1180

Chapter 27

1.   Gebhard, R. L. et al. (1992). Thyroid hormone differentially augments biliary sterol secretion in the rat. I: The isolated-perfused liver model. *The Journal of Lipid Research, 33*, 1459–1466.

2.   Flaws, B., & Sionneau, P. (2001).*The treatment of modern western medical diseases with Chinese medicine: A textbook and clinical manual* (p. 123). Boulder, CO: Blue Poppy Press.

3.   Chen, J., & Chen, T. (2008). *Chinese herbal formulas and applications: Pharmacological effects & clinical research* (p. 206). City of Industry, CA: Art of Medicine Press.

4.   Fu Jian Zhong Yi Yao (1986). *Fujian Chinese Medicine and Herbology, 17*(3), 48.

5.   Ibid, p. 371.

Chapter 28

1.   Yaylali, O. et al. (2009). Does hypothyroidism affect gastrointestinal motility? *Gastroenterology Research and Practice, 2009*, Article ID 529802. doi: 10.1155/2009/529802

2.   Maclean, W., & Lyttleton, J. (2002). *Clinical handbook of internal medicine: The treatment of disease with traditional Chinese medicine. Volume 2: Spleen and stomach* (p. 164). Penrith, Australia: University of Western Sydney.

3.   Chen, J., & Chen, T. (2008). *Chinese herbal formulas and applications: Pharmacological effects & clinical research* (p. 174). City of Industry, CA: Art of Medicine Press.

4.   Ibid, p. 1209.

5.   Zhe Jiang Zhong Yi Za Zhi (1966). *Zhejiang Journal of Traditional Chinese Medicine, 1*(17).

Chapter 29

1.   Maclean, W., & Lyttleton, J. (2002). *Clinical handbook of internal medicine: The treatment of disease with traditional Chinese medicine. Volume 2: Spleen and stomach* (p. 212). Penrith, Australia: University of Western Sydney.

2.   Meredith C. Roath, MD, Jack A. DiPalma, MD, *Genetics of Gastroenterology: What You Need to Know Part 1*, Consultant360, February, 2012, Volume 52, Issue 2, www.consultant360.com/article/genetics-gastroenterology-what-you-need-to-know-part-1

3.   Ibid, p. 222.

4.   Chen, J., & Chen, T. (2008). *Chinese herbal formulas and applications: Pharmacological effects & clinical research* (p. 1071). City of Industry, CA: Art of Medicine Press.

5.   Ibid, p. 257.

6.   Zong Lan Xu. (2001). *Pocket handbook of Chinese herbal prescriptions* (p. 286). Miami, FL: Waclion International, Inc.

Chapter 30

1.   Graettinger, J. S. et al. (1959). A correlation of clinical and hemodynamic studies in patients with hypothyroidism with and without congestive heart failure. *Journal of Clinical Investigation, 38*(8), 1316–1327. doi: 10.1172/JCI103906

2.   Maclean, W., & Lyttleton, J. (2002). *Clinical handbook of internal medicine: The treatment of disease with traditional Chinese medicine. Volume 2: Spleen and stomach* (p. 484). Penrith, Australia: University of Western Sydney.

3.   Zong Lan Xu. (2001). *Pocket handbook of Chinese herbal prescriptions* (p. 166). Miami, FL: Waclion International, Inc.

4.   Chen, J., & Chen, T. (2008). *Chinese herbal formulas and applications: Pharmacological effects & clinical research* (p. 879). City of Industry, CA: Art of Medicine Press.

Appendix 2

1.   Deng Ming-Dao (1983). *The Wandering Taoist.* San Francisco: Harper & Row.

Appendix 3

1.   Becker, C., Bopp, T., & Jonuleit, H. (2012). Boosting regulatory T cell function by CD4 stimulation enters the clinic. *Frontiers in Immunology, 3,* 164. doi: 10.3389/fimmu.2012.00164

2.   Ibid.

3.   Shan, M. et al. (2013). Mucus enhances gut homeostasis and oral tolerance by delivering immuno-regulatory signals. *Science, 342*(6157), 447–453. doi: 10.1126/science.1237910

4.   Chung, C. Y. et al. (2013). Dendritic cells: Cellular mediators for immunological tolerance. *Clinical and Developmental Immunology, 2013,* Article ID 972865. doi: 10.1155/2013/972865

5.   Cone, R. E. et al. (1996). Elevation of intracellular cyclic AMP induces an anergic-like state in Th1 clones. *Cellular Immunology, 173*(2), 246–251.

6.   Khramova, D. S. et al. (2009). Abrogation of the oral tolerance to ovalbumin in mice by citrus pectin. *Nutrition, 25*(2): 226–232. doi: 10.1016/j.nut.2008.08.004

7.   Matysiak-Budnik, T. et al. (2003). Gastric Helicobacter infection inhibits development of oral toler-ance to food antigens in mice. *Infection and Immunity, 71*(9), 5219–5224. doi: 10.1128/IAI.71.9.5219-5224.2003

8.   Oliveira, F. M. et al. (1998). Coupling of palmitate to ovalbumin inhibits the induction of oral toler-ance. *Brazilian Journal of Medical and Biological Research, 31*(11), 1421–1424.

9.   Paparo, L. et al. (2014). The influence of early life nutrition on epigenetic regulatory mechanisms of the immune system, *Nutrients, 6*(11), 4706–4719. doi: 10.3390/nu6114706

10.   Calder, P.C. (2010). Omega-3 fatty acids and inflammatory processes. *Nutrients, 2*(3), 355–374. doi: 10.3390/nu2030355

11.   Plunkett, C.H., & Nagler, C. R. (2017). The Influence of the microbiome on allergic sensitization to food. *The Journal of Immunology, 198*(2), 581–589. doi: 10.4049/jimmunol.1601266

12.   Liu, Y. et al. (2011). Ursolic acid promotes robust tolerance to cardiac allografts in mice. *Clinical and Experimental Immunology, 164*(2), 282–288. doi: 10.1111/j.1365-2249.2011.04333.x

13. Dharmananda, S. (n.d.). Treatments for thyroid diseases with Chinese herbal medicine. Retrieved from http://www.itmonline.org/arts/thyroid.htm

14. Wang, H. et al. (2012). Dietary flavonoid naringenin induces regulatory T cells via an aryl hydrocarbon receptor mediated pathway. *Journal of Agricultural and Food Chemistry, 60*(9), 2171–2178. doi: 10.1021/jf204625y

15. Goldhammer, E. et al. (2005). Exercise training modulates cytokines activity in coronary heart disease patients. *International Journal of Cardiology, 100*(1), 93–99. doi: 10.1016/j.ijcard.2004.08.073

16. Nicklas, B. J., & Brinkley, T. E. (2009). Exercise training as a treatment for chronic inflammation in the elderly. *Exercise & Sport Sciences Reviews, 37*(4), 165–170. doi: 10.1097/JES.0b013e3181b7b3d9

17. Petersen, A. W., & Pedersen, B. K. (2005). The anti-inflammatory effect of exercise. *The Journal of Applied Physiology, 98,* 1154–1162. doi:10.1152/japplphysiol. 00164.2004

Index

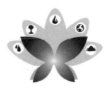

ABOUT THE AUTHOR

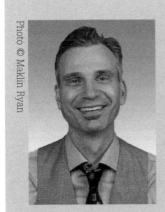

Photo © Maklin Ryan

Marc Ryan, LAc is a graduate of Cornell University and a licensed acupuncturist and herbalist in the state of California who practices functional medicine. After suffering from his own battle with Hashimoto's and discovering an alternative approach to healing it, he decided to devote his life to doing everything he could to help others find hope, help and healing.

Since 2013, Marc has spent thousands of hours researching, working with and talking to over 2,000 Hashimoto's patients.

www.hashimotoshealing.com

Hay House Titles of Related Interest

YOU CAN HEAL YOUR LIFE, the movie, starring Louise Hay & Friends
(available as a 1-DVD program, an expanded 2-DVD set, and an online streaming video)
Learn more at www.hayhouse.com/louise-movie

THE SHIFT, the movie,
starring Dr. Wayne W. Dyer
(available as a 1-DVD program, an expanded 2-DVD set,
and an online streaming video)
Learn more at www.hayhouse.com/the-shift-movie

Fat for Fuel: A Revolutionary Diet to Combat Cancer, Boost Brain Power, and Increase Your Energy,
by Dr. Joseph Mercola

*Medical Medium Thyroid Healing: The Truth behind Hashimoto's, Graves', Insomnia,
Hypothyroidism, Thyroid Nodules & Epstein-Barr,* by Anthony William

*The Telomere Miracle: Scientific Secrets to Fight Disease, Feel Great, and
Turn Back the Clock on Aging,* by Ed Park

*The Truth about Cancer: What You Need to Know about
Cancer's History, Treatment, and Prevention,* by Ty Bollinger

All of the above are available at www.hayhouse.co.uk.